Intellectual and Developmental Disabilities

Intellectual and Developmental Disabilities provides a unique contribution not currently available in the professional literature by addressing the experiences and perspectives of families living with or raising a child with a disability. Designed for family therapists, social workers, and other helping professionals, it provides empirically based, practical information for working with families experiencing intellectual and developmental disabilities of a loved one. This book also provides important information for navigating the various professional systems of care with which these families interface: health care providers, early childhood intervention teams, educational systems, the legal system, and financial planners.

Briana S. Nelson Goff, PhD, LCMFT, is a professor in the School of Family Studies and Human Services at Kansas State University. Dr. Nelson Goff received dual Bachelors of Science degrees in psychology and life science and a Master of Science degree in marriage and family therapy, all from Kansas State University. She completed a doctoral degree in marriage and family therapy from Texas Tech University.

Nicole Piland Springer, PhD, LMFT, is an associate professor of practice in community, family, and addiction sciences and the director of the Center for Family Systems Research and Intervention and the Family Therapy Clinic at Texas Tech University. Dr. Piland Springer received a Bachelor of Arts in psychology, a Master of Science degree in human development and family studies, and a doctoral degree in marriage and family therapy from Texas Tech University.

Intellectual and Developmental Disabilities

A Roadmap for Families and Professionals

Edited by Briana S. Nelson Goff and Nicole Piland Springer

Routledge
Taylor & Francis Group
NEW YORK AND LONDON

First edition published 2018
by Routledge
711 Third Avenue, New York, NY 10017

and by Routledge
2 Park Square, Milton Park, Abingdon, Oxon, OX14 4RN

Routledge is an imprint of the Taylor & Francis Group, an informa business

Library of Congress Cataloging-in-Publication Data
Names: Nelson Goff, Briana S., editor. | Springer, Nicole Piland, editor.
Title: Intellectual and developmental disabilities: a roadmap for families and professionals / edited by Briana S. Nelson Goff and Nicole Piland Springer.
Other titles: Intellectual and developmental disabilities (Nelson Goff)
Description: First edition. | New York: Routledge, 2017. | Includes bibliographical references and index.
Identifiers: LCCN 2017029013 | ISBN 9781138672451 (hbk : alk. paper) | ISBN 9781138672468 (pbk : alk. paper) | ISBN 9781315562490 (ebk)
Subjects: | MESH: Intellectual Disability | Family | Developmental Disabilities | Caregivers | Child | Adolescent | Adult
Classification: LCC RC455 | NLM WS 107.5.R5 | DDC 362.2–dc23
LC record available at https://lccn.loc.gov/2017029013

ISBN: 978-1-138-67245-1 (hbk)
ISBN: 978-1-138-67246-8 (pbk)
ISBN: 978-1-315-56249-0 (ebk)

Typeset in Galliard
by Deanta Global Publishing Services, Chennai, India

Contents

About the Editors viii
Preface ix
Acknowledgments xi

PART I
Foundations for Understanding Developmental, Intellectual, and Other Disabilities 1

1 **Intellectual and Developmental Disabilities: An Introduction and Overview** 3
BRIE TURNS, PHD, BRIANA S. NELSON GOFF, PHD, MARILYN MASTERSON, PHD, RN, JESSICA D. CLESS, MS, AND ADAM W. CLESS, MS

2 **A Systemic and Contextual Lens of Disability: Family Stress, Ambiguous Loss, and Meaning Making** 17
NICOLE PILAND SPRINGER, PHD, BRIE TURNS, PHD, AND MARILYN MASTERSON, PHD, RN

3 **Discovering Resilience: Moving Forward on the Journey** 32
THOMAS KNESTRICT, EDD

4 **Advice to New Parents from Parents: Reflecting on the Journey** 46
JESSICA D. CLESS, MS, ELLEN BODINE, BS, ASHLEY EDELMAN, BS, LAURA FARKAS, BS, ADAM W. CLESS, MS, BRIANA S. NELSON GOFF, PHD, AND NICOLE PILAND SPRINGER, PHD

PART II
Perspectives, Contributions, and Lived Experiences of Individuals with IDD and Their Families on the Journey 59

5 Understanding and Supporting Identity Formation and Meaning Making 61
KAMI L. GALLUS, PHD AND JENNIFER L. JONES, PHD

6 Perspectives from Mothers: Recognizing Their Strengths and Contributions beyond Caregiving 76
JESSICA D. CLESS, MS AND CHRISTYNE STEPHENSON, MS

7 Perspectives from Fathers: Recognizing Their Strengths and Contributions beyond Breadwinning 90
GAIL E. BENTLEY, PHD, MATTHEW D. BROWN, PHD, AND JASON B. WHITING, PHD

8 The Sibling Experience: More than My Brother's Keeper 104
CAROLYN SHIVERS, PHD

9 Grandparents: Meaningful Contributors to a Changing Family Landscape 117
SANDRA WOODBRIDGE, PHD AND LAURIE BUYS, PHD

PART III
Navigating Professional Systems of Care: From Birth to Adolescence 131

10 The Medical Perspective: Developing Health Literacy in Families 133
KAREN SUMMAR, MD, MS

11 Allied Health Professionals: Enhancing Potential through Early Childhood Intervention and Therapies 148
JENNIFER J. BEKINS, MS

12 The Education System: Building Partnerships and Inclusive Communities 158
GRACE FRANCIS, PHD AND SARAH NAGRO, EDD

PART IV
Preparing for the Future: The Transition to Adulthood and Beyond 171

13 Special Needs Financial Planning: Optimizing Resources for the Future 173
MITZI K. LAUDERDALE, JD, CFP®, MICHAEL C. WALTHER II, CPA/PFS, CFP®, CFA®, AND NICOLE PILAND SPRINGER, PHD

14 Meaningful Employment: Fostering Opportunities for Adults with IDD to Thrive 188
JENNIFER L. JONES, PHD AND KAMI L. GALLUS, PHD

15 Special Needs Legal Concerns: Guidelines for Families and Guardians 201
MICHELE K. GOLDBERG, JD

16 When the Journey Ends: Parental Caregiving and Later Life Planning 216
ELIZABETH A. PERKINS, PHD AND LIEKE VAN HEUMEN, PHD

Index 229

About the Editors

Briana S. Nelson Goff, PhD, LCMFT, is a Professor in the School of Family Studies and Human Services at Kansas State University. Dr. Nelson Goff received dual bachelors of science degrees in psychology and life science and a master of science degree in marriage and family therapy, both from Kansas State University. She completed a doctoral degree in marriage and family therapy from Texas Tech University. Dr. Nelson Goff and her husband have two children, Dalton and Gracyn. Dalton was diagnosed with Down syndrome at birth.

Nicole Piland Springer, PhD, LMFT, is an Associate Professor of Practice in Community, Family, and Addiction Sciences, and the Director of the Center for Family Systems Research and Intervention and the Family Therapy Clinic at Texas Tech University. Dr. Piland Springer received a bachelor of arts in psychology, a master of science degree in human development and family studies, and a doctoral degree in marriage and family therapy from Texas Tech University. Dr. Piland Springer has two children, Travis and Katarina. Katarina received a series of preliminary in utero diagnoses of cystic hygroma, hydrops fetalis, and intrauterine growth retardation, but was ultimately diagnosed with Down syndrome during the second trimester of the pregnancy via amniocentesis.

Drs. Nelson Goff and Piland Springer were doctoral students at Texas Tech University and, since 2010, have collaborated on research, workshops, and educational programs at their respective universities, as well as co-presented at national conferences. Their national research study focuses on the positive aspects of having a child with Down syndrome, titled, "*My Kid Has More Chromosomes than Yours!: The Journey to Hope and Resilience in Parenting a Child with Down Syndrome.*"

Preface

We started our doctoral program together at Texas Tech University in 1995. Little did we know after completing our degrees and starting our careers that just over a decade later we would be reconnected in another way, through an extra 21st chromosome. We had very different pregnancy experiences—Nicole faced a series of difficult prenatal testing appointments and diagnoses, some of which were not typically compatible with life, along with recommendations from medical professionals to "terminate the inevitable." Briana had a relatively uneventful pregnancy with Dalton, but soon after he was born, the doctor told her and her husband (first-time parents) that she suspected their son had Down syndrome. Several months after Katarina was born, one of Nicole's academic mentors mentioned their common experience with Down syndrome. An email followed from Nicole to Briana titled: *Something Unique in Common*. It is from that email that their research and ultimately this book was born.

After several discussions, and the awareness of the privilege we both held as educators, clinicians, and researchers, we decided to launch a national study on the experiences of parenting a child with Down syndrome (DS), with an emphasis on positive parenting experiences. We contacted several DS organizations to recruit parents, with plans to obtain 150–200 parents, particularly married couples, to participate in the research study. What started out as a small study, ended up with almost 650 parents completing the online survey! It was exciting, emotional, and thrilling to read the parents' comments and stories in the survey. While we have conducted several analyses with this data set, we believed a practical, but research-based resource for professionals and families was missing in the field. After further discussion and a conference presentation that caught the attention of a publishing company book editor, this book opportunity emerged.

Although our personal experience is with Down syndrome, we wanted to ensure that this book would be relevant across a variety of intellectual and developmental disabilities. We acknowledge that there are many other intellectual and development disability (IDD) areas we could have included, but we attempted to ensure the information contributed to this edited volume would be applicable to a broader audience. We sought contributions from a variety of professional areas and are thrilled with the resulting chapters in this book. In developing this book, we wanted it to be a tool that could be useful to family members and caregivers of individuals with intellectual and developmental disabilities, in addition to serving as a resource for professionals from a variety of areas: disability advocates, healthcare service providers, school personnel, and anyone who is personally or professionally connected to an individual with IDD.

We also expect it to be a resource for families across the life span. It is not intended to be a book to sit and read from cover to cover. There are certain chapters that may be most beneficial to new parents and prospective parents. Other chapters may be helpful in preparing for anticipated life transitions. We also invited several professionals to share their perspectives, from the "inside," as medical, educational, and employment providers, as well as financial planning and legal advisors, as these systems of care can be overwhelming for parents and caregivers. We hope that by hearing directly from the viewpoint of professionals, parents, and families of individuals with IDD, readers will feel like they have allies and co-navigators on this journey.

Finally, we hope our readers will personally and professionally benefit from this book and recognize the "labor of love" that it was for us, as co-parents on this journey. We have learned so much from the contributors to the chapters in our role as editors. While we have made some of the referenced transitions ourselves and faced similar experiences described in these pages, each individual family's experience is unique, sometimes difficult, and often exceptional. We hope your exceptional and wonderful moments on the journey far outnumber the challenges—and that you discover the resilience within your family and the joy that comes with all meaningful journeys.

Acknowledgments

Nicole: I would like to express my heartfelt gratitude for the many people who have crossed my path and supported me throughout my educational, personal, and professional journey, but more specifically for the "Sherpas" who have made themselves available, just prior to and since Katarina's birth. There are too many of you to name individually, but I trust you will know who you are, and I want you to know how indebted I am to you. I am particularly grateful for Travis who gave me the opportunity to become a mother. You are an amazing young man in-the-making and an incredible brother to Katarina. And to Katarina, you have demonstrated such bravery in your medical challenges and have beat the odds. Thank you for inviting us on this journey.

Briana: Words cannot express my appreciation to my family, friends, colleagues, and the professionals with whom we have interacted over the past decade since DS entered our lives. To my husband, Craig, who is my constant reinforcement and strength. And to Dalton, who is the reason for this journey, and Gracyn, who gets to tag along; you both will make this world a better place for individuals with disabilities.

And finally, we want to specifically thank the parents who paused on their DS journey to participate in our original research study and everyone on the research team who has assisted with our project. The parents paved the way for us to give voice to the experiences of families living with DS. But also, the stories shared by parents became the catalyst for us to step into our professional journey for helping families raising a loved one with IDD. The following statement was formulated after initial qualitative analyses were conducted on the responses provided by parents on their DS journey, in an effort to capture the "essence" of their lived experiences:

> The initial impact of receiving a Down syndrome diagnosis is often characterized by shock, fear, and grief. However, the intense emotional responses are considered "normal" given the circumstances of adjusting to a different life than was originally dreamed of for one's child. Parenting a child with Down syndrome seems to require a process of readjusting expectations, seeking out

resources, and identifying a new dream; but doesn't mean surrendering any and all expectations for the child or the family. This parenting journey is filled with challenges like any other parenting experience, but is often described as life changing in a very positive and meaningful way. Children with Down syndrome are often described as, "joy, happiness, unconditional love, a gift or a blessing." The biggest challenge associated with this parenting journey is related to interactions with medical professionals and systems of care. There continues to be a narrow range of information provided to parents upon diagnosis, inaccurate or largely discouraging descriptions of DS, a lack of sensitivity by the ones delivering the news, and a lack of systematic support offered to families. Ultimately, there are no guarantees with any child, and parenting one born with DS is truly more similar than different than raising a "typical" child; and at times even better than one could imagine.

(Springer, McCallum, Pounds, & Nelson Goff, 2011)

Part 1

Foundations for Understanding Developmental, Intellectual, and Other Disabilities

1 Intellectual and Developmental Disabilities

An Introduction and Overview

Brie Turns, PhD, Briana S. Nelson Goff, PhD, Marilyn Masterson, PhD, RN, Jessica D. Cless, MS, and Adam W. Cless, MS

Introduction

> Brent is a shy 13-year-old who lives a relatively quiet life with his single mother, Stacy. Brent rarely ventures out in public aside from attending school, which has recently increased his anxiety. From as early as he could remember, he experienced being bullied by peers, ridiculed by teachers, and having trouble understanding why he did not have many friends. Brent often hears his mother discussing his "autism" and how he is "different" from others. He has few interactions with extended family members, and despite his diagnosis, they continually think of him as a quiet and awkward recluse who needs "better parenting" from his mother. His school counselor provides a daily check-in for Brent to ensure he understands his classwork and is not being bullied. Stacy, Brent's mother, has been working two jobs since Brent's father left when he was five years old. Stacy's family members do not fully understand the extent of Brent's condition and have recently stopped inviting Stacy and Brent to family functions. As a young man lacking the necessary support from his family and school, he has gradually descended into isolation and depression. Noticing his behavior, his school counselor recommended an autism support group for Brent to attend in order learn about his diagnosis and make friends.

Brent's school and family life is not an isolated incident, but rather, a common experience for families and individuals diagnosed with an intellectual or developmental disability (IDD). Families with a member who has an IDD diagnosis or other special needs encounter unique issues that families with typically developing children may not experience (Werner *et al.*, 2009). Family resources are important as family members begin to understand the diagnosis and affiliated symptoms of their loved one's condition, both acute and chronic health problems; access community support services and resources, including medical, financial, educational, social, and other programs; and plan for the stages and challenges that are a part of coping with the demands faced by families with a member with special needs (Flaherty, Masters, & Glidden, 2000; Glidden, Billings, & Jobe, 2006). As can be seen in the previous case vignette, while greater demands on family resources and higher stress levels may be associated with having a family member with an IDD diagnosis, developing support networks and expanding resources can reduce the stress and negative effects that are often assumed to be part of the experiences of families with IDD and related special needs (Nelson Goff, High *et al.*, 2016).

Definition of Terms

Throughout the years, a significant shift has occurred from classifying and defining *mental retardation* specifically towards using the term intellectual disability (Schalock, Luckasson, & Shogren, 2007), with the former term now regarded as inappropriate and obsolete. There have been changes in the construct from a person-oriented approach to a more inclusive contextual, sociological framework (Schalock *et al.*, 2007). Previously, the term *disability* was used to describe an individual's limitations or deficits; more recently, the term encompasses the individual's ability to perform certain roles or functions within the broader social context (DePloy & Gilson, 2004). Disability is not considered a fixed personal trait or characteristic but instead addresses the interaction between an individual and his or her environment, including the resources and supports available to the individual within the social context (Chapireau, 2005; Schalock *et al.*, 2007).

According to the World Health Organization (WHO, 2001), three components are used to classify disability; body function and structure, activity, and participation levels. These components also include how an individual interacts with his or her environment. In other words, the needs of an individual are based on how functional that person is in the context of society; if the disease or condition is limiting the functionality of that person, then the needs will be greater, increasing the likelihood the individual is experiencing difficulties with a specific disability. Disability is defined through social contexts; this social process of defining different ability levels becomes important in understanding the impact on individuals with IDD and related special needs (Chapireau, 2005).

The process of defining and classifying terminology is challenging and complex in nature. Ambiguity and uncertainty are common with defining disability, as well as placing individuals within a specific disability category or group. Each area of disability has variations in cause and functional level, as well as timing of diagnosis and changes in the needs of the individual that may occur over time and across the life span (Hallahan & Kauffman, 2000). Despite these challenges, defining and classifying the terminology associated with disability is paramount to providing universal descriptors and language that will assist individuals with developing effective strategies for creating more universal acceptance and recognition within the social context (Chapireau, 2005).

While there are a variety of conditions that can be defined by the term *disability*, for our purposes, we will limit our review to primarily IDD research and literature. We present the National Institutes of Health (NIH, 2010) definitions to provide a starting description of IDD for the purposes of this edited volume of work:

> *Intellectual disability* refers to a group of disorders characterized by a limited mental capacity and difficulty with adaptive behaviors such as managing money, schedules and routines, or social interactions. Intellectual disability originates before the age of 18 and may result from physical causes, such as autism or cerebral palsy, or from nonphysical causes, such as lack of stimulation and adult responsiveness.
>
> (NIH, 2010, p. 1)

> *Developmental disability* is a severe, long term disability that can affect cognitive ability, physical functioning, or both. These disabilities appear before age 22 and are likely to be lifelong. The term "developmental disability" encompasses intellectual disability but also includes physical disabilities. Some developmental disabilities may be solely physical, such as blindness from birth. Others involve both physical and intellectual disabilities stemming from genetic or other causes, such as Down syndrome and fetal alcohol syndrome.
>
> (NIH, 2010, p. 1)

As mentioned previously, there is significant variation in the level of an individual's needs based on the broad variety of what are described as special needs or disabilities. In addition, depending on the condition of the individual, there are changes that the family can come to expect as the individual transitions into different stages across the life span. While having a family member with intellectual disability and related special needs may present unique challenges, it is important to recognize that the experiences of individuals and their families often vary and depend on a variety of individual, contextual, and biopsychosocial factors that will affect the health, stability, and well-being of the individual and the family (WHO, 2001).

There are numerous intellectual disability diagnoses, as well as developmental disabilities. It was not our intent to exclude any particular groups, as each IDD area has its own unique characteristics; however, because of the limited space, it was necessary to limit the focus to some of the more common IDD categories. For this reason, we provided more detailed descriptions of three primary IDD areas: autism spectrum disorders (ASD), cerebral palsy (CP), and Down syndrome (DS). The descriptions of these areas below are not exhaustive but provide an overview of key diagnostic criteria, treatments, and similarities and differences between these three areas of IDD. In addition, we specifically focused on intellectual and developmental disabilities in this book because of the unique challenges and situations individuals and families face with these particular diagnoses. We acknowledge that there are many additional areas we could have included, as well as focus on other physical, psychological, and cognitive disabilities; however, for our purposes, it was important to narrow the focus to intellectual and developmental disabilities.

Autism Spectrum Disorders

An autism spectrum disorder (ASD) is a lifelong, childhood neurological disorder. Recent prevalence rates estimate that one in 68 children are diagnosed with

ASD (Christensen *et al.*, 2016). As indicated by the name, individuals with ASD can exhibit a *spectrum* of behaviors in two primary areas: social communication and social interaction, and restricted, repetitive patterns of behavior, interests, or activities (American Psychiatric Association [APA], 2013; Harstad *et al.*, 2015). The first diagnostic criterion are often displayed by language impairments, ranging from complete lack of speech to language delays, echoed speech, or overly literal language (APA, 2013). Individuals may also have delays in social-emotional reciprocity, including inability to engage with others, deficits in nonverbal communication, such as lack of eye contact, or impairments in understanding and responding to social cues (APA, 2013). For the second criterion, restricted, repetitive patterns of behavior, interests, or activities, individuals must display at least two of the four categories: (a) stereotyped or repetitive movements, use of objects or speech, (b) insistence on sameness, strict adherence to schedules/routines, or ritualized patterns of verbal or nonverbal behavior, (c) highly restricted interests that are abnormal in intensity, and (d) high or low reactivity to sensory input, for example, excessive smelling of objects (APA, 2013). These symptoms are present from early childhood and impair the individual's everyday functioning (APA, 2013).

Treatment for ASD

To date, there are no known medical cures for an ASD diagnosis. However, researchers and clinicians have made great advancements in identifying treatments that help individuals with ASD manage, and oftentimes, overcome many of the tendencies and symptoms associated with their diagnosis, such as behavior, sensory, and communication needs. It is out of the scope of this chapter to review all of the treatments for individuals with ASD, and we do not consider this selected treatment list exhaustive or exclusive.

Behavior and Communication. Treatment approaches designed to assist diagnosed individuals with behavior and communication deficits provide structure, direction, and organization for the child in addition to family participation (National Research Council [NRC], 2001). Applied Behavior Analysis (ABA) is one of the most widely accepted treatments and is used in schools and treatment clinics around the world (Cooper, Heron, & Heward, 2007). ABA encourages desired behaviors and discourages negative behaviors. The basic principles of ABA arose from the work of B. F. Skinner (1938), who contended that behavior was determined by a process called "selection by consequences," meaning that individuals engage in behaviors that produce desirable outcomes and behaviors that do not produce desirable outcomes will decrease over time, or disappear completely. Various types of ABA include Discrete Trial Training, Early Intensive Behavioral Intervention, Pivotal Response Training, and Verbal Behavior Intervention (Centers for Disease Control and Prevention [CDC], 2015a). Practitioners of ABA are typically credentialed by the Behavior Analyst Certification Board (BACB) and are referred to as Board-Certified Behavior Analysts (BCBA; BACB, n.d.).

Medications. Although there are no medications that can cure ASD or even treat the main symptoms, there are a variety of medications that may be prescribed to assist individuals with related symptoms (i.e., medications for seizures, depression, improving attention, irritability). This list is not considered to be exhaustive or exclusive, but commonly prescribed medications for individuals with ASD include Selective Serotonin Re-uptake Inhibitors (SSRIs), tricyclics, psychoactive or anti-psychotic medications, stimulants, anti-anxiety medications, and anticonvulsants (National Institutes of Health [NIH], 2016).

Cerebral Palsy

Cerebral palsy (CP) is a neurodevelopmental condition caused by abnormal development or damage to the portion of the developing brain that affects muscle movement (CDC, 2015b; National Institute of Neurological Disorders and Stroke [NINDS], n.d.). While CP cannot be diagnosed by a chromosomal test, it is most commonly diagnosed because of motor difficulties observed in the child, due to delays in reaching age-appropriate developmental milestones, and is often diagnosed in the first three years of life (CDC, 2015c). Although specifically defining and classifying CP has varied over the years, CP is considered to be a group of developmental disorders impacting movement and posture that are attributed to disturbances in the brain during fetal development, at birth, or immediately after birth (Bax, Goldstein, Rosenbaum, Leviton, & Paneth, 2005). Problems with body movement, muscle coordination, and balance are the issues most associated with CP; however, these motor impairments are often accompanied by disturbances in sensation, cognition, communication, perception, and behavior (Bax *et al.*, 2005).

The prevalence of CP is estimated to be approximately one in 323 (Christensen *et al.*, 2014). CP may be congenital (due to brain damage before or during birth), which accounts for 85–90% of all CP cases, or acquired after birth, resulting primarily from injuries (e.g., child abuse or other injuries) or infections (e.g., meningitis) (CDC, 2015b). It was previously believed that birth difficulties subsequent to a prolonged second stage of labor contributed to the majority of cerebral palsy diagnoses. Researchers now suggest that this accounts for only 10% of the total incidences of CP (Menkes & Flores-Sarnat, 2006). Other major risk factors for CP include low birth weight (Lie, Groholt, & Eskild, 2010), infections prior to and during pregnancy (Streja *et al.*, 2013; Wu *et al.*, 2013), and multiple births (Odding, Roebroeck, & Stam, 2006). Approximately 50–65% of individuals diagnosed with CP have a co-existing developmental or intellectual disability (CDC, 2016; Enkelaar, Ketelaar, & Gorter, 2008).

In addition to motor impairments, individuals with CP face numerous health problems, including respiratory problems, such as dysphagia (difficulty swallowing) and pneumonias, and feeding problems. Gastroesophageal reflux (GERD), skeletal malformations, seizures, and malnutrition as well as mobility difficulties contribute to these risks (Braverman, 2001; Gerdung *et al.*, 2016). Visual impairments and seizure disorders are also common (Bruck *et al.*, 2001; Kirby *et al.*, 2011; Liptak *et al.*, 2001; Odding *et al.*, 2006). Seizure disorders occur in approximately 21–67% of individuals with CP, with the highest incidence found in those with severe mobility impairment (Christensen *et al.*, 2014).

Life expectancy for those with CP is similar to that in the general population, unless severe impairments are present (Strauss, Shavelle, Reynolds, Rosenbloom, & Day, 2007). As individuals with CP age, health problems often include pain, additional sensory problems, and decreased mobility and ability to feed themselves (Erkin, Culha, Ozel, & Kirbiyik, 2010; Jahnsen, Villien, Aamodt, Stanghelle, & Holm, 2004). Most individuals with CP will experience declines in mobility across their life spans. In fact, problems associated with mobility and nutrition often exacerbate other health problems and contribute most to the morbidity and mortality of individuals with CP. The inability to walk independently is significant because severe impairments in independent movement negatively impact life expectancy, as those with minimal to no mobility rarely survive to age 60 (Strauss, Ojdana, Shavelle, & Rosenbloom, 2004). Support for both the individuals with CP and their families is necessary throughout the life span.

Treatment for CP

Treatments for the symptoms of CP include early intervention, supportive therapies, medications, and surgery (NINDS, n.d.). Primary treatments for those with CP involve specific exercises from physical, occupational, and speech therapies, which not only add to quality of life but also prevent problems in oxygenation and skin integrity, both of which become more significant as the person ages (Crawford & Harris, 2016; Farage, Miller, Elsner, & Maibach, 2008). For example, positional changes are imperative if individuals with CP are not independently mobile. Individuals need to be provided with physical supports for their posture, including specialized wheelchairs or standing boards, which will improve mobility and lung expansion. Speech-language pathologists can assist the individual with CP to develop skills to reduce drooling and to aid in chewing and swallowing (see Chapter 11 for information on early childhood intervention and therapies). Dental problems are common and are related to gastroesophageal reflux disease (GERD), poor nutrition, difficulties in eating, and infections (Braverman, 2001; Guare *et al.*, 2012). Caregivers often need instruction on assisting the individual with teeth cleaning, regardless of whether s/he eats by mouth (Jan & Jan, 2016). All treatments should include parents or caregivers as well as individuals with CP when they are developmentally able to understand and participate in these services and personal care.

There are also newer treatments available that include therapies to combat limb spasticity, a common phenomenon in those with CP, which results in changes in mobility. This has been treated in the past with botulism; however, the long-term benefits are negligible (Huntley & Bradley, 2017). Other programs that may be beneficial for gross motor function include adaptive riding in hippotherapy and riding simulation, as well as adaptive water therapies (Angsupaisal *et al.*, 2015; Lee, Kim, & Na, 2014; Ryu *et al.*, 2016). Stem cell therapy is also being explored for the treatment of patients with CP, but these studies, albeit promising, remain in clinical trials (Chen *et al.*, 2013).

Down Syndrome

Down syndrome (DS) is a genetic condition in which a person is born with an extra copy of chromosome 21 (National Down Syndrome Congress [NDSC], 2014). It is the most common chromosomal disorder, occurring in approximately one in every 700 babies born in the United States (Parker *et al.*, 2010). There are no known causes of DS, and although the chances of having a child with DS increases with maternal age, it does not vary by race, ethnicity, socioeconomic status, or other demographic variables (NDSC, 2014).

Down syndrome is unique because a diagnosis can be obtained in utero or postpartum, providing a relatively quick and definitive diagnosis of this genetic condition (National Down Syndrome Society [NDSS], 2012). Two types of tests can be performed prenatally, screening tests and diagnostic tests, which occur at different points in the pregnancy. Prenatal screenings estimate the chance of the fetus having DS or other problems; however, these tests are often confused with diagnostic tests (e.g., chorionic villus sampling and amniocentesis), which do provide a definitive diagnosis with almost 100% accuracy (NDSC, 2014; NDSS, 2012). Prenatal screenings involve a blood test of the mother and an ultrasound/sonogram, and while they do provide a probability of a fetus having a chromosomal abnormality, they do not provide a definite diagnosis (Global Down Syndrome Foundation and National Down Syndrome Congress, 2012). For a diagnosis after the birth of the baby, a blood test or *karyotype* is conducted to examine the baby's cells to determine whether there is an extra 21st chromosome—in other words, there are three copies of the 21st chromosome instead of the usual pair (NDSS, 2012). Initially, the baby is examined for physical traits that are common in individuals with DS, including low muscle tone, a small nose, small stature (height), small skin folds on the inner corners and an upward slant of the eyes, space between the large and second toes, and a single deep crease across the center of the palm, but the blood test provides the definitive diagnosis of DS (NDSC, 2014; NDSS, 2012).

People with DS are at an increased risk for various health conditions, such as sleep apnea, heart defects, thyroid disease, and anemia (Bull, 2011). Life expectancy for individuals with DS has dramatically increased over the last 50 years, increasing from an expected ten years of age in 1960 to 47 years in 2007 (Presson *et al.*, 2013), with some individuals with DS living well into later life stages. Because of the longer life expectancy, many individuals with DS are seeking employment and higher education, thus creating new opportunities and achievements that previously have not been possible for this population of individuals with IDD.

Treatment for Down Syndrome

Most individuals with DS experience mild to moderate cognitive and physical developmental delays, as well as specific health problems. While there is not a treatment for DS, there are a number of therapies as well as health guidelines that are important for individuals with DS. Early intervention services are critical for babies with DS and include speech and language therapy, physical therapy, occupational therapy, and other activities and exercises that address developmental delays (NDSS, 2013; see Chapter 11 on early intervention services for additional information). Specific healthcare guidelines for individuals with DS include regular medical tests, such as tests for thyroid function and celiac disease, as well as specific therapies and other complementary and alternative treatments that may be available (Bull, 2011; NDSS, 2013; see Chapter 10 for additional information about healthcare for individuals with IDD). Although individuals with DS may be at risk for certain health problems and medical issues, establishing a comprehensive medical team can contribute to a healthy, long life.

Families of Individuals with IDD

Almost every study prior to the 1980s indicated poor outcomes for families of children with IDD and focused on a deficit framework that explored the negative factors associated with disability as a life stressor (Hodapp, 2007). Recent studies point to more positive experiences for parents of children with IDD, rather than any negative pathology being created because of the disability (Cunningham, 1996). More recently, researchers have investigated the general experiences parents and families have when raising a child with an IDD diagnosis. In general, families raising a child with ASD seem to experience more distress and negative effects than families raising a child with another IDD. For example, several authors have stated that parents' level of stress is higher in parents of children with ASD than in parents of children with other IDDs, including DS and CP (e.g., Dabrowska & Pisula, 2010; Eisenhower, Baker, & Blacher, 2005; Hodapp, Ly, Fidler, & Ricci, 2001). Parents raising a child with ASD also report significantly higher levels of depression and anxiety than parents of children with DS (Hamlyn-Wright, Draghi-Lorenz, & Ellis, 2007).

Although parents of children with ASD seem to report the most negative impact compared to parents of children with other IDDs, parents of children with IDD may experience more challenges, in general, than families of typically developing children. Several researchers have found that parents of children with DS reported slightly lower stress and better coping scores than families with other IDDs, including ASD and CP (Eisenhower *et al.*, 2005), but they may experience higher levels of stress and poorer coping than families with typically developing children (Hodapp *et al.*, 2001; Sanders & Morgan, 1997). Corrice and Glidden (2009) found that differences between parents of children with DS and parents of children with other IDDs disappeared when age (maternal and child) and child behaviors were held constant (Corrice & Glidden, 2009; Glidden, Grein, & Ludwig, 2014).

Even though there appears to be a mixture of experiences reported by parents of children with IDD, support systems and coping strategies for families are crucial. Siklos and Kerns (2006) found that parents of children with ASD and parents of children with DS reported similar needs, but differed in the types of support they needed. Parents of children with ASD reported more needs related to professionals working with their child, while parents of children with DS reported needing more school supports, community programming, and friendship opportunities for their child. Others have addressed support and coping between mothers and fathers and across different life span stages. Davis and colleagues (2010) explored quality of life differences between mothers and fathers and across different ages of children with CP. While they did not find any differences in their qualitative study across age groups or between mothers and fathers, they did indicate that caring for a child with CP affects parents' physical, social, financial, and family well-being as well as freedom and independence. The parents also indicated that they felt unsatisfied with the availability of services for their child and their family and the level of support received from the programs and services that are available (Davis *et al.*, 2010). Other researchers have indicated different levels of stress and coping at different life span stages (Nelson Goff, Monk *et al.*, 2016; Woodman, 2014), but results are varied across different studies. Thus, it may not be the presence of an IDD diagnosis in a child that has the most impact, positively or negatively, but rather various individual characteristics, as well as family resources, strengths, and experiences that may be most critical for understanding how families are affected when a member has an intellectual or developmental disability.

Conclusion

The current chapter has reviewed information on three areas of IDD: autism spectrum disorders, cerebral palsy, and Down syndrome. We provided information about the unique features of each of these areas of intellectual or developmental disability, as well as treatments for symptoms and problems associated with each one. Finally, we provided a brief review of the literature on the impact of having a child with ASD, CP, or DS on families. While some research indicates more impairment for parents of children with ASD, the research comparing across different IDD groups is limited, and research on IDD in families in general needs further development, with more robust methodologies and more diverse samples. The conclusions that can be made suggest that the experiences of parents and families are as unique as the individuals with IDD themselves. It is also important to recognize the positive experiences and generally low levels of problems or symptoms reported by parents of children with IDD in several of the studies (see Eisenhower *et al.*, 2005; Nelson Goff, Monk *et al.*, 2016; Woodman, 2014).

Families of individuals with IDD must respond to the needs of the individual, which may require additional resources, such as time, finances, and social support that may vary across the individual's life span (Nelson Goff, Monk e*t al.*, 2016). This is of particular importance to recognize as their life span extends into adulthood and later life years, which brings a variety of experiences around independence, transitions, and later life caregiving for individuals with IDD (Nelson Goff, High *et al.*, 2016). Thus, while caring for a child with IDD can have challenges, it is clear that there is value in recognizing the unique and positive aspects of having a child with IDD. Regardless of the level of impairment or type of disability, families often experience a unique and balanced quality of life that is difficult to describe or classify in clear or traditional ways. Thus, as you continue through this book, keep in mind the unique perspectives of each family and each individual with IDD that shapes and defines their experiences with the world—and the experience of the world with each of them.

References

American Psychiatric Association. (2013). *Diagnostic and statistical manual of mental disorders* (5th ed.). Washington, DC: American Psychiatric Pub.

Angsupaisal, M., Visser, B., Alkema, A., Meinsma-van der Tuin, M., Maathuis, C. G., Reinders-Messelink, H., & Hadders-Algra, M. (2015). Therapist-designed adaptive riding in children with cerebral palsy: Results of a feasibility study. *Physical Therapy*, *95*(8), 1151–1162. doi:10.2522/ptj.20140146

Bax, M., Goldstein, M., Rosenbaum, P., Leviton, A., & Paneth, N. (2005). Proposed definition and classification of cerebral palsy. *Developmental Medicine and Child Neurology*, *47*(8), 571–576. doi:10.1017/S001216220500112X

Behavior Analyst Certification Board (n.d.). *Board-certified behavior analysts.* Retrieved from http://bacb.com/bcba/

Braverman, J. (2001). Respiratory problems in individuals with cerebral palsy: Recognition, management, and prevention. *Exceptional Parent*, *31*(6), 56–58. Retrieved from http://www.eparent.com/

Bruck, I., Antoniuk, S. A., Spessatto, A., de Bem, R. S., Hausberger, R. S., & Pacheco, C. G. (2001). Epilepsy in children with cerebral palsy. *Arquivos de Neuro-Psiquiatria*, *59*(1), 35–39. doi:10.1590/S0004-282X2001000100008

Bull, M. J. (2011). Clinical report: Health supervision for children with Down syndrome. *Pediatrics*, *128*(2), 393–406. doi:10.1542/peds.2011-1605

Centers for Disease Control and Prevention. (2015a). *Autism spectrum disorder: Treatment.* Retrieved from https://www.cdc.gov/ncbddd/autism/treatment.html

Centers for Disease Control and Prevention. (2015b). *Cerebral palsy: Causes and risk factors of cerebral palsy.* Retrieved from https://www.cdc.gov/ncbddd/cp/causes.html

Centers for Disease Control and Prevention (2015c). *Cerebral palsy: Screening and diagnosis of cerebral palsy.* Retrieved from https://www.cdc.gov/ncbddd/cp/diagnosis.html

Centers for Disease Control and Prevention. (2016). *Cerebral palsy: Data & statistics for cerebral palsy.* Retrieved from https://www.cdc.gov/ncbddd/cp/data.html

Chapireau, F. (2005). The environment in the international classification of functioning, disability and health. *Journal of Applied Research in Intellectual Disabilities*, *18*(4), 305–311. doi:10.1111/j.1468-3148.2005.00269.x

Chen, G., Wang, Y., Xu, Z., Fang, F., Xu, R., Fan, L., & Liu, H. (2013). Neural stem cell-like cells derived from autologous bone mesenchymal stem cells for the treatment of patients with cerebral palsy. *Journal of Translational Medicine*, *11*(21), 1–11. doi:10.1186/1479-5876-11-21

Christensen, D. L., Baio, J., Van Naarden Braun, K., Bilder, D., Charles, J., Constantino, J. N., Daniels, J., Drukin, M. S., Fitzgerald, R. T., Kurzius-Spencer, M., Lee, L.-C., Pettygrove, S. Robinson, C., Schulz, E., Wells, C., Wingate, M. S., Zahorodny, W., & Yeargin-Allsopp, M. (2016). Prevalence and characteristics of autism spectrum disorder among children aged 8 years—Autism and Developmental Disabilities Monitoring Network, 11 sites, United States, 2012. *Morbidity and Mortality Weekly Report (MMWR) Surveillance Summaries*, *65*(3), 1–23. doi:10.15585/mmwr.ss6503a1

Christensen, D, Van Naarden Braun, K., Doernberg, N. S., Maenner, M. J., Arneson, C. L., Durkin, M. S., Benedict, R. E., Kirby, R. S., Wingate, M.S., Fitzgerald, R., & Yeargin-Allsopp, M. (2014). Prevalence of cerebral palsy, co-occurring autism spectrum disorders, and motor functioning—Autism and Developmental Disabilities Monitoring Network, USA, 2008. *Developmental Medicine and Child Neurology*, *56*(1), 59–65. doi:10.1111/dmcn.12268

Cooper, J. O., Heron, T. E., & Heward, W. L. (2007). *Applied behavior analysis* (2nd ed.). Upper Saddle River, NJ: Pearson.

Corrice, A. M., & Glidden, L. M. (2009). The Down syndrome advantage: Fact or fiction? *Journal on Intellectual and Developmental Disabilities*, *114*(4), 254–268. doi:10.1352/1944-7558-114.4.254-268

Crawford, A., & Harris, H. (2016). Caring for adults with impaired physical mobility. *Nursing*, *46*(12), 36–41. doi:10.1097/01.NURSE.0000504674.19099.1d

Cunningham, C. (1996). Families of children with Down syndrome. *Down Syndrome Research & Practice*, *4*(3), 87–95. Retrieved from https://www.down-syndrome.org/perspectives/66/?page=1

Dabrowska, A., & Pisula, E. (2010). Parenting stress and coping styles in mothers and fathers of pre-school children with autism and Down syndrome. *Journal of Intellectual Disability Research*, *54*(3), 266–28. doi:10.1111/j.1365-2788.2010.01258.x

Davis, E., Shelly, A., Waters, E., Boyd, R., Cook, K., & Davern, M. (2010). The impact of caring for a child with cerebral palsy: Quality of life for mothers and fathers. *Child: Care, Health and Development*, *36*(1), 63–73. doi:10.1111/j.1365-2214.2009.00989.x

DePloy, E., & Gilson, S. F. (2004). *Rethinking disability: Principles for professional and social change*. Belmont, CA: Thompson Brooks/Cole.

Eisenhower, A. S., Baker, B. L., & Blacher, J. (2005). Preschool children with intellectual disability: Syndrome specificity, behaviour problems, and maternal well-being. *Journal of Intellectual Disability Research*, *49*(9), 657–671. doi:10.1111/j.1365-2788.2005.00699.x

Enkelaar, L., Ketelaar, M., & Gorter, J. W. (2008). Association between motor and mental functioning in toddlers with cerebral palsy. *Developmental Neurorehabilitation*, *11*(4), 276–282. doi:10.1080/17518420802581164

Erkin, G. E., Culha, C., Ozel, S., & Kirbiyik, E. G. (2010). Feeding and gastrointestinal problems in children with cerebral palsy. *International Journal of Rehabilitation Research*, *33*(3), 281–224. doi:10.1097/MRR.0b013e3283375e10

Farage, M. A., Miller, K. W., Elsner, P., & Maibach, H. I. (2008). Functional and physiological characteristics of the aging skin. *Aging Clinical & Experimental Research*, *20*(3), 195–200. doi:10.1007/BF03324769

Flaherty, E., Masters, E., & Glidden, L. (2000). Positive adjustment in parents rearing children with Down syndrome. *Early Education and Development*, *11*(4), 407–422. doi:10.1207/s15566935eed1104_3

Gerdung, C. A., Tsang, A., Yasseen, A. S., Armstrong, K., McMillan, H. J., & Kovesi, T. (2016). Association between chronic aspiration and chronic airway infection with pseudomonas aeruginosa and other gram-negative bacteria in children with cerebral palsy. *Lung*, *194*(2), 307–314. doi:10.1007/s00408-016-9856-5

Glidden, L. M., Billings, F. J., & Jobe, B. M. (2006). Personality, coping style and well-being of parents rearing children with developmental disabilities. *Journal of Intellectual Disability Research, 50*(12), 949–962. doi:10.1111/j.1365-2788.2006.00929.x

Glidden, L. M., Grein, K. A., & Ludwig, J. A. (2014). The Down syndrome advantage: It depends on what and when you measure. *American Journal on Intellectual and Developmental Disabilities, 119*(5), 389–404. doi:10.1352/1944-7558-119.5.389

Global Down Syndrome Foundation and National Down Syndrome Congress. (2012). *Down syndrome prenatal testing pamphlet, English.* Retrieved from http://www.downsyndrometest.org/down-syndrome-prenatal-testing-pamphlet-english/

Guare, R. O., Ferreira, M. C., Leite, M. F., Rodrigues, J. A., Lussi, A., & Santos, M. T. (2012). Dental erosion and salivary flow rate in cerebral palsy individuals with gastroesophageal reflux. *Journal of Oral Pathology and Medicine, 41I*(5), 367–371. doi:10.1111/j.1600-0714.2011.01112.x

Hallahan, D., & Kauffman, J. (2000). *Exceptional learners* (8th ed.). Boston, MA: Allyn & Bacon.

Hamlyn-Wright, S., Draghi-Lorenz, R., & Ellis, J. (2007). Locus of control fails to mediate between stress and anxiety and depression in parents of children with a developmental disorder. *Autism, 11*(6), 489–501. doi:10.1177/1362361307083258.

Harstad, E. B., Fogler, J., Sideridis, G., Weas, S., Mauras, C., & Barbaresi, W. J. (2015). Comparing diagnostic outcomes of autism spectrum disorder using "DSM-IV-TR" and "DSM-5" criteria. *Journal of Autism and Developmental Disorders, 45*(5), 1437–1450. doi:10.1007/s10803-014-2306-4

Hodapp, R. M. (2007). Families of persons with Down syndrome: New perspectives, findings, and research and service needs. *Mental Retardation and Developmental Disabilities Research Reviews, 13*(3), 279–287. doi:10.1002/mrdd.20160

Hodapp, R. M., Ly, T. M., Fidler, D. J., & Ricci, L. A. (2001). Less stress, more rewarding: Parenting children with Down syndrome. *Parenting, 1*(4), 317–337. doi:10.1207/S15327922PAR0104_3

Huntley, J. S., & Bradley, L. J. (2017). The evidence base for botulinum toxin injection for the treatment of cerebral palsy-related spasticity in the lower limb: The long-term effects. In S. Alshryda, J. S. Huntley, & P. A. Banaszkiewicz (Eds.), *Paediatric orthopaedics: An evidence-based approach to clinical questions* (pp. 369–373). New York, NY: Springer.

Jahnsen, R., Villien, L., Aamodt, G., Stanghelle, J., & Holm, I. (2004). Musculoskeletal pain in adults with cerebral palsy compared with the general population. *Journal of Rehabilitation Medicine, 36*(2), 78–84. doi:10.1080/16501970310018305

Jan, B. M., & Jan, M. M. (2016). Dental health of children with cerebral palsy. *Neurosciences, 21*(4), 314–318. doi:10.17712/nsj.2016.4.20150729

Kirby, R. S., Wingate, M. S., Van Naarden, B. K., Doernberg, N. S., Arneson, C. L., Benedict, R. E., Mulvihill, B., Durkin, M. S., Fitzgerald, R. T., Maenner, M.J., Patz, J. A., & Yeargin-Allsopp, M. (2011). Prevalence and functioning of children with cerebral palsy in four areas of the United States in 2006: A report from the Autism and Developmental Disabilities Monitoring Network. *Research in Developmental Disabilities, 32*(2), 462–469. doi:10.1016/j.ridd.2010.12.042

Lee, C. W., Kim, S. G., & Na, S. S. (2014). The effects of hippotherapy and a horse riding simulator on the balance of children with cerebral palsy. *Journal of Physical Therapy Science, 26*(3), 423–425. doi:10.1589/jpts.26.423

Lie, K. K., Groholt, E-K., & Eskild, A. (2010). Association of cerebral palsy with Apgar score in low and normal birthweight infants: Population based cohort study. *BMJ*, *341*, c4990. doi:10.1136/bmj.c4990

Liptak, G. S., O'Donnell, M., Conaway, M., Chumlea, W. C., Worley, G., Henderson, R. C., Fung, E., Stallings, V.A., Samsong-Fang, L., Calvert, R., Rosenbaum, P., & Stevenson, R. D. (2001). The health status of children with moderate to severe cerebral palsy. *Developmental Medicine & Child Neurology*, *43*(6), 364–370. doi:10.1111/j.1469-8749.2001.tb00223.x

Menkes, J. H., & Flores-Sarnat, L. (2006). Cerebral palsy due to chromosomal anomalies and continuous gene syndromes. *Clinics in Perinatology*, *33*(2), 481–501. doi:10.1016/j.clp.2006.03.001

National Down Syndrome Congress. (2014). *Down syndrome informational brochure*. Retrieved from http://www.ndsccenter.org/new-and-expectant-parents/

National Down Syndrome Society. (2012). *The NDSS brochure*. Retrieved from http://www.ndss.org/Resources/Publications/Printed-Materials/

National Down Syndrome Society. (2013). *A promising future together: A guide for new and expectant parents*. New York, NY: Author. Retrieved from http://www.ndss.org/Resources/Publications/Printed-Materials/

National Institute of Neurological Disorders and Stroke. (n.d.). *Cerebral palsy information page*. Retrieved from https://www.ninds.nih.gov/Disorders/All-Disorders/Cerebral-Palsy-Information-Page

National Institutes of Health. (2010). *Fact sheet: Intellectual and developmental disabilities*. Retrieved from https://report.nih.gov/nihfactsheets/Pdfs/IntellectualandDevelopmentalDisabilities(NICHD).pdf

National Institutes of Health. (2016). *Autism spectrum disorder: Medication treatment*. Retrieved from https://www.nichd.nih.gov/health/topics/autism/conditioninfo/Pages/medication-treatment.aspx

National Research Council, Division of Behavioral and Social Sciences and Education, Youth and Families Board on Children, Cognitive and Sensory Sciences Board on Behavioral, and Committee on Educational Interventions for Children with Autism. (2001). *Educating children with autism* (1st ed.). Washington, DC: National Academy Press.

Nelson Goff, B. S., High, J., Cless, A., Koblitz, K., Staats, N., & Springer, N. (2016). Special needs in families. In C. A. Price, K. R. Bush, & S. J. Price (Eds.), *Families and change: Coping with stressful events and transitions* (5th ed., pp. 79–94). Thousand Oaks, CA: Sage.

Nelson Goff, B. S., Monk, J. K., Malone, J., Staats, N., Tanner, A., & Springer, N. (2016). Comparing parents of children with Down syndrome at different life span stages. *Journal of Marriage and Family*, *78*, 1131–1148. doi:10.1111/jomf.12312

Odding, E., Roebroeck, M. E., & Stam, H. J. (2006). The epidemiology of cerebral palsy: Incidence, impairments and risk factors. *Disability and Rehabilitation*, *28*(4), 183–191. doi:10.1080/09638280500158422

Parker, S. E., Mai, C. T., Canfield, M. A., Rickard, R., Wang, Y., Meyer, R. E., Anderson, P., Mason, C. A., Collins, J. S., Kirby, R. S., & Correa, A. (2010). Updated national birth prevalence estimates for selected birth defects in the United States, 2004–2006. *Birth Defects Research Part A: Clinical and Molecular Teratology*, *88*(12), 1008–1016. doi:10.1002/bdra.20735

Presson, A. P., Partyka, G., Jensen, K. M., Devine, O. J., Rasmussen, S. A., McCabe, L. L., & McCabe, E. R. (2013). Current estimate of Down syndrome population prevalence in the United States. *Journal of Pediatrics, 163*(4), 1163–1168. doi:10.1016/j.jpeds.2013.06.013

Ryu, K., Ali, A., Kwon, M., Lee, C., Kim, Y., Lee, G., & Kim, J. (2016). Effects of assisted aquatic movement and horseback riding therapies on emotion and brain activation in patients with cerebral palsy. *Journal of Physical Therapy Science, 28*(12), 3283–3287. doi:10.1589/jpts.28.3283

Sanders, J. L., & Morgan, S. B. (1997). Family stress and adjustment as perceived by parents of children with autism or Down syndrome: Implications for intervention. *Child & Family Behavior Therapy, 19*(4), 15–32. doi:10.1300/J019v19n04_02

Schalock, R. L., Luckasson, R. A., & Shogren, K. A. (2007). The renaming of mental retardation: Understanding the change to the term intellectual disability. *Intellectual and Developmental Disabilities, 45*(2), 116–124. doi:10.1352/1934-9556(2007)45[116: TROMRU]2.0.CO;2

Siklos, S., & Kerns, K. A. (2006). Assessing need for social support in parents of children with autism and Down syndrome. *Journal of Autism and Developmental Disorders, 36*(7), 921–933. doi:10.1016/j.ridd.2005.09.003

Skinner, B. F. (1938). *The behavior of organisms: An experimental analysis.* Oxford, UK: Appleton-Century.

Strauss, D. J., Ojdana, K., Shavelle, R., & Rosenbloom, L. (2004). Decline in function and life expectancy of older persons with cerebral palsy. *NeuroRehabilitation, 19*(1), 69–78. Retrieved from http://content.iospress.com/articles/neurorehabilitation/nre00216

Strauss, D., Shavelle, R., Reynolds, R., Rosenbloom, L., & Day, S. (2007). Survival in cerebral palsy in the last 20 years: Signs of improvement? *Developmental Medicine & Child Neurology, 49*(2), 86–92. doi:10.1111/j.1469-8749.2007.00086.x

Streja, E., Miller, J. E., Bech, B. H., Greene, N., Pedersen, L. H., Yeargin-Allsopp, M., Van Naarden Braun, K., Schendel, D. E., Christensen, D., Uldall, P., & Olsen, J. (2013). Congenital cerebral palsy and prenatal exposure to self-reported maternal infections, fever, or smoking. *American Journal of Obstetrics and Gynecology, 209*(4), 332.e1–332.e10. doi:10.1016/j.ajog.2013.06.023

Werner, S., Edwards, M., Baum, N., Brown, I., Brown, R. I., & Isaacs, B. J. (2009). Family quality of life among families with a member who has an intellectual disability: An exploratory examination of key domains and dimensions of the revised FQOL survey. *Journal of Intellectual Disability Research, 53*(6), 501–511. doi:10.1111/j.1365-2788.2009.01164.x

Woodman, A. C. (2014). Trajectories of stress among parents of children with disabilities: A dyadic analysis. *Family Relations, 63*(1), 39–54. doi:10.1111/fare.12049

World Health Organization. (2001). *International classification of functioning, disability, and health—ICF.* Geneva, Switzerland: Author. Retrieved from http://www.who.int/classifications/icf/en/

Wu, C. S., Pedersen, L. H., Miller, J. E., Sun, Y., Streja, E., Uldall, P., & Olsen, J. (2013). Risk of cerebral palsy and childhood epilepsy related to infections before or during pregnancy. *PLoS One, 8*(2), e57552. doi:10.1371/journal.pone.0057552

2 A Systemic and Contextual Lens of Disability

Family Stress, Ambiguous Loss, and Meaning Making

Nicole Piland Springer, PhD, Brie Turns, MS, PhD, and Marilyn Masterson, PhD, RN

Introduction

This chapter will describe past and current theoretical perspectives for understanding family stress and coping, with an emphasis on key elements of adaptation, grief processes, and meaning making for those raising and/or caring for a loved one with an intellectual and developmental disability (IDD). An overview of family stress (McCubbin & Patterson, 1983) and chronic illness health models (McDaniel, Hepworth, & Doherty, 1992; Rolland, 1994) will be provided. In addition, the application of the ambiguous loss theory, developed by Pauline Boss in the 1970s–1980s, will be described as it has direct relevance to the experiences of parents facing a disability diagnosis of their child (Bentley, 2011; Boss, 1999, 2002, 2006; O'Brien, 2007). However, for some disabilities, like cerebral palsy or autism spectrum disorder (ASD), a chronic sorrow model may be more applicable (Masterson, 2010). Relevant background literature as it applies to IDD will be provided, as well as a description of how these theories or models can be applied in professional interactions with families.

Viewing the person living with IDD in the context of a family system, while also considering the strengths and resources within his/her social and professional-provider community, is essential. It is within the larger community where a variety of providers interface with the family and their loved one, from birth and across the life span. There are many chapters within this textbook that will cover the specific resources available to families (i.e., early childhood intervention, legal and financial services, the educational system, supportive employment), the benefits of those resources, and the challenges families face with regards to access and potential barriers to certain resources.

Family Systems, Stress, and Adaptation

Based on a family systems orientation, significant value is placed on the interactions between family members, as well as the relationship between families and larger social systems (von Bertalanffy, 1968). Thus, as systemic providers, individuals with IDD are not viewed as living in isolation, and family members and professionals within their lives are considered as having a bi-directional influence on their well-being. Therefore, family stress and coping is also viewed from a relationally focused perspective. When families are faced with typical life stressors, in addition to the unique factors associated with raising a child or caring for an adult with IDD, sometimes families are forced to make changes in their relationships that are new or unfamiliar to them, ultimately creating disequilibrium (Price, Bush, & Price, 2016; von Bertalanffy, 1968). More specifically, the emotional, relational, and diagnosis-specific influences often require a shift in the system, which some family systems can negotiate more successfully than others. Regaining homeostasis can be achieved, and part of the role of helping professionals is to assist families with this process.

Early Theories of Family Stress and Crisis

Adaptation to stress has been explored in families facing a variety of life stressors; however, the study of families and IDD from a relational or systemic perspective is relatively under-studied (Brown, 2012; Nelson Goff *et al.*, 2016; Parker, 2016). The primary aim of this chapter is to provide a variety of conceptual frameworks and relevant findings from existing research for enhancing your role as the helping professional in the lives of these families. One of the early models for understanding family stress and crisis was the ABC-X model (Hill, 1949). This model takes into account the (a) stressor event (*A*), (b) resources available (*B*), and (c) the family's perceptions (*C*), which can culminate into a crisis (*X*) (Hill, 1949). In this model, the stressor event may be the IDD diagnosis itself, with the available resources and perceptions of the diagnosis factoring into whether the family experiences a crisis.

The simplicity of this model has its advantages, but one particular limitation of this model is that families do not function within a single moment in time or in response to a single stressor. Hill's (1949) original model was later expanded by McCubbin and Patterson (1983) to include a pre-crisis, crisis, and post-crisis stage for understanding adaptation. McCubbin and Patterson's Double ABC-X model helps to capture the family's functioning over time and takes into account (*aA*) new stressors, (*bB*) resources, and (*cC*) perceptions, as well as (*xX*) level of adaptation. In addition, Boss (2002) expanded these models to include the influence of contextual factors experienced by the family. The degree of family stress that is experienced depends upon the accumulation of both elements of external context (i.e., cultural, historical, developmental factors) and internal context (i.e., family structure, psychological characteristics, beliefs/philosophy). This theoretical model puts the family's situation into context to better understand the relationships between internal and external contextual factors and the various family system components that lead to coping, adaptation, and resilience in individuals and families with IDD. Studies that highlight these systemic models for understanding relational dynamics with families experiencing IDD as a stressor event will be presented next.

The Double ABC-X Model and IDD Research

Most recently, a few studies have applied the Double ABC-X model to research on IDD in families. Parker (2016) examined the relationship between hope, coping, life satisfaction, and relational adjustment. The sample in his study included married couples raising a child diagnosed with Down syndrome (DS); which was deemed the identified (x) stressor. This study is one of the few studies that has attempted to examine the couple as a dyad using the Actor-Partner Interaction Model (APIM; Kenny, Kashy, & Cook, 2006). Ultimately, the study yielded few significant findings due in part to a small sample size, but did establish that male hope was positively associated with both male and female relational adjustment. More specifically, a positive association between hope and satisfaction with life for both fathers and mothers was identified. In addition, male satisfaction with life had a positive association with female relational adjustment. Similarly, in a sample of mothers of children with DS, Cless, Nelson Goff, and Durtschi (2017) found that mothers' hope mediated the association between coping and relationship quality. These findings, in the context of the Double ABC-X model, support the assumptions of the model by considering perceptions of hope (cC) and the role of coping (cC) as a resource in managing the demands of raising a child with DS, which in turn influences relational adjustment (xX) or adaptation.

Ramisch (2012) applied the Double ABC-X model for therapists to evaluate and guide treatment with couples raising a child with ASD. Therapists are encouraged to view numerous stressors, such as obtaining the correct diagnosis, problem behaviors, facing an unknown future, financial instability, and negative reactions of family members and society as the (aA) pile-up of stressors. The (bB) resources for couples raising a child with ASD can include individual resources (i.e., education), family system resources (i.e., marital satisfaction), informal social support (i.e., social agencies), and formal support services (i.e., counseling and respite). Different (cC) coping mechanisms, such as problem- and emotion-focused coping, that are often used by parents raising a child with ASD should also be noted by mental health professionals. Ramisch (2012) warned against the improper use of some emotion-focused coping techniques, such as avoiding people or substance use as an escape. The couple's (xX) adaptation to life changes may impact their stress levels. For example, if one parent quits his/her job to care for the child, that parent may have trouble with social isolation or lack of adult contact following the transition.

Although these studies serve as examples of applying family stress theory to research variables of interest within sub-populations of those living with IDD, they do not specifically address the diagnosis process, the course of illness (when applicable), or the ongoing demands faced by caregivers of those with IDD. Thus, we will now turn our attention to models that take into consideration the systemic role of illness and disability for better understanding and meeting the needs of families living with IDD.

Families, Chronic Illness, and Disability

There are a couple of models that more specifically address the role of the illness and disability factors, which serve as ways to understand and support families on their journey. These frameworks developed out of a sub-specialty of providers who value the holistic approach to care and particularly the role of the family and medical/healthcare providers in relation to health outcomes. The sub-specialty of Marriage and Family Therapy (MFT), referred to as Medical Family Therapy, or MedFT, has evolved as a result of the clinical, research, and training contributions of professionals from multiple disciplines (Hodgson, Lamson, Mendenhall, & Crane, 2014; McDaniel *et al.*, 1992; Rolland, 1994). MedFT specifically values the position of working with patient-families in conjunction with the patient's medical or healthcare team in an effort to enhance patient health outcomes, patient-family functioning, and provider-patient communication, to name a few (Hodgson & Lamson, 2016). Over the past two decades, many medical settings have moved toward an integrated delivery of care, calling for greater collaboration between mental health and medical providers, or incorporating mental health providers directly within the medical setting, also referred to as co-located care (Hodgson *et al.*, 2014). Although not all families living with IDD need mental health intervention, mental health needs should be assessed along with illness or disability-related needs given the elevated levels of stress and barriers to resources and coping which can develop for these families.

An overview of key chronic illness models will be highlighted below with specific emphasis on the application of those models for families living with IDD. John Rolland's (1994) Family Systems Illness model takes into consideration the following factors: Developmental stage, illness course or anticipated trajectory, and family functioning. His work highlighted the importance of assessing family responses in relation to the onset, course, outcome, and level of incapacitation regarding the identified patient's illness (Rolland, 1984). Some of the challenges in caring for a loved one with IDD is the unknown trajectory of the child's development, acquiring an accurate or official diagnosis, the additional stressors of medical or health-related problems affiliated with a diagnosis, and the demands on the family in seeking intervention or treatment for those conditions. Moreover, the natural developmental life transitions, which co-occur at the parental, sibling, and/or the familial levels simultaneously require attention.

For example, a couple might be faced with the birth of their newborn child diagnosed with Down syndrome (DS), which includes many unknowns with regards to future medical intervention needed for a congenital heart defect, while needing to build a medical team of early intervention specialists, also supporting their oldest child's transition to school, and adjusting to the demands of new jobs without extended family support due to a recent move. Thus, it is important for professionals to consider the family development as a whole, as well as the disability and illness factors influencing and being influenced by the family's development, resources, and available supports.

McDaniel *et al.* (1992) highlighted key areas of assessment for families facing childhood chronic illness. Some questions they encourage providers to ask include: "What beliefs and meanings do family members bring to the child's health problems? How are the family relationships being attended to? How are the siblings functioning? and How are the parents relating to health professionals?" (McDaniel *et al.*, 1992, p. 221). Although not all intellectual disabilities entail chronic illness, families are still required to attend to demands associated with the disability that families of typically developing children do not. Thus, these questions serve as a valuable assessment tool in determining a family's response to their loved one's IDD.

Some additional components of assessment involve exploring the level of acceptance regarding the child's illness or disability, "putting the illness in its place," supporting open communication, and navigating medical and school professional relationships (McDaniel *et al.*, 1992, p. 226). McDaniel and Pisani (2012) emphasized the role of family dynamics and disability, the importance of considering the mix of physical and intellectual challenges across disorders/diagnoses, not losing sight of the contextual view of disability, identifying environmental deficiencies, and acknowledging the role of all caregivers within and beyond the immediate family. In addition, the role of spirituality has become a valued element to address in patient care, which serves as an important component of meaning making (Wright, Watson, & Bell, 1992). The role of meaning making for families will be discussed in other chapters throughout the book (see Chapters 4 and 5 for related discussions).

Grief and Loss: Facing Ambiguity About the Future

Another area for consideration in working with individuals, couples, and families is the role of emotions, but particularly the role of grief and loss. The reality is no parent expecting his/her first child, or any child, wants to consider the possibility of becoming a parent to a child with a chronic/lifelong, medical, congenital, or developmental condition. The prevalence of birth defects varies considerably, but data are available by state in the 2016 Congenital Malformations Surveillance Report, which includes prevalence rates for 47 congenital defects per 10,000 live births (Kirby & Browne, 2016). Despite the positive expectations of parents and grandparents to welcome a perfectly healthy baby into the family, in 2015, approximately 7.6% of children from birth to 17 years old were identified as having a disability in the United States (Krause, 2017). Even though families are often thrust into a reality that most would not want to face, many parents are still able to reflect on the positive nature of their experiences. This mother described the benefit of knowing other parents on a similar journey:

> Because of my son's disability, I have been able to meet and become close to many parents taking on the same role as myself. Without parents in our lives, our children would not become the adults we strive for them to be. It is a club. A private organization that requires a secret handshake of sorts. We nod to each other with the same knowledge. We love to see our children come together as friends, but it's the parents [...] friendships that keep all of us going. We are not alone.
>
> (Springer, McCallum, Pounds, & Nelson Goff, 2011)

Some parents also report they are better people as a result of their child's presence in their life. An example of this is illustrated in the following parent reflection:

> I have learned so much from him and will continue to learn along our journey. I am a better person because of him. He has strengthened my soul [...] my outlook on life. *He is truly an amazing child!*
>
> (Springer *et al.*, 2011)

Ultimately, many parents learn to embrace the unexpected and find meaning in unique ways (Hampton, 2012; Soper, 2007; Springer, 2015), and yet some families remain affected by grief in an ongoing manner (Masterson, 2010). As helping professionals, we are charged with the task of supporting families in whatever ways they are impacted by their child's disability, positively or negatively. But, it is particularly important that professionals recognize the elements of ambiguous loss when families are challenged by their situation.

Ambiguous Loss and Families Living with IDD

Ambiguous loss theory by Boss (1999, 2006, 2007) is rooted in the assumption that individuals and families are most challenged when they are faced with situations that include a range of psychological presence/physical absence or psychological absence/physical presence, combined with the level of boundary ambiguity for those affected by the situation. So, for example, in the case of a traumatic brain injury (TBI), a child or teen is physically present, but is psychological absent (to greater or lesser degrees), based on the severity of the injury. How the family navigates the new roles and responsibilities following the TBI, and the level of boundary ambiguity that results, is considered valuable for understanding the family's ability to make meaning of and function within their altered life. Boss (1999, 2006) emphasized that the disability-specific characteristics are not of greatest influence, but rather the ambiguity of the situation that affects perceived stress and challenges for family functioning.

Two studies have applied ambiguous loss to families living with an IDD diagnosis, one with a sample of mothers and another with a sample of fathers. Bentley (2011), in her study on fathers raising a child with DS (see Chapter 7 on father perspectives for more details on this study), utilized a mixed-method analysis and applied ambiguous loss as a way of understanding the lived experience of fathers adjusting to their child's DS diagnosis. In another mixed-method study, O'Brien (2007) examined the role of *identity ambiguity* for mothers of children with ASD and reviewed the specific ways that parenting a child with ASD contributed to the experience of ambiguous loss. She highlighted that "the severity of a child's disability has not been consistently linked to family functioning" (O'Brien, 2007, p. 135).

More specifically, O'Brien identified the following factors inherent to ASD: (a) lack of clarity in the diagnosis, (b) difficulty in predicting outcomes, (c) day-to-day variability in functioning, (d) appearance of health, and (e) loss of relationships (O'Brien, 2007). She reported that some mothers in her study shared about the unpredictable nature of their child's functioning, which left them "off-balance" in terms of not being able to anticipate their child's progress or behaviors, due to the ambiguity of the situation. In addition, some mothers reflected that they found themselves in a process of comparing expectations about their child prior to receiving the ASD diagnosis. This process is likely an important element for those facing an ASD diagnosis versus those with a diagnosis at birth, like DS. Families raising a child with an ASD may begin life with the perception that their child is typically developing, but then embark on life following the diagnosis that often comes several months or even years later.

In terms of the quantitative findings from O'Brien (2007), depressive symptoms and level of stress were not related to the severity of the child's ASD symptoms; thus, O'Brien suggested that distress of mothers in her sample was directly related to identity ambiguity rooted in ambiguous loss. Whereas parents of children with DS also describe an emotional process following the diagnosis of their child (Nelson Goff *et al.*, 2013), they do not have the experience of first perceiving the child as neurotypical. Moreover, parents of children with DS have the benefit of being exposed to the physical characteristics common to DS at birth, or shortly thereafter (National Down Syndrome Congress [NDSC], 2014a; National Down Syndrome Society [NDSS], 2012). Perhaps their grief process is still rooted in ambiguity and tied to some of the same factors outlined above by O'Brien, but parents of children with DS are more abruptly thrust into the experience of adjusting to an unexpected reality, in contrast to families facing an ASD diagnosis. This is captured best by the following response from a parent of a child with DS who reflected on the question about her most negative experience when facing her child's diagnosis. "I believed all my dreams were shattered. They were not, I have new dreams now" (Springer *et al.*, 2011). Future research is needed to more fully understand the particular process for parents of moving from 'shattered dreams' to discovering 'new dreams.' Researchers need to seek answers to the question: How or what is different about the process for parents who are struggling to make meaning or having difficulty with creating new or alternative dreams? One explanation might be related to the role of chronic sorrow (Olshansky, 1962; Masterson, 2010).

Chronic Sorrow and Congenital Disabilities

Chronic sorrow was first introduced as an observation by Olshansky (1962) and described as a pervasive, never-ending, and ongoing type of grief experienced by parents, particularly mothers, who gave birth to infants with identifiable congenital disabilities. Olshansky (1962) believed these feelings occurred whether the child lived with or away from the parents. Factors such as personality traits, ethnicity, religion, social class, and other variables (Olshansky, 1962) were not related to how this sorrow was perceived. These emotions occurred with any disability, but they were more common among parents who had children who were "severely or moderately retarded – whose children would be considered retarded in any society and in any cultural group" (Olshansky, 1962, p. 191). Current research about chronic sorrow experienced by parents of adult children who have congenital disabilities is limited. As children live longer with more severe disabilities and with a possible corresponding increase in the severity of intellectual disabilities, it is important to determine how chronic sorrow is recognized and whether it may be expressed differently. There are some similarities between grief and chronic sorrow, and while chronic sorrow may be considered a type of grief, it is different from grief. Grief, in general, entails many different expressions and emotions, and while parents of children with disabilities experience this grief on many levels and at different points across the life span, chronic sorrow appears to be, as described by Olshansky (1962), ongoing, pervasive, and at a depth that may not be expressed to others unless they also face a similar situation.

Masterson (2010) highlighted the nature of chronic sorrow in her study, which involved semi-structured interviews with mothers of children with multiple disabilities, including DS, schizophrenia, and cerebral palsy. She reported that all were willing and perhaps even eager to share their perspectives and feelings about their child's disability. Most often, mothers mentioned the sorrow occurring at times of normative developmental milestones for other children of similar ages, particularly those developmental milestones that their child would never meet, or would meet much later, in addition to times when their child's accomplishments would not be recognized by others (Masterson, 2010). These were considered to be recurrent losses, which may be a key factor distinguishing grief from chronic sorrow.

Another consideration for when chronic sorrow may apply is when families are faced with extremely rare and more debilitating diagnoses, or when parents are never able to acquire a diagnosis (Dellve, Samuelsson, Tallborn, Fasth, & Hallberg, 2006; National Organization for Rare Disorders, 2016). Sometimes, just having a name for something brings value to families who are then able to explore intervention and treatment options, even if the condition is not "curable." Moreover, belonging to community support groups or disability-specific organizations offers opportunities to connect with others, online or in person, who are on a similar journey and possibly further along on the journey. In this respect, families can provide key resources to new families just beginning on the path; however, in cases with rare disorders or more severe conditions, access to community groups may be difficult or may not even be available.

Principles for Practice

Family stress and illness models provide a foundation of concepts and guidance for understanding families, but it is necessary to not lose sight of the nuances any family might possess or unique characteristics they might exhibit. A contextual and systemic view, which assesses for individual, relational, and environmental factors, as well as disability-related influences, is essential (McDaniel & Pisani, 2012). It is important to recognize that many families want to share about their experiences, so it may be appropriate to ask questions and invite the family's story. Some families can celebrate their reality and embrace it fully, while others have great difficulty seeing beyond the present moment and might feel hopeless about the future. Some families find acceptance relatively soon after the diagnosis (Nelson Goff *et al.*, 2013), while other families remain constrained by the persistent nature of grief associated with the life not lived, and enduring recurrent stressors and challenges of everyday demands of caring for a loved one with a severe IDD or chronic special needs (Masterson, 2010).

While most families with IDD are resilient, it may be beneficial to consider what ways the family might be stuck and unable to move forward, when they show signs of difficulty (O'Brien, 2007). It is important to help them recognize their strengths, but also to seek help and support in facing the stressors and situations affecting them. Families can benefit from the perspective of a neutral, but supportive outside party when they are struggling in a way that is creating a significant level of distress, when they have reached a point where they are unable to navigate the problem successfully, or when the attempts they have made to resolve the problem have not produced the outcome they desire.

From Grief to Meaning Making

How parents and families make meaning of a situation is a unique process during their IDD journey, particularly because families are often thrust into the unexpected, or the ways in which the diagnosis impacts the child's functioning can remain ambiguous for extended periods of time. There are significant unknowns about what the future holds for their loved one, which can be particularly heightened during the diagnosis period (Nelson Goff *et al.*, 2013). Avoid making assumptions about a family's grief, loss, and meaning making process (O'Brien, 2007). Grief does not usually result in closure and is not a linear process; grief responses may subside at some points along the journey, only to be activated by new challenges or the other typical life experiences all families face. New challenges can occur at developmental transitions for any family member, not just transitions associated with the loved one with IDD.

Ultimately, meaning making is a social experience that occurs within relationships, between parents of individuals with IDD, and between parents and their typically developing children, extended family, co-workers, and friends. And, sometimes, the social experience occurs between parents and complete strangers in the checkout line at the grocery store, where those almond eyes with "brushfield spots" are recognized by another family member familiar with the physical features common in individuals with DS (NDSC, 2014a). Appreciating the beauty of this unique aspect of DS, during such an encounter, becomes an opportunity for meaning making. Thus, how society views and engages families living with IDD, from the point of diagnosis and beyond, is a piece we will turn our attention to in an effort to bring awareness to the changing social climate that families today are experiencing, compared to only 40–50 years ago, when families were encouraged to institutionalize their loved one at birth (National Council on Disability [NCD], 2012).

A Changing Culture: A New Identity Rooted in Ability

The evolution of terms or references applied to those with an IDD diagnosis is one that addresses the long-standing social stigma against those living with either a physical or intellectual difference or disability. Over the past few decades, there has been a strong and consistent movement away from labels such as *retard* or *retarded*, *handicapped*, and even *disabled*, to the use of person-first language (National Center on Birth Defects and Developmental Disabilities, 2017) or operating from a more strengths-based lens, which assumes the perspective about those living with an IDD diagnosis as possessing *abilities*, not *disabilities* (Abilities Not Disabilities, n.d.). Many advocacy groups have introduced these more functional and positive frameworks in direct opposition to the historical deficit lens, which has ultimately contributed to the inception of slogans like "We're more alike than different" (NDSC, 2014b). There have also been campaigns to "Spread the Word to End the Word," which specifically has called for people worldwide to make a pledge to not use the words *retard* or *retarded*, which are deemed derogatory and offensive (Special Olympics, 2017).

Despite these advocacy efforts, families living with disabilities in the varied forms continue to face stigma and discrimination on their IDD journey. Fortunately, progress has been made largely due to the efforts of many determined families, professionals, and communities touched by the lives of those living with an IDD diagnosis. There is still a need for ongoing efforts to break through stereotypes and rejection in support of inclusion, acceptance, and equal opportunities for persons living with an IDD diagnosis (NCD, 2012). Some parents have even spearheaded efforts to create business, service, and intervention opportunities in response to the limited resources available for their own children at the time of their diagnosis or when facing a related need. A couple of examples of this are GiGi's Playhouse—Down Syndrome Achievement Centers, with 24 locations nationally and one center located in Mexico (GiGi's Playhouse, 2016), and the Global Down Syndrome Foundation, which is "dedicated to improving the lives of individuals with Down syndrome through research, medical care, education and advocacy" (Global Down Syndrome Foundation [GDSF], 2017). Moreover, in 2015, A&E TV debuted the first of its kind documentary series, *Born This Way*, which follows families and their loved ones with DS pursuing their dreams (A&E Television Networks, 2017). The cast of this Emmy award-winning show has shared in their journey of dating, employment, and seeking independence, and their third season will be airing in late 2017.

Where We Have Come From, Where We Are Headed

The shift from a deficit lens toward a strengths-based approach to understanding families who are more successful on the IDD journey began through the efforts of many professionals who have contributed to theory development, resilience research, and intervention-based service delivery as is highlighted within and across chapters throughout this book. Continued advocacy at local, state, national, and global levels is bringing recognition of the positive impact having a child with IDD has on families. The next chapter, by Thomas Knestrict, highlights the application of a resilience framework based on research that gained rich, descriptive reflections from parents raising a loved one with a variety of diagnoses (Knestrict & Kuchey, 2009).

In addition to resilience research in the academic realm, conducted by those invested in the field of families and disabilities as part of their life work, many courageous parents have given voice to their personal experiences by publishing inspiring books to bring attention to the powerful, and yet sometimes painful journey of raising a child with an IDD diagnosis. Some of those books include reflections written by parents which focus on the ways in which their children have changed their lives (Beck, 1999; Groneberg, 2008; Hampton, 2012; Soper, 2007, 2009; Stallings & Cook, 1997). The availability of greater access to online support and resources, more balanced and accurate disability-related information, and increased media exposure to inspiring stories has allowed families to gain a more encouraging glimpse into their future through other families, as they are just beginning their IDD journey, which was not available a generation ago.

Conclusion

Children come into the world in all shapes, colors, sizes, and abilities and yet expectant parents may shockingly learn of the special or unique characteristics of their child in utero either via a pre-natal diagnosis, or when complications arise during delivery, shortly after birth, or weeks, months or even years later. The reality is, parenting is a challenging job that does not come with a manual and requires "on the job" training. Ultimately, there are no guarantees in life, and birthing a typical child is simply an illusion that temporarily serves to protect parents from the reality of future unknowns. Some children are born with a diagnosis or given a label, but many inherit one at some point during their lifetime (e.g., attention-deficit disorder, depression and suicidal ideation, dyslexia, addiction, post-traumatic stress disorder, cancer). What if parents were handed those labels at their child's birth? The joy and the excitement of that new life would be greatly tainted by the future reality, instead of being able to embrace the celebration of life.

The experiences that happen on the journey we call life include only the guarantee that in order for parents to love and care for another human, the willingness to risk experiencing pain, loss and hardship, and sometimes death is required. But as you will hear directly from those who have walked along the IDD journey, many have learned to embrace the reality they have landed in by re-claiming dreams for the child they now have, and do so with grace, courage, and perseverance. Springer (2015) spoke to her experience of meaning making and the essence of embracing a pre-natal diagnosis, after pursuing reproductive assistance to ensure a successful pregnancy following several miscarriages:

> We are all faced with opportunities in life that we can learn to accept, or we can become paralyzed. I had a choice—I could either focus on the ways in which our little girl would be "less able" and remain stuck in the grief for the baby I expected, or I could await the beauty of what she had to offer the world [...] From the moment we were told our daughter had an extra chromosome, I knew I was being invited on a journey that would take me to the

depths of my fears, the edges of my faith, and expand my capacity to give and receive love [...] and for that, I am grateful!

(Springer, 2015, pp. 32–33)

Key Messages from This Chapter

- **For individuals with IDD and their families**: Several family stress and chronic illness models can be utilized for understanding family functioning in relation to IDD, as well as applying ambiguous loss to understanding boundary ambiguity in families.
- **For professionals**: Meaning making and the types and severity of grief experienced by individuals with IDD and their families can vary tremendously. Professionals may interface with a family at any phase on their IDD journey, normalize the grief, highlight their strengths, and encourage them when they feel overwhelmed by their current situation. Helping families capitalize on their strengths will help them move toward greater resilience on their IDD journey.
- **For policy makers**: The research trend toward a strengths-based framework is in line with the social inclusion trends of many national (and global) disability awareness campaigns and disability-specific advocacy groups, with continued efforts toward inclusion and equal opportunities for those with IDD. Policies are needed that reduce negative stereotypes and stigmas while promoting the strengths and abilities of individuals with IDD.

References

Abilities Not Disabilities. (n.d.). *Abilities not disabilities.* Retrieved from http://abilitiesnotdisabilities.org/

A&E Television Networks. (2017). *Born this way.* Retrieved from http://www.aetv.com/shows/born-this-way

Beck, M. (1999). *Expecting Adam: A true story of birth, rebirth and everyday magic.* New York, NY: Berkley Publishing Group.

Bentley, G. (2011). *The upside of Down syndrome and fathering: An exploration of hope, satisfaction and coping* (Unpublished doctoral dissertation). Texas Tech University, Lubbock, TX.

Boss, P. (1999). *Ambiguous loss: Learning to live with unresolved grief.* Cambridge, MA: Oxford Press University.

Boss, P. (2002). *Family stress management: A contextual approach.* Thousand Oaks, CA: Sage.

Boss, P. (2006). *Loss, trauma, and resilience: Therapeutic work with ambiguous loss.* New York, NY: W. W. Norton.

Boss, P. (2007). Ambiguous loss theory: Challenges for scholars and practitioners. *Family Relations*, *56*(2), 105–111. doi:10.1111/j.1741-3729.2007.00444.x

Brown, M. (2012). *Dyadic coping, relationship satisfaction, and parenting stress among parents of children with an autism spectrum disorder: The role of couple relationship* (Unpublished doctoral dissertation). Texas Tech University, Lubbock, TX.

Cless, J., Nelson Goff, B. S., & Durtschi, J. A. (2017). *Hope, coping, and relationship quality in mothers of children with Down syndrome.* Manuscript submitted for publication.

Dellve, L., Samuelsson, L., Tallborn, A., Fasth, A., & Hallberg, L. R.-M. (2006). Stress and well-being among parents of children with rare diseases: A prospective intervention study. *Journal of Advanced Nursing, 53*(4), 392–402. doi:10.1111/j.1365-2648.2006.03736.x

GiGi's Playhouse—Down Syndrome Achievement Centers. (2016). *GiGi's locations.* Retrieved from https://gigisplayhouse.org/locations

Global Down Syndrome Foundation. (2017). *About the Global Down Syndrome Foundation.* Retrieved from http://www.globaldownsyndrome.org/

Groneberg, J. G. (2008). *Road Map to Holland: How I found my way through my son's first two years with Down syndrome.* New York, NY: New American Library.

Hampton, K. (2012). *Bloom: Finding beauty in the unexpected—A memoir.* New York, NY: William Morrow.

Hill, R. (1949). *Families under stress.* New York, NY: Harper.

Hodgson, J., & Lamson, A. (2016, September). *Medical family therapy in primary care: Research updates.* Presentation at the meeting of the American Association for Marriage and Family Therapy, Indianapolis, IN.

Hodgson, J., Lamson, A., Mendenhall, T., & Crane, D. R. (Eds.) (2014). *Medical family therapy: Advanced applications.* New York, NY: Springer.

Kenny, D. A., Kashy, D. A., & Cook, W. L. (2006). *Dyadic data analysis.* New York, NY: Guilford.

Kirby, R., & Browne, M. L. (Eds.) (2016). Major birth defects from population-based birth defects surveillance programs in the United States, 2009–2013. *Special Issue: 2016 Congenital Malformations Surveillance Report: A Report from the National Birth Defects Prevention Network, 106*(11), 863–988. Retrieved from https://www.nbdpn.org/ar.php#2016

Knestrict, T., & Kuchey, D. (2009). Welcome to Holland: Characteristics of resilient families raising children with severe disabilities. *Journal of Family Studies, 2*(4), 227–244. doi:10.5172/jfs.15.3.227

Krause, L. (2017). *2016 disability statistics annual report.* Durham, NH: University of New Hampshire. Retrieved from https://disabilitycompendium.org/sites/default/files/user-uploads/2016_AnnualReport.pdf

McCubbin, H. I., & Patterson, J. M. (1983). The family stress process: The Double ABC-X model of adjustment and adaptation. In H. I. McCubbin, M. B. Sussman, & J. M. Patterson (Eds.), *Social stress and the family* (pp. 7–37). New York, NY: Haworth Press.

McDaniel, S. H., Hepworth, J., & Doherty, W. J. (1992). *Medical family therapy: A biopsychosocial approach to families with health problems.* New York, NY: Basic Books.

McDaniel, S. H., & Pisani, A. (2012). Family dynamics and chronic disabilities. In R. C. Talley & J. E Crews (Eds.). *Multiple dimensions of caregiving and disability: Research, practice, policy* (pp. 11–28). New York, NY: Springer.

Masterson, M. (2010). *Chronic sorrow in mothers of adult children with cerebral palsy: An exploratory study* (Unpublished doctoral dissertation). Kansas State University, Manhattan, KS.

National Center on Birth Defects and Developmental Disabilities. (2017). *Communicating with and about people with disabilities.* Retrieved from https://www.cdc.gov/ncbddd/disabilityandhealth/pdf/disabilityposter_photos.pdf

National Council on Disability. (2012). *Deinstitutionalization: Unfinished business, companion paper to unfinished business toolkit.* Retrieved from http://www.ncd.gov/rawmedia_repository/NCD_UnfinishedBusiness_Paper_FINAL508.pdf

National Down Syndrome Congress. (2014a). *Down syndrome informational brochure.* Retrieved from http://www.ndsccenter.org/new-and-expectant-parents/

National Down Syndrome Congress. (2014b). *More alike awareness campaign: We're more alike than different.* Retrieved from http://www.ndsccenter.org/more-alike-awareness-camp/

National Down Syndrome Society. (2012). *The NDSS brochure.* Retrieved from http://www.ndss.org/Resources/Publications/Printed-Materials/

National Organization for Rare Disorders. (2016). *National Organization for Rare Disorders.* Retrieved from https://rarediseases.org/

Nelson Goff, B. S., Monk, J. K., Staats, N., Malone, J., Tanner, A., & Springer, N. (2016). Comparing parents of children with Down syndrome at different life span stages. *Journal of Marriage and Family, 78,* 1131–1148. doi:10.1111/jomf.12312

Nelson Goff, B. S., Springer, N., Foote, L. C., Frantz, C., Peak, M., Tracy, C., Veh, T., Bentley, G. E., & Cross, K. A. (2013). Receiving the initial Down syndrome diagnosis: A comparison of prenatal and postnatal parent group experiences. *Intellectual and Developmental Disabilities, 51,* 446–457. doi:10.1352/1934-9556-51.6.446

O'Brien, M. (2007). Ambiguous loss in families of children with autism spectrum disorders. *Family Relations, 56,* 135–146. doi:10.1111/j.1741-3729.2007.00447.x

Olshansky, S. (1962). Chronic sorrow: A response to having a mentally defective child. *Social Casework, 43,* 190–193.

Parker, T. (2016). *Raising a child with Down syndrome: A dyadic analysis of resiliency, coping, and relational adjustment* (Unpublished doctoral dissertation). Texas Tech University, Lubbock, TX.

Price, C. A., Bush, K. R., & Price, S. J. (Eds.) (2016). *Families and change: Coping with stressful events and transitions* (5th ed.). Thousand Oaks, CA: Sage.

Ramisch, J. (2012). Marriage and family therapists working with couples who have children with autism. *Journal of Marital and Family Therapy, 38*(2), 305–316. doi:10.1111/j.1752-0606.2010.00210.x

Rolland, J. (1984). Toward a psychosocial typology of chronic and life-threatening illness. *Family Systems Medicine, 2,* 245–262. doi:10.1037/h0091663

Rolland, J. (1994). *Family, illness & disability: An integrative treatment model.* New York, NY: Basic Books.

Soper, K. L. (2007). *Gifts: Mothers reflect on how children with Down syndrome enrich their lives.* Bethesda, MD: Woodbine House.

Soper, K. L. (2009). *Gifts 2: How people with Down syndrome enrich the world.* Bethesda, MD: Woodbine House.

Special Olympics. (2017). *R-word: Spread the word to end the word.* Retrieved from http://www.r-word.org/

Springer, N. P. (2015). The path of the unexpected: Deliberately conceived, perfectly created! *Family Therapy Magazine, 14*(4), 28–31. Retrieved from http://www.aamft.org/magazine/JulyAugust2015/

Springer, N., McCallum, S., Pounds, M., & Nelson Goff, B. (2011, March). *Resilience and hope: Embracing life with Down syndrome.* Poster presented at the Texas Association of Marriage and Family Therapy Annual Conference, San Antonio, TX.

Stallings, G., & Cook, S. (1997). *Another season: A coach's story of raising an exceptional son*. New York, NY: Little, Brown and Company.
von Bertalanffy, L. (1968). *General system theory: Developments, foundations, applications*. New York, NY: George Braziller.
Wright, L., Watson, W., & Bell, J. (Eds.) (1992). *Beliefs: The heart of healing in families and illness*. New York, NY: Basic Books.

3 Discovering Resilience
Moving Forward on the Journey

Thomas Knestrict, EdD

Introduction

This chapter will address the theoretical framework for understanding resilience and pertinent research that highlights individual and family factors essential to resilience in families living with a loved one who has an intellectual or developmental disability (IDD). The role of developmental and ecological factors will be addressed. A specific focus on families who are rhythmic and regenerative, who have found ways to make meaning of their loved one's disability in positive ways, and who have an inherent tenacity about how they approach life will be provided. In addition, principles for practice and considerations for future resilience research with this population will be highlighted.

Reflections on "Welcome to Holland" (Kingsley, 1987)

Emily Pearl Kingsley (1987) wrote a now famous essay in which she described the experience of having a child with special needs. She explained that it is like preparing for a once in a lifetime trip to Italy. You learn the language. You plan the trip. Finally, the day arrives and as you are flying to your special destination the pilot comes on the public address and announces that there has been a change in flight plan. You are no longer going to Italy. You will now land in Holland. "Holland? I was looking forward to my trip to Italy." But, as Kingsley explains, Holland is not a bad place, it is just a *different* place. In fact, Holland has windmills, tulips, and Rembrandts! No better and no worse than Italy would have been. But, still, it's not what you were imagining. She ends the essay by stating:

> But [...] if you spend your life mourning the fact that you didn't get to Italy, you may never be free to enjoy the very special, the very lovely things [...] about Holland.
>
> (Kingsley, 1987)

I have always been interested by the wide and varied response to this essay. Some parents I have worked with over the years have stated that this essay captures their feelings exactly. Other parents have told me that the essay and the suggestion that the birth of their child is anything but a blessing offends them. This essay and the responses to it were the genesis of the research into the area of families who are raising children with an IDD diagnosis and gaining insight into the development of resilience in these parents. I have often wondered, why do some parents report feeling blessed, while others report feeling angry or overwhelmed? How could some parents, when dealing with significant differences with their child, seem so grateful and happy, while others report feeling cursed and sad? Why do some parents thrive, while others struggle to accept the diagnosis and move forward? These are some of the questions resilience research attempts to answer. The findings of this research have led many to realizations that have caused them to rethink traditional views concerning families who are raising children with an IDD diagnosis and, more broadly, the constructs of disability and difference.

Resilience Research

Individual Resilience

The study of resilient families and their characteristics and dimensions has been a rich area of research for the past 20 years. Research topics have been wide and varied and include resilience of families with conditions such as asthma (Svavarsdottir, McCubbin, & Kane, 2000), families with children facing serious illness such as cancer (McCubbin, Balling, Possin, Frierdich, & Bryne, 2002), as well as families dealing with alcoholism or extreme poverty (Walsh, 2015). However, parent and family resilience research in the area of raising children with an IDD diagnosis has not been as thoroughly examined (Greeff & van der Walt, 2010).

Resilience can be viewed as one's ability to respond to adverse life events and overcome the aftermath of crisis, or "to withstand and rebound from adversity" (Walsh, 2015, p. 14). Initial efforts to uncover resilience characteristics began with research into individual resilience (Werner, 1993, 1995). The focus of this work was to isolate the characteristics that differentiated resilient from less resilient individuals. The results of these early studies formed a theoretical framework for understanding individual resilience by creating lists of resilience factors evident in those individuals identified as resilient in longitudinal studies (Werner, 1993). Werner found that more resilient children developed internal protective factors that insulated them in spite of significant risk factors. They were found to be more active, affectionate and cuddly at one year of age. She also reported that resilient toddlers were more verbal and were advanced in their language development. At 10 years old, these children scored higher on practical problem-solving skills and had developed a special talent that they took pride in and received praise from others for their accomplishments. These skills remained stable throughout the 30-year study (Werner, 2005).

Parental and Family Resilience

The findings of individual resilience studies are not always easily generalized and are somewhat limited in scope. Hence, family resilience, and more specifically, parental resilience research was born. Subsequent studies have identified resilience as a set of characteristics possessed by families (McCubbin & McCubbin, 1988) and others describe it as a flexible process (Walsh, 2015). McCubbin and McCubbin (1988) created a theoretical framework for understanding the different and more dynamic qualities of family resilience by identifying three family types: ***balanced***, ***midrange***, and *extreme*, with the former being the most viable, as the name suggests (McCubbin & McCubbin, 1988). Within this family type, there were two characteristics identified as important in the formation of ***balanced families***, based on McCubbin and McCubbin's research. These characteristics were referred to as *rhythmic* and *regenerative*, which will be described in more detail next.

Rhythmic families. Rhythmic families are those who establish rules, rituals, and routines in their home (Hastings & Taunt, 2002). Rules, rituals, and routines are defined as a communicated sense of what is expected of children by the parents (Knestrict, 2007). Rituals are defined as family efforts to consistently establish and practice routines with the purpose of creating family togetherness, regularity, and predictability (McCubbin & McCubbin, 1988). Research suggests that families who are able to establish these rules, rituals, and routines are better able to develop feelings of closeness, and ultimately bonding, which creates predictability (Luster & Okagaki, 2005), which also resulted in greater family satisfaction, closeness, and flexibility. Family rhythm provides families the space and the time to reflect on the meaning of their life, family, and often on the concept of disability itself (Knestrict & Kuchey, 2009).

Walsh (2015) provided a similar construct for understanding resilience in families. This research has helped to establish the importance of three key factors which contribute to a family becoming resilient. This framework is based on the following domains: (a) belief systems, which includes meaning making, positive outlook, and transcendence/spirituality; (b) organizational processes, which include adaptation, connectedness, and resources; and (c) communication, which includes clear information, emotional sharing, and problem-solving (Walsh, 2015, p. 19).

The role of belief systems and particularly meaning making has also been referred to as ***reconfiguration*** (Knestrict & Kuchey, 2009). It has been suggested that a rhythmic family, who establishes rules, rituals, and routines in their household, will create time and space for reflection, which may contribute to a reconstruction of the parents' understanding of their child and the concept of disability itself. Knestrict and Kuchey (2009) found that this reflection process is captured in parent narratives, which they referred to as a *criterion reference*, meaning that the child is no longer being compared to typically developing children. Parents are only comparing their child in terms of growth over time; thus, parents view the concept of disability as simply a difference within their child, instead of possessing a deficit perspective.

The role of spiritual belief systems has also been examined by contributors to resilience research (see Ciarrocchi, Dy-Liacco, & Deneke, 2008; Miltiades & Pruchno, 2002; Speraw, 2006; Walsh, 2003). These studies suggest that faith may simply be having hope for the future or holding an optimistic view. But, it is often more traditionally seen and expressed as a belief in something larger than the self. Many families rely upon this hope, and it is believed that hope can facilitate creating space for reflection that often leads to a feeling of peace and acceptance (Allen & Marshall, 2010).

Regenerative families. Regenerative families are defined by their hardiness and coherence, which is the measure of how well a family develops coping strategies for dealing with family problems (McCubbin, McCubbin, & Thompson, 1987), and coherence is manifested as the family's emphasis on loyalty, pride, faith, trust, respect, caring and shared values. This typology also includes family hardiness (McCubbin *et al.*, 1987), which is characterized by an internal sense of control of life events and hardships, a sense of meaningfulness in life and involvement in activities, as well as a commitment to learn and explore new and challenging experiences (McCubbin *et al.*, 2002). The combination of these characteristics within balanced families is thought to describe resilience in families and is consistent with Walsh's second and third domains: organizational processes and communication (Walsh, 2015). Walsh (2003, 2015) has suggested that the resilient family must possess certain organizational qualities, such as flexibility, connectedness, communication, and the ability to locate and utilize resources to be able to rebound in the face of challenging situations.

Hastings and Taunt (2002) described the importance of the family's formation of positive perceptions of their child with a severe disability and a positive perception of the family circumstances. Such positive perceptions seem to aid the family in adapting to the changes that arise within a family raising a child with an IDD diagnosis. In their study, they asked parents to report on the positive impact the child with a disability had on them, their family, as well as extended family members. They also asked parents to report on their feelings about their child's future. In response to the first question, parents reported multiple positive effects on themselves and their families, including improved family dynamics, increased confidence, assertiveness, and strengthened religious faith. In response to the second question, parents expressed some anxiety about the future but generally were hopeful. King, Baxter, Rosenbaum, Zwaigenbaum, and Bates (2009) found that positive parental perceptions of their family's health were significantly correlated to parental reports of family satisfaction.

There has been extensive research documenting the effects of a positive perspective in coping with life stressors, in general (King *et al.*, 2009; Nelson Goff *et al.*, 2016). Highly resilient families have been found to hold a more optimistic view of life (Bayat, 2007; Beavers & Hampson, 1990). Walsh (2015) described the concept of *positive illusions*, which may be beneficial in the development of resilience. Taylor and colleagues (2000) related a story about a family who was told that their child had only a 10% chance of surviving an illness (Taylor, Kemeny, Reed, Bower, & Gruenewald, 2000). The parents immediately began to say that someone has to be in that 10%—why not them? This positive bias can fuel efforts that can increase resilience and maximize the chances of success (Walsh, 2015).

Criterion Reference: Construction of Meaning Through an Ecological Model

Resilience is a complex equation that demands a systemic, developmental, and contextual lens. Bronfenbrenner (1979) originally theorized a developmental model that was structured in separate eco-systems. The family rested within the inner most system called the micro-system. The meso-system holds within it the micro-system much like the Russian nesting dolls. Each subsequent system, moving out from the family into the next larger system, holds each of the previous systems. According to Bronfenbrenner (1979), these various ecological systems interact with each other to influence the development of resilience of individuals, parents, and the family.

This ecological approach is central to understanding the development of resilience in parents raising children with an IDD diagnosis because of the innumerable ecological variables that can affect the development of resilience (Hodapp & Ly, 2005; Luster & Okagaki, 2005). Studying resilience from this ecological point of view allows us to understand where the supports are located, how each system interacts with and supports the family, and where interventions may be most beneficial. For example, in their qualitative study of 20 families raising children with an IDD diagnosis, Knestrict and Kuchey (2009) found that money was the most consistent variable for the development of resilience in families. In this study, the authors lived with these families for a 24-hour period, conducted structured interviews with each parent pair, and subsequently conducted focus groups to uncover the details of the daily life experiences of these families. From this study, they were able to begin to identify some of the ecological variables involved. The context that the ecological framework provides allowed for a clearer understanding of the contextual nuances and subtle variance in the experiences of families with an individual with an IDD diagnosis.

It seems that more resources, including financial resources and greater family income, allowed families to live in places that more substantially supported families to attend schools with quality support services, to purchase insurance policies, and to obtain supplemental therapy and services. In addition, families described accessing additional professionals to help them meet the needs of their family. All of these elements assisted families in reducing the stressors in their lives and allowed them more time to reflect, reconfigure, and develop more positive and hopeful outlooks (Knestrict & Kuchey, 2009). Part of developing a positive outlook on disability appears to be the ability of parents to reconstruct their understanding of disability, which is more likely when key resources are available and accessed by families (Hastings & Taunt, 2002).

Bogden and Taylor (1994) described the process of developing a positive outlook when he talked about moving beyond the terms and definitions provided by a perspective of pathology toward a contextual meaning of the individual. In the eyes of resilient parents, they no longer saw the "disabled child"—they saw their child first. This was evident in the research by Knestrict and Kuchey (2009). The comments made by a mother whose child had a condition called Idiodycentric

15, a rare genetic disorder causing severe developmental delays, global apraxia, and "autism-like" behaviors (Batshaw, Roizen, & Lotrecchiano, 1997):

> Christine is a beautiful child with lots and lots of strengths. She loves to climb and she loves to color. She can sing and play and dance. She is also quite the artist. She has significant issues physically and cognitively but she is a beautiful child.
>
> (Knestrict & Kuchey, 2009, p. 236)

The following comments are from a family whose child was diagnosed with bipolar disorder and severe emotional disturbance. Their comments reflect the acceptance of their son, who often has to be restrained because of threatening behaviors to himself and the other children in the family:

> You know we have to deal with a whole lot with Johnny. But in the end, he is our son. We see him as a gift from God. A gift! We are honored to be given this gift and we love him more than life itself.
>
> (Knestrict & Kuchey, 2009, p. 236)

These families are able to see the child first and the disability second. This "criterion referenced view" differs from the "norm referenced view" of less resilient families. Resilient families tend not to compare their family or child to others or to "typical" families. This manifested itself in the Knestrict and Kuchey (2009) study as positive feelings expressed about the child and family derived not from a comparison but from an appreciation of the child and his/her abilities. An entirely different construction of reality was documented within less resilient families. These families were less able to see their child in a criterion referenced way and were still making comparisons to typically developing children. For example, one family was raising a child with a comparatively mild developmental disability, accompanied by some issues with sensory integration and speech problems. This mother stated:

> Sometimes I just feel like all I do is take care of Quentin. I don't have any time for myself. I get so angry with him for not being able to use a toilet I could scream. Sometimes I do scream and yell at him. I think and think and think about what to do for Quentin next, what about school? When will he talk more clearly? Will he play baseball like our neighbors' kids? Will he have friends?
>
> (Knestrict & Kuchey, 2009, p. 237)

Knestrict and Kuchey (2009) found that resilient families are free to form positive attitudes around their child and the disability. One family had a child with a severe genetic disorder called 22q3 Deletion Syndrome (Batshaw *et al.*, 1997). This condition is manifested by the absence of speech, limited muscle tone and the ability to walk, sit up or talk. He must be fed, bathed, and diapered, requiring a high level of commitment for daily care. However, the parents of this child were filled with joy when they talked about him. When asked what was loveable about their son, the father said, "He's the happiest kid you would ever want to meet. Our house is always full of laughter. He is just very sweet" (Knestrict & Kuchey, 2009, p. 237).

Another parent described how she and her husband were not going to change the family to accommodate their daughter who had a disability. They acknowledged the challenges ahead but saw a value in the strength of assimilating her into the already existing values, expectations and unconditional love that was already there. Their daughter was going to have to adjust to being a part of this family, as is. This represents a reverse logic that seems to benefit parents and families and establishes an environment of inclusion in addition to a refusal to alter the existing family framework to accommodate "the special need."

Tenacity, Regenerativity, and Family Hardiness

In addition to the unique and specific meaning created within families of children with an IDD diagnosis, research has also found that more resilient families share a tenacity that manifests itself in the manner in which they advocate for their child and their family as a whole (McCubbin *et al.*, 1987; Walsh, 2003, 2015). One mother in the Knestrict and Kuchey (2009) study spoke of the difficulty in securing services for her child with a disability. At one point in time, the family lost their insurance coverage, and as soon as this occurred, they lost their access to therapy and other support services. To reinstate services, it took numerous phone calls, letters, and emails to re-establish their child's services. The mother stated, "I was not going to let them take this away from my daughter. I was going to do what I had to do to get the services she deserved." As described previously, McCubbin and McCubbin (1988) called this characteristic *regenerative*, when families begin to view their child and their life differently. One family in the Knestrict and Kuchey (2009) study, whose youngest child was diagnosed with autism at two years old, shared the following story about the day a neighbor told her to start looking at the diagnosis differently:

> I remember calling a friend the day after he was diagnosed [...] and I was crying and I was very, very upset. She said "Are you going to let that word change your relationship with your son? Snap out of it! Knock it off! Do what you have to do for your kid because [autism] is just a word." I needed to hear that. It was the best advice I had gotten. Feeling sad and depressed was a waste of my time. I'm done with that. Now I have things to do!
>
> (p. 238)

Another mother, who was 76 years old, had raised and cared for her 39-year-old daughter since birth. She described what she was told by the doctor after her child was born, which changed her perspective for the rest of her life:

> The doctor sat down by my bed to talk with me. He told me that Karen was mongoloid [...] that's what they called Down syndrome in those days.

> He told me that it would be better for Karen and the family if we put Karen away in a home for the rest of her life. Well, I thought [...] this was my child I'm not gonna do that. In fact, when my husband went home to tell our sons about their sister and about what the doctor had said, the boys told Pat "That's our sister. You bring her home." We were going to love her just like anybody else. It's always been that way.
>
> (Knestrict & Kuchey, 2009, p. 3)

In summary, Knestrict and Kuchey (2009) found that resilient families who have experienced this process had the time to talk with each other about family issues and the realities of their specific family situation and experiences with IDD; to organize their life, their days, and their schedules; to search for services and resources; and to spend time with all of their children, not just the child with an IDD diagnosis. These circumstances allowed the families to configure a new understanding of their circumstances and create a new framework for understanding their child's abilities and future (Woodgate, Ateah, & Secco, 2008).

In contrast, families who did not experience this process were distracted from this type of reflection. There was a constant search for services, follow up phone calls, and seeking resources. Several of the families in the Knestrict and Kuchey (2009) study found it impossible for both parents to continue working outside of the home. In all of these cases, the mother quit her job to become the primary caregiver for the child/children. But with less income and fewer financial resources, these families experienced economic stressors, making the act of reflection difficult. The presence of a child with special needs became the center of the family's life—all other events became secondary.

Knestrict and Kuchey (2009) suggested that this reconstructive process was not accessible for all families, as specific markers may be observed in families who are able to reconstruct a criterion referenced perspective. The most obvious marker was the tendency of resilient parents to not compare their child to typically developing children. They were able to see the beauty and the potential of their child and compare their progress only within the context of their child's life. It was also observed as a process that occurred at different rates and in different ways for families. This reconstruction of a criterion reference perspective hinged upon having time to reflect on the global meaning of "the family" as well as a different understanding of disability. Establishing a global meaning of family refers to the way in which a resilient parent places their family and their family's challenges in an ecological framework. They begin to think of their family not as a "family with a child with a disability" but simply as a "family."

Principles for Practice: Moving Toward Resilience

Professionals supporting parents who are raising children with IDD should be aware of the importance of reflection and reconfiguration (Knestrict & Kuchey, 2009). They also should be able to facilitate supports and processes that provide parents with the opportunity to reflect and reconfigure (Russell, 2005).

Traditionally, this type of support is expert driven, originating from a medical model (Hibbard & Greene, 2013). Parents rely upon a doctor to diagnose their child and prescribe medicine and therapy, which will guide the family toward improved health. This medical model discounts the participation of the parent and devalues the input of the family, leaving the family at the mercy of the experts (Hibbard & Greene, 2013). Since evidence shows that important work is done internally within the family (i.e., reconfiguration, rhythmic, and regenerative processes), it makes sense to explore options that place the parents at the center of problem-solving and the therapeutic process. Behavior change that entails a positive and empowered outlook by parents is essential in the development of resilience (Walsh, 2015).

DiClemente and Prochaska (1998) described a six-stage model for changing behavior. Each stage, ranging from *pre-contemplation* to *maintenance*, is described as process-oriented, involving unique tasks that must be resolved before the person moves on to the next stage toward maintenance of the new behavior. The process of change is dynamic and is represented in this model by stages of change (Klöckner, 2017). The individual or family looking to change is not static either, requiring targeted, staged, and matched interventions. It is clear that the future of family change models lies in these staged, matched, and customized interventions that require a great deal of participation by the individual or family members (Harvey, Fowles, Xi, & Terry, 2012). This higher level of parent participation or *patient activation* (Hibbard, & Greene, 2013; Salyers *et al.*, 2009) creates a climate that the family is invested in and engaged with and creates higher levels of autonomy and feelings of self-efficacy (Rollnick, Heather, & Bell, 1992). However, the use of the term *patient* is often seen as part of the old pathology model (Taylor *et al.*, 2000); a preferred term is *parent activation*, which serves to de-emphasize the previous medical model that valued the expert's ability to exclusively diagnose and prescribe rather than engage families in their own care (Hibbard & Greene, 2013). It seems an additional step needs to be developed to facilitate these initial moments of the parent-provider relationship.

It is critical that professionals work to put parents in the center of the process and communicate to parents that they have the ability to guide the family where they want to go, not where someone else believes they should go. This autonomy is seen as a facilitator of the reconfiguration process (Knestrict & Kuchey, 2009), and suggests that the more empowered the family is, the more they look for answers within their control and the less dependent they are on locating and finding outside resources. Families who look within their family first and are less dependent on others, including professionals, to locate resources, are more likely to embrace change and develop resilience (Hibbard & Greene, 2013).

The Future of IDD and Family Resilience Research

There are three primary areas that should inform our research of IDD, special needs, and family resilience. First, it is important to develop a new framework for understanding these families and observe them from a perspective that does not see them as defective or broken—and that helps them gain a more positive view of themselves, as well (Knestrict & Kuchey, 2009). Second, it is necessary to approach resilience from an ecological perspective using a qualitative research inquiry to elicit richly descriptive voices from families of individuals with an IDD diagnosis, including their individual and collective experiences (Bronfenbrenner, 1979; Chenail & Maione, 1997). It is also important to gain information and input from all members of the family, especially the individual with an IDD diagnosis. Finally, professionals and researchers need to establish ways to lead parents toward reconfiguration and a criterion referenced perspective (Chenail & Maione, 1997; Knestrict & Kuchey, 2009).

There is a convergence of literature that currently de-emphasizes differences while at the same time valuing the similarities of families of all kinds. This way of thinking is linked to disability studies in general and seeks to de-pathologize the disability and de-medicalize the pathology framework (Bogden & Taylor, 1994). A new perspective is warranted, one that places the parents in the center of their loved one's care. This perspective is known as *patient activation* (Hibbard & Greene, 2013; Robinson, 2010), but for this context, could be called *parent activation*. What matters most is empowering individuals and families to manage their own health or the health of their loved one (Todd & Higgins, 1998).

An ecological framework (Bronfenbrenner, 1979; Hodapp & Ly, 2005) is crucial to understand parent and family resilience in any future research or clinical support models. The contextual richness of families makes generalizing large portions of resilience research difficult. However, using the ecological model and studying the interactions between systems allows for an understanding of not only the phenomena being observed, but the contextual factors as well. The interactions of the family, the parents, and the children within the meso-system (i.e., environments just outside of the home), the exo-system (i.e., community based environments, agencies, support providers), and the macro-system (i.e., political climate) gives a complete, contextualized portrait of the family as a unit and the circumstances it interfaces with daily. This approach provides rich, contextualized data for the researcher (Chenail & Maione, 1997). Ultimately, the movement away from a deficit model to a resource model of intervention is crucial for empowering families to develop and sustain resilience (Walsh, 2015).

Evidence suggests the central importance of this movement involves family empowerment (Hastings & Taunt, 2002), patient activation (Hibbard & Greene, 2013), reconfiguration (Knestrict & Kuchey, 2009), and discovering the ways in which families can develop other balanced family type characteristics (McCubbin & McCubbin, 1988). These themes should be further investigated in order to better ensure adequate support of families with loved ones diagnosed with an IDD diagnosis. In addition, it is necessary that parents create time and space for reflection and reconfiguration, as their family develops and they face the challenges—and benefits—of raising a child with an IDD diagnosis. Finally, it is necessary for professionals to approach parents in supportive and beneficial ways, from a respectful and parent-centered perspective, that encourages parent activation and values the position that views parents as the navigators of their family along their journey with IDD.

Conclusion

This chapter began with a reference to the essay entitled "Welcome to Holland" (Kingsley, 1987). The story began with the metaphor of a trip to Italy as a way of describing what it feels like when expecting a child. But, when the flight plan changes and a parent is re-routed, there is disappointment or loss of that dream vacation. The change in plans, and specifically parenting a child born with a difference, requires a change over the course of one's entire life. However, the mother in the poem adjusts to this new reality. She discovers new people and new experiences that she never expected. It is obvious that the mother has adjusted to the realities of her life and what is required of her. I would attribute this to the beginnings of reconfiguration, in that she discovers "Holland has Rembrandts!" (Kingsley, 1987).

Five years after the birth of his son with a significant genetic disorder that would change the course of their lives, a father once shared:

> At first, I felt like I had lost my passport and I was stranded in Holland. I didn't want to be there. It was cold, different, and foreign. But I watched my son grow into this amazing kid. Will he play football? No. But can he read? Yes. Can he love me? Yes! Can we love him? Yes! He is my amazing son! Now, I have a passport and I can go anywhere I want to go. I will always depart from Holland, but because of my new way of thinking about my son, my life, the world, I'm free. I'm blessed.
>
> (Knestrict & Kuchey, 2009, p. 7)

This quote captures the essence of adjusting to the reality of an unexpected turn by way of developing a criterion referenced perspective following significant life-changing events, which serves as a lived example of resilience and moving forward on this journey.

Key Messages from This Chapter

- **For individuals with IDD and their families**: Resilience is a process that involves several components. Part of developing a positive outlook on IDD appears to be the ability of parents to reconstruct their understanding of disability. In addition, families who are able to develop both rhythmic (i.e., establish rules, rituals, and routines) and regenerative (i.e., develop coping strategies to deal with challenges) characteristics are able to achieve resilience and positive outcomes for all family members.
- **For professionals**: Professionals should work from an ecological perspective and begin to view the family as part of a larger interactive system that is contextually sensitive.

Professionals need to have a strengths-based approach to working with families and view the development of resilience as a process requiring reflection and time to process through the changes families face. Professionals should also emphasize the importance of rules, rituals, and routines in an effort to structure family life to be more predictable and to provide parents time to reflect.

- **For policy makers**: Policy should be viewed from an ecological perspective understanding that macro-system legislation affects the micro-system events that families experience. In addition, creating ways to increase ease of accessing resources within benefit programs, which ultimately reduces financial stressors, will help families to have a greater capacity to find meaning and problem-solve more successfully as a family caring for a loved one with an IDD diagnosis.

References

Allen, D., & Marshall, E. S. (2010). Spirituality as a coping resource for African American parents of chronically ill children. *MCN: The American Journal of Maternal/Child Nursing*, *35*(4), 232–237. doi:10.1097/NMC.0b013e3181de3f76

Batshaw, M. L., Roizen, N. J., & Lotrecchiano, G. R. (1997). *Children with disabilities* (4th ed.). Baltimore, MD: Paul H. Brookes.

Bayat, M. (2007). Evidence of resilience in families of children with autism. *Journal of Intellectual Disability Research*, *51*(9), 702–714. doi:10.1111/j.1365-2788.2007.00960.x

Beavers, W. B., & Hampson, R. B. (1990). *Successful families: Assessment and intervention*. New York, NY: Norton.

Bogden, R., & Taylor, S. (1994). *The social meaning of mental retardation*. New York, NY: Teacher College Press.

Bronfenbrenner, U. (1979). *The ecology of human development: Experiments by nature and design*. Cambridge, MA: Harvard University Press.

Chenail, R.J., & Maione, P. (1997). Sense making in clinical qualitative research. *The Qualitative Report*, *3*(1), 1–10. Retrieved from http://www.nova.edu/ssss/QR/QR3-1/sense.html

Ciarrocchi, J. W., Dy-Liacco, G. S., & Deneke, E. (2008). Gods or rituals? Relational faith, spiritual discontent, and religious practices as predictors of hope and optimism. *Journal of Positive Psychology*, *3*(2), 120–136. doi:10.1080/17439760701760666

DiClemente, C. C., & Prochaska, J. O. (1998). Toward a comprehensive, transtheoretical model of change: Stages of change and addictive behaviors. In W. R. Miller & N. Heather (Eds.), *Treating addictive behaviors* (2nd ed., pp. 3–24). New York, NY: Plenum Press.

Greeff, A. P., & van der Walt, K.-J. (2010). Resilience in families with an autistic child. *Education and Training in Autism and Developmental Disabilities*, *45*(3), 347–355. Retrieved from http://www.jstor.org/stable/23880109

Harvey, L., Fowles, J. B., Xi, M., & Terry, P. (2012). When activation changes, what else changes? The relationship between change in Patient Activation Measure (PAM) and employees' health status and health behaviors. *Patient Education and Counseling*, *88*(2), 338–343. doi:10.1016/j.pec.2012.02.005

Hastings, R. P., & Taunt, H. M. (2002). Positive perceptions in families of children with developmental disabilities. *American Journal on Mental Retardation, 107*(2), 116–127. doi:10.1352/0895-8017(2002)107 0116:PPIFOC 2.0.CO;2

Hibbard, J. H., & Greene, J. (2013). What the evidence shows about patient activation: Better health outcomes and care experiences; fewer data on costs. *Health Affairs, 32*(2), 207–214. doi:10.1377/hlthaff.2012.1061

Hodapp, R., & Ly, T. M. (2005). Parenting children with developmental disabilities. In T. Luster & L. Okagaki (Eds.), *Parenting: An ecological perspective* (pp.177–201). Mahwah, NJ: Lawrence Erlbaum.

King, G., Baxter, D., Rosenbaum, P., Zwaigenbaum, L., & Bates, A. (2009). Belief systems of families of children with autism spectrum disorders or Down syndrome. *Focus on Autism and Other Developmental Disabilities, 24*(1), 50–64. doi: 10.1177/1088357608329173

Kingsley, E. P. (1987). *Welcome to Holland.* Retrieved from http://firefliesofhope.typepad.com

Klöckner, C. A. (2017). A stage model as an analysis framework for studying voluntary change in food choices—The case of beef consumption reduction in Norway. *Appetite, 108*, 434–449. doi:10.1016/j.appet.2016.11.002

Knestrict, T. (2007). *Rules, rituals and routines* [Video production]. Chicago, IL: Learning Seed/Magna.

Knestrict, T., & Kuchey, D. (2009). Welcome to Holland: Characteristics of resilient families raising children with severe disabilities. *Journal of Family Studies, 2*(4), 227–244. doi:10.5172/jfs.15.3.227

Luster, T., & Okagaki, L. (Eds.). (2005). *Parenting: An ecological perspective* (2nd ed.). Mahwah, NJ: Lawrence Erlbaum.

McCubbin, H., & McCubbin, M. (1988). Typologies of resilient families: Emerging roles of social class and ethnicity. *Family Relations, 37*(3), 247–254. doi:10.2307/584557

McCubbin, H., McCubbin, M., & Thompson, A. (1987). FHI: The Family Hardiness Index. In H. McCubbin & A. Thompson (Eds.), *Family assessment inventories for research and practice* (pp. 125–132). Madison, WI: University of Wisconsin.

McCubbin, M., Balling, K., Possin, P., Frierdich, S., & Bryne, B. (2002). Family resiliency in childhood cancer. *Family Relations, 51*(2), 103–111. doi:10.1111/j.1741-3729.2002.00103.x

Miltiades, H. B., & Pruchno, R. (2002). The effect of religious coping on caregiving appraisals of mothers of adults with developmental disabilities. *The Gerontologist, 42*(1), 82–91. doi:10.1093/geront/42.1.82

Nelson Goff, B., Monk, J. K., Staats, N., Malone, J., Tanner, A., & Springer, N. (2016). Comparing parents of children with Down syndrome at different life span stages. *Journal of Marriage and Family, 78*, 1131–1148. doi:10.1111/jomf.12312

Robinson, K. (2010). Care coordination: A priority for health reform. *Policy, Politics, & Nursing Practice, 11*(4), 266–274. doi:10.1177/1527154410396572

Rollnick, S., Heather, N., & Bell, A. (1992). Negotiating behavior change in medical settings: The development of brief motivational interviewing. *Journal of Mental Health, 1*(1), 25–37. doi:10.3109/09638239209034509

Russell, T. (2005). Can reflective practice be taught? *Reflective Practice: International and Multidisciplinary Perspectives, 6*(2), 199–204. doi:10.1080/14623940500105833

Salyers, M. P., Matthias, M. S., Spann, C. L., Lydick, J. M., Rollins, A. L., & Frankel, R. M. (2009). The role of patient activation in psychiatric visits. *Psychiatric Services*, *60*(11), 1535–1539. doi:10.1176/ps.2009.60.11.1535

Speraw, S. (2006). Spiritual experiences of parents and caregivers who have children with disabilities or special needs. *Issues in Mental Health Nursing*, *27*(2), 213–230. doi:10.1080/01612840500436974

Svavarsdottir, E. K., McCubbin, M. A., & Kane, J. H. (2000). Well-being of parents of young children with asthma. *Research in Nursing & Health*, *23*(5), 346–358. doi:10.1002/1098-240X(200010)23:5 346::AID-NUR2 3.0.CO;2-W

Taylor, S. E., Kemeny, M. E., Reed, G. M., Bower, J. E., & Gruenewald, T. L. (2000). Psychological resources, positive illusions, and health. *American Psychologist*, *55*(1), 99–109. doi:10.1037/0003-066X.55.1.99

Todd, E. S., & Higgins, S. (1998). Powerlessness in professional and parent partnerships. *British Journal of Sociology of Education*, *19*(2), 227–236. doi:10.1080/0142569980190205

Walsh, F. (2003). Family resilience: A framework for clinical practice. *Family Process*, *42*(1), 1–18. doi:10.1111/j.1545-5300.2003.00001.x

Walsh, F. (2015). *Strengthening family resilience* (3rd ed.). New York, NY: Guilford.

Werner, E. E. (1993). Risk, resilience and recovery: Perspectives from the Kauai longitudinal study. *Development and Psychopathology*, *5*, 503–515. doi:10.1017/S095457940000612X

Werner, E. E. (1995). Resilience in development. *Current Directions in Psychological Science*, *4*(3), 81–84. doi:10.1111/1467-8721.ep10772327

Werner, E. (2005). Resilience and recovery: Findings from the Kauai longitudinal study. *Focal Point: Research, Policy, and Practice in Children's Mental Health*, *19*(1), 11-14. Retrieved from https://www.pathwaysrtc.pdx.edu/pdf/fpS0504.pdf

Woodgate, R. L., Ateah, C., & Secco, L. (2008). Living in a world of our own: The experience of parents who have a child with autism. *Qualitative Health Research*, *18*(8), 1075–1083. doi:10.1177/1049732308320112

4 Advice to New Parents from Parents

Reflecting on the Journey

Jessica D. Cless, MS, Ellen Bodine, BS, Ashley Edelman, BS, Laura Farkas, BS, Adam W. Cless, MS, Briana S. Nelson Goff, PhD, and Nicole Piland Springer, PhD

Introduction

Having a child with a disability can be a source of great joy for parents, and it can also lead to moments of stress and frustration that are challenging for families. Parents of children with an intellectual or developmental disability (IDD) most often take primary responsibility in responding to the needs of their child, which may include providing care for medical conditions, coping with educational challenges, managing financial issues, and dealing with social stigmas in larger society that may create strain for parents (Glidden, Billings, & Jobe, 2006). Literature has demonstrated time and again the risks associated with parenting a child with an IDD diagnosis, to include caregiving stress and poorer physical health (Gallagher & Whiteley, 2013), lower levels of marital satisfaction (Quittner *et al.*, 1998), and poorer family functioning (Al-Krenawi, Graham, & Gharaibeh, 2011). Fewer studies have focused on prevention of these stressors or positive aspects of parenting a child with an IDD diagnosis.

Since parents of children with an IDD diagnosis often face stressors that parents of typically developing children do not, receiving support from the IDD community has been shown to be helpful to remediate stress (Shilling *et al.*, 2013). While research literature has identified positive coping strategies meant to combat stressors specific to families living with a loved one with IDD, few studies have been conducted that present advice that parents of children with an IDD diagnosis would share with other parents facing the same or a similar diagnosis. In this chapter, we review literature that demonstrates the importance of parent-to-parent support in the IDD community, as well as studies available which utilize parents' voices, providing wisdom and advice to new parents. We conclude this chapter with data from a study in which parents of children with Down syndrome (DS) lend their own voices to contribute to the empirical literature on this topic.

The Role of Advice

Parent-to-Parent Support

The role of parent-to-parent support has been identified as helpful in various studies of parents of children with disabilities (Kerr & McIntosh, 2000; Law, King, Stewart, & King, 2002; Singer *et al.*, 1999; Solomon, Pistrang, & Barker, 2001). Parents of children with disabilities who engage in supportive relationships with other parents whose children have disabilities have reported many benefits of receiving this support, such as having an ally who has gone or is going through a similar situation from which they receive practical advice (Ainbinder *et al.*, 1998). Furthermore, receiving practical advice regarding how to cope with having a child with a disability may protect against feelings of insecurity and helplessness for parents (Taanila, Järvelin, & Kokkonen, 1998). As technology has advanced, support from parents over the internet has even been identified as a possible resource for parents of children with IDD to connect with others in their same situation (Baum, 2004). This technology provides a vehicle for parents when they are separated by geography but connected via their child's diagnosis, particularly when faced with more rare conditions.

In one study, which compared parents who received the IDD diagnosis of DS prenatally to those who received the diagnosis post-natally, both groups identified support networks, including support from other parents, extended family members, friends, and neighbors as positive and helpful in the process of initially coping with the diagnosis (Nelson Goff *et al.*, 2013). While parent-to-parent support has surely been identified as helpful for parental well-being, literature has focused on this support in the setting of support groups. Research on the content of recommendations and advice that parents of children with disabilities may be receiving from these support groups or in other settings in which they are connected with other parents of children with disabilities is limited.

The literature that explores parent-to-parent advice regarding raising a child with IDD has come primarily from the DS community. These studies have focused on the early diagnosis of DS. In one study, researchers found that parents' description of the DS varied from very positive to very negative (Gilmore, 2006). These parents also gave advice to genetic counselors working with new parents of children with DS, in which many parents recommended that the similarities between children with DS and typically developing children should be shared with parents, as well as noting that parents should be educated using a variety of methods such as stories, videos, and connecting with other parents of children with the same diagnosis (Hippman, Inglis, & Austin, 2012). In another study, parents of a child with DS shared advice they would offer to other parents expecting a child with DS to include loving the child, experiencing joy in the child's milestones, but also in the negative experiences that will inevitably become a part of their journey (Skotko, Levine, & Goldstein, 2011). In the spirit of this study and to expand the literature that offers advice from parents themselves, the current study, which included a large sample of parents raising children with DS, explored the themes of advice that parents offer new parents of a child living with DS.

Research Methods

Study Participants

The purpose of this study was to give voice to advice from parents of children living with DS. Participants were recruited via both regional and national DS groups including the National Down Syndrome Congress (NDSC; ndsccenter.org), the Down Syndrome Guild of Greater Kansas City (kcdsg.org), Band of Angels (bandofangels.com), and the Council for Exceptional Children (cec.sped.org). In order to recruit participants, the NDSC passed recruitment information to affiliate groups, which then distributed the information to their local listservs. In this way, potential participants around the United States were contacted with information about the study as well as a link to participate in the web-based survey.

In total, 651 parents of children with DS completed the survey, which was comprised of both quantitative measures and open-ended questions. Of these participants, 435 parents provided a response to the question, "What advice would you have for other families who are preparing for a child with Down syndrome?", which was the focus of the current study. Thus, the final sample size for the analysis was $n = 435$ parents. Most participants were female (83%), Caucasian (86.7%), and currently married or remarried (85%). Many parents were employed full-time (46.7%), and had completed a college degree or higher (61.8%). Finally, parents were representative of higher socioeconomic statuses, with 63.7% of parents in the sample reported an annual household income over $70,000. Full demographic information is reported in Table 4.1.

Data Analysis Procedures

Grounded theory analysis and thematic coding (see Braun & Clarke, 2006) were used to analyze the parent responses. One graduate research assistant and three undergraduate research assistants first independently engaged in open coding of parent responses to this question (see Holton, 2007). Once all parent responses had been openly coded by individual research team members, the team met to engage in consensus coding in order to share open codes, share perceptions and reactions, and resolve any discrepancies across coders. Multiple codes were allowed to be assigned to a single response in an attempt to grasp the fullness and multifaceted nature of the parents' responses. Upon reaching consensus for each of the codes, the team met again to group together similar and related codes to form categories, or themes. Over 40 codes were initially identified in the data. Upon further examination, similar codes were then combined by the research team to establish themes. Overarching themes were organized from most to least prevalent, and later reorganized by the research team to group similar codes into themes. Within these themes, similar codes were seen as having the same basic sentiment present in the overarching theme, but perhaps articulating a more specific idea. The four most prevalent codes identified as themes that described a group of other similar codes will be described next.

Table 4.1 Descriptive Statistics (n = 435 Parents of Children with Down syndrome)

Variables	*n (M)*	*% (SD)*	*Range*
Sex			
Female	371	85.3	–
Male	64	14.7	–
Age	(41.8)	(9.6)	19–87
Race			
Caucasian	377	86.7	–
Hispanic	19	4.4	–
African American	4	1	–
Other	29	6.7	–
Relationship Status			
Married/Remarried	370	85	–
Dating/Engaged/Living Together	21	4.8	–
Separated/Divorced	26	6	–
Employment			
Employed Full-time	203	46.7	–
Employed Part-time	82	18.9	–
Full-time Homemaker	105	24.1	–
Unemployed	30	7	–
Retired	15	3.4	–
Education			
Less than High School	7	1.6	–
Completed High School	18	4.1	–
Some College	92	21.1	–
Completed College	152	34.9	–
Postgraduate Degree	117	26.9	–
Total Number of Children	(2.81)	(1.8)	1–22
Age of Child with DS	(9.43)	(9.1)	1–55

Due to missing data, not all demographics sum to 100%.

Study Results

The four primary themes identified from the data analysis were: putting the child first, parent education, parent attitude, and parent advocacy (see Table 4.2). These themes and codes are hereafter described along with examples of respondent quotes. These themes address the major points of advice offered by parents of children with DS, which may be relevant for parents of children with various forms of IDD.

Theme One: Putting the Child First

The most prevalent idea identified in the data (n = 164) was the recommendation to put the child with DS before his or her diagnosis, or in other words, to put the child first. This sentiment was simply described in a quote from a mother of a 24-year-old son with DS, “Prepare for a child, Down syndrome is only a factor.” Putting the child first was determined to be associated with several other codes,

Table 4.2 Advice Codes (n = 435 Parents)

Code	*n*	*Code*	*n*
Child first	164	Parent attitude	–
Love child for who they are	90	Positive outlook	99
Focus on child strengths	13	One day at a time	46
Don't compare to others	8	Patience	39
No limitations	70	Tough skin	26
Don't underestimate child	14	Open-minded	23
Parent education	109	Celebrate milestones	17
Cautious education	66	Parent advocacy	60
Early intervention	47		
Focus on positive materials	4		
Get involved with DS community	140		
Research medical professionals	17		

and was therefore grouped together as an overall theme of "Child First." Another code included the idea that new parents should love the child for who they are ($n = 90$), to focus on the strengths the child holds as opposed to their weaknesses ($n = 13$), and to not compare the child to others ($n = 8$). One mother of a 14-month-old baby girl diagnosed with DS said, "Don't compare. Just love your child for who [they are]." Another mother of a two-year-old son emphasized the child's strengths, stating "I would advise parents to focus on their child's strengths and their child's dreams, rather than focusing on their child's weaknesses and their own dreams for their child."

The sentiment of placing the child before his or her diagnosis was also echoed in the suggestion by many parents ($n = 70$) that new families should not place limitations on their child but instead "have high expectations" because "the sky's the limit for what [children with DS] can learn and accomplish" (mother of a 15-year-old boy). Along with not placing limitations on children with DS, participants also suggested that new parents should not underestimate children with DS ($n = 14$). One mother of a two-year-old son with DS said, "Don't ever underestimate ability (no matter what challenges you face)!" This piece of advice may be pertinent to parents of children across IDD diagnoses, as recognizing and focusing on the child outside of his/her disability may help parents to enjoy the child for who s/he is apart from the perceived deficits related to the particular diagnosis.

Theme Two: Parent Education

Parents seeking education was a key factor of advice for respondents who wanted to share with new parents ($n = 109$). Some parents were more specific in their advice to gain education surrounding the DS diagnosis; however, many participants ($n = 66$) warned that parents should be cautious when becoming educated about DS. A minority of parents suggested that parents should focus only on positive materials ($n = 4$), but most suggested a more balanced education. One female respondent of an in-utero child with DS shared the following:

> Research the info to learn the possibilities of what you might have to face, just so you know what to look out for, but don't focus too much on the negatives or you could scare yourself to death! Remember you are having a BABY, not a syndrome. All babies come into the world and face their own challenges, it's a lucky dip how healthy or smart they will be, all the diagnosis is really is a heads up to prepare you for what may come.

Apart from the recommendation that parents seek education in a general sense, many participants also recommended specific avenues for parents in order to become educated. One such education-related theme was the recommendation for parents to learn by getting involved in the DS community ($n = 140$). One mother of a 19-year-old son with DS said, "Reach out to other families who have a child with [DS]. Get connected to a [DS] group. You will learn so much from their collective experiences." Another mother of a two-year-old daughter shared the following:

> Get support from your local Down syndrome group, and participate. We have a great time with our group and have met so many friends through the group. The online networks have also been helpful in that I can get answers to questions very quickly from people who have dealt with the same issues I have!

Another point of education that parents described as important was early childhood intervention programs (see Chapter 11 for more information about these programs). In order to help children reach their goals and capitalize on their strengths, many parents ($n = 47$) stated that early intervention was a key to success. "Get educated about early intervention services—good ones really help" (mother of a two-year-old boy). Another mother of a two-year-old girl stated:

> Be patient and start early with intervention and therapy. We learned so much about development through the MRDD (Mental Retardation and Developmental Disabilities) therapist and how to help [our child] with different techniques, etc. Don't be afraid to ask [or] seek help with anything!

Yet another specific education-related suggestion from respondents ($n = 17$) was to research medical professionals. One parent shared, "Find a pediatrician and a team of doctors with experience with children with DS *and* who are empathic." In this way, parents of children with DS seem to recognize the importance of not only self-education, but also seeking out others who are educated and informed of best practices related to the diagnosis. Lastly, several specific educational books and poems were recommended by participants, including *The Holland Poem* by Emily Perl Kingsley ($n = 10$), *Gifts: Mothers Reflect on How Children with Down Syndrome Enrich Their Lives* by Kathryn Lynard Soper ($n = 4$), and *Choosing Naia: A Family's Journey* by Mitchell Zuckoff ($n = 1$). One quote that exemplifies several of these educational elements was shared by a father of a seven-year-old daughter:

> Research; go online and get as much information as you possibly can so that you can better understand what DS is. Go to as many informational meetings as possible; Down Syndrome Guild is a good place to start to find a 'new parent' meeting where you are able to meet other parents either going through the same thing, or who have recently had a child with DS [...] Know that there are other people in your community with experience to help you get through the initial shock and/or despair.

For parents of children with DS and other IDD diagnoses, it seems as though engaging with these materials for positive support may not only be helpful in terms of education and as a sort of "introduction" to parenting a child with IDD, but also normalizing and perhaps a type of psychological aid in processing through the initial reactions and emotions related to learning about their child's diagnosis.

Theme Three: Parent Attitude

Over half of all respondents gave advice concerning a specific aspect of parent attitude, particularly emphasizing that having a positive attitude during the parenting experience really aided them in parenting a child with IDD. Having a positive attitude includes demonstrating a positive outlook in difficult situations, which was found to be the highest indicator ($n = 99$). Parents also noted that taking one day at a time ($n = 46$), having patience ($n = 39$), striving to have a tough skin in all situations ($n = 26$), being open-minded ($n = 23$), and celebrating all milestones ($n = 17$) of their child were all aspects of having a positive attitude. One mother of a three-year-old girl with DS stated:

> Hang in there [...] it's not really all that bad. There is HOPE. Their child will walk, will talk, will do most things that typical kids do. It just might be done a little differently or take a little longer. Focus on the things they CAN do [...] not what they can't. You are not alone.

The diagnosis of DS can at times be difficult to manage; however, many parents noted that taking one day at a time and having patience can help the parenting process and positivity. One mother of an 11-year-old daughter stated, "Try not to worry about things that have not happened. Don't borrow trouble and take one day at a time. It is like raising any other child." This advice focuses on parent attitude, but also highlights the important coping strategy of staying focused in the present rather than letting future worries overcome their functioning.

Striving to have a tough skin was yet another piece of advice that was described to be beneficial to the parenting process. Because society does not always understand or recognize the diagnosis of DS, this can cause situations in which parents are faced with negative behaviors toward their child. The advice of incorporating the "tough skin" response into parent attitude was given as a way to respond to these situations. One mother of an eight-year-old child shared:

> Don't listen to people who don't know what they are talking about. There is still a lot of misinformation and misunderstanding out there about Down syndrome. Some people will say some really stupid things in the process of trying to help you [...] you may want to talk to other parents of children with Down syndrome, or you may not be ready for that yet, but whatever you do, don't let people feel sorry for you or fill your head with horror stories.

Being open minded to all the possibilities that your child can accomplish is also a very important aspect to keep in mind for positivity. Children with IDD can accomplish many great things, and they should never be limited on what they can or cannot do. One father of a ten-year-old boy stated:

> Don't look at the negatives. Always keep an open mind. Those dreams are still there, they have only been slightly modified. Remember this is your child and they love you unconditionally. There will be bad days but the good days will out-number them.

Finally, parents must remember to celebrate their child's milestones and children with DS deserve the same amount of celebration. Oftentimes it is more difficult for children with DS to achieve certain milestones than their typically developing peers, highlighting the importance that parents celebrate these milestones to increase positivity in the parenting process. One mother of a three-year-old boy stated:

> Overall enjoy your little one. Their milestones are so much more heartfelt because of what it took to get there but to enjoy the journey. There is nothing wrong with taking life a little slower, that is what our children teach us and it is a much more peaceful place.

Theme Four: Parent Advocacy

The final theme reported by parents was advocacy for their child. Advocacy is a vital aspect of parenting a child with DS and other IDD. Many parents gave advice acknowledging this role (n = 60), indicating this was an important tool in parenting a child with DS because this helped their child to receive services, as well as education and general rights that their child deserved. Advocating for their child might include reaching out to other families for support and resources, being proactive by seeking out education about the diagnosis and educational laws, and sharing information with others in the community. Parents emphasized the importance of advocating on their child's behalf because children with IDD are just like any other child and deserve the same amount of respect, love, and care as other children. One mother of a 20-year-old daughter with DS stated:

> Be an advocate for your child. Stay up on all the new developments in the Down [syndrome] world. I remember what the geneticist told us: "She is more normal than not! She has more normal chromosomes than not. So, take her home and love her." Treat your child as you would any of your other children.

One father of a seven-year-old boy with DS explains what advocacy means to him:

> Educate yourself about the condition and the educational laws, because no one will advocate for your child like you. Don't ever give up on your child, he or she is a person in the fullest sense. Celebrate all achievements. Frequently remind yourself of everything your child can do, not what they cannot. Most of all love your child.

Principles for Practice

This study described results that contribute to existing literature on parent-to-parent support and advice in the special needs community by amplifying the voices of parents of children with DS in order to identify resources that may be helpful for new parents of a child with DS. This study may also address the current gap in literature on positive and prevention-related literature regarding the experience of parenting a child with IDD. Overall themes of putting the child first, parents seeking education, and parents considering their own attitude and advocating for their child were the primary points of advice from parents of children with DS, which have implications for both the DS community as well as for parents of children with other forms of IDD. For helping professionals across disciplines working with parents and families with a child with special needs, utilizing parent advice as a resource may be helpful to remediate stress and frustration that may arise from parenting a child with DS in several ways.

Acquire a Child First Stance

Considering the overarching advice of putting the child before his or her diagnosis, professionals can draw many takeaways. First, professionals working with families with children with IDD should follow this advice themselves by putting the child first even in the helping role. Not only may this give the professional the opportunity to model this positive behavior for parents, but it also may help professionals to actively form a mindset in which the child as a person is always recognized, even in consideration of his or her disability. Asking questions about the child as a person to include his or her own interests, likes and dislikes, and goals for the future may be helpful for professionals when interacting with the child, or to ask these questions of parents. Focusing on the child as a child, first, may also be helpful for professionals to remind parents, especially when it comes to normal stresses and challenges that all parents may face at some point.

Encourage Parent Education and Advocacy

Regarding parent education—a realm in which many helping professionals are already situated—professionals may work to directly provide the parents themselves with knowledge and training, or they may work within an organization that coordinates care with educational services the child is receiving elsewhere.

Of course, professionals working with children and parents with DS should have a reasonable level of education regarding the IDD diagnosis, how it can affect the family, and various resources (both local and national) that parents can access in order to more effectively manage stressors when they arise. Helping professionals can serve a key role in encouraging parents to seek their own education, either through recommending educational materials such as books, documentaries, films, or websites that may be beneficial for parents to consult. Professionals might also frame parent education as a way for parents to become an advocate for their child, balancing this advocacy with the encouragement that as each child is unique, parents will always be the expert on their own child. In this way, helping professionals have the unique opportunity, not only to learn together with parents, but to normalize any reactions to materials they access, and empower parents through knowledge and advocacy.

The Power of Positivity

In line with the advice of keeping a positive attitude, helping professionals can aid parents in multiple ways. Professionals working directly with parents, such as therapists, social workers, or support group leaders, may fill the role of listener and normalizer for parents in order to lend a supportive ear; which may help parents to release some of the stress and anxiety that may be barring them from staying positive. Helping professionals may also assist in keeping positivity in perspective by encouraging parents to articulate the things that they appreciate about their child, or the positive aspects of their life that they would have not otherwise known had it not been for the presence of the child with IDD. Positive affect has been identified as an important factor for parents of children with IDD (Baker, Blacher & Olsson, 2005; Gupta & Singhal, 2004; Heiman, 2002), and in one study was a moderator for parent total stress (Song *et al.*, 2014). In helping parents preserve positive attitude and affect, helping professionals may indirectly help to reduce overall stress that parents of children with IDD may experience.

As professionals work with parents and families with a child with IDD, they may model this advice-focused approach through refocusing any anxieties to the present or even acknowledging the inevitable sense of uncertainty that the future holds for all of us. Professionals may also help parents to plan for the future of their child, which may help parents feel more secure and have the capacity to focus on taking things one day at a time, encouraging patience for themselves as parents, and for their child.

Conclusion

This chapter has provided an overview of the role of advice and parent-to-parent support in the IDD community, as well as presented and summarized themes from a qualitative study of parents of children with Down syndrome. Future studies may wish to continue to utilize the voices of parents of children with special needs in identifying advice, points of resilience, and the positive aspects of parenting a child with IDD. In providing a greater presence of literature on these areas of parenting a child with IDD, additional resources for parents may become available and societal views of this population may shift to become more positive and affirming. Professionals could also make practical and effective use of this literature to help support parents who are raising a child with IDD in multiple ways that are not dominated by professional opinion alone; but rather, with professional opinion that utilizes the voices of parents who have actually experienced raising a child with IDD. Finally, policy makers could also benefit from literature in this area because it sheds light on the kinds of resources and support families who have a child with a disability might need. Additionally, this type of literature could help clarify what resources the government might be able to specifically provide to better support these families.

Key Messages from This Chapter

- **For individuals with IDD and their families**: New parents of children with IDD may feel more empowered in their role through seeking education, maintaining a positive attitude, and acting as advocates for their child. Parents also may benefit from seeing their child with IDD as a child first, not allowing the diagnosis to be the only part of their child's identity.
- **For professionals**: As professionals work with individuals with IDD and their families, they should recognize the parents' role as potential sources for information regarding the uniqueness of their child. Professionals may benefit from listening to information from parents, not only to understand what is recommended in the IDD community as best practices, but also to more deeply connect with the experiences of these families.
- **For policy makers**: From the voices of the parents in this study, policy makers should examine the experiences and advice of parents of children with IDD, as they are often the key parent advocates and educators on behalf of their child. In this study, parents' advice often included recommending self-education and advocacy for their child, which may imply that parents must step in as advocates on their child's behalf, possibly filling a gap or a need that is not being met by professionals. Policy makers, therefore, should seek to understand the experiences of parents that lead them into the advocacy role to identify areas for growth.

References

Ainbinder, J. G., Blanchard, L. W., Singer, G. H. S., Sullivan, M. E., Powers, L. K., Marquis, J. G., & Santelli, B. (1998). A qualitative study of parent to parent support for parents of children with special needs. *Journal of Pediatric Psychology*, *23*(2), 99–109. doi:10.1093/jpepsy/23.2.99

Al-Krenawi, A., Graham, J. R., & Gharaibeh, F. A. (2011). The impact of intellectual disability, caregiver burden, family functioning, marital quality, and sense of coherence. *Disability and Society*, *26*(2), 139–150. doi:10.1080/09687599.2011.543861

Baker, B. L., Blacher, J., & Olsson, M. B. (2005). Preschool children with and without developmental delay: Behaviour problems, parents' optimism and well-being. *Journal of Intellectual Disability Research*, *49*, 575–590. doi:10.1111/j.1365-2788.2005.00691.x

Baum, L. S. (2004). Internet parent support groups for primary caregivers of a child with special health care needs. *Pediatric Nursing*, *30*(5), 381–388. Retrieved from http://www.pediatricnursing.net/issues/index.html

Braun, V., & Clarke, V. (2006). Using thematic analysis in psychology. *Qualitative Research in Psychology*, *3*(2), 77–101. doi:10.1191/1478088706qp063oa

Gallagher, S., & Whiteley, J. (2013). The association between stress and physical health in parents caring for children with intellectual disabilities is moderated by children's challenging behaviours. *Journal of Health Psychology*, *18*(9), 1220–1231. doi:10.1177/1359105312464672

Gilmore, L. (2006). Perceptions of Down syndrome in the Australian community. *Journal on Developmental Disabilities*, *12*(1), 59–70. Retrieved from http://oadd.org/journal/volume-12-number-1-supplement-2-down-syndrome-expanding-areas-of-study/

Glidden, L. M., Billings, F. J., & Jobe, B. M. (2006). Personality, coping style and well-being of parents rearing children with developmental disabilities. *Journal of Intellectual Disability Research*, *50*(12), 949–962. doi:10.1111/j.1365-2788.2006.00929.x

Gupta, A., & Singhal, N. (2004). Positive perceptions in parents of children with disabilities. *Asia Pacific Disability Rehabilitation Journal*, *15*(1), 22–35. Retrieved from http://english.aifo.it/disability/apdrj/apdrj104/positive-perceptions.pdf

Heiman, T. (2002). Parents of children with disabilities: Resilience, coping, and future expectations. *Journal of Developmental and Physical Disabilities*, *14*(2), 159–171. doi:10.1023/A:1015219514621

Hippman, C., Inglis, A., & Austin, J. (2012). What is a "balanced" description? Insight from parents of individuals with Down syndrome. *Journal of Genetic Counseling*, *21*, 35–44. doi:10.1007/s10897-011-9417-2

Holton, J. A. (2007). The coding process and its challenges. In A. Bryant & K. Charmaz (Eds.), *The Sage handbook of grounded theory* (pp. 265–289). Thousand Oaks, CA: Sage.

Kerr, S. M., & McIntosh, J. B. (2000). Coping when a child has a disability: Exploring the impact of parent-to-parent support. *Child: Care, Health, and Development*, *26*(4), 309–322. doi:10.1046/j.1365-2214.2000.00149.x

Law, M., King, S., Stewart, D., & King, G. (2002). The perceived effects of parent-led support groups for parents of children with disabilities. *Physical & Occupational Therapy in Pediatrics*, *21*(2-3), 29–48. doi:10.1080/J006v21n02_03

Nelson Goff, B. S., Springer, N., Foote, L. C., Frantz, C., Peak, M., Tracy, C., & Cross, K. A. (2013). Receiving the initial Down syndrome diagnosis: A comparison of prenatal and postnatal parent group experiences. *Intellectual and Developmental Disabilities*, *51*(6), 446–457. doi:10.1352/1934-9556-51.6.446

Quittner, A. L., Espelage, D. L., Opipari, L. C., Carter, B., Eid, N., & Eigen, H. (1998). Role strain in couples with and without a child with a chronic illness: Associations with marital satisfaction, intimacy, and daily mood. *Health Psychology*, *17*(2), 112–124. doi:10.1037/0278-6133.17.2.112

Shilling, V., Morris, C., Thompson-Coon, J., Ukoumunne, O., Rogers, M., & Logan, S. (2013). Peer support for parents of children with chronic disabling conditions:

A systematic review of quantitative and qualitative studies. *Developmental Medicine & Child Neurology*, *55*(7), 602–609. doi:10.1111/dmcn.12091

Singer, G. H., Marquis, J., Powers, L. K., Blanchard, L., DiVenere, N., Santelli, B., Ainbinder, J. G., & Sharp, M. (1999). A multi-site evaluation of parent to parent programs for parents of children with disabilities. *Journal of Early Intervention*, *22*(3), 217–229. doi:10.1177/105381519902200305

Skotko, B. G., Levine, S. P., & Goldstein, R. (2011). Having a son or daughter with Down syndrome: Perspectives from mothers and fathers. *American Journal of Medical Genetics*, *155*, 2335–2347. *doi:*10.1002/ajmg.a.34293

Solomon, M., Pistrang, N., & Barker, C. (2001). The benefits of mutual support groups for parents of children with disabilities. *American Journal of Community Psychology*, *29*(1), 113–132. doi:10.1023/A:1005253514140

Song, J., Mailick, M. R., Ryff, C. D., Coe, C. L, Greenberg, J. S., & Hong, J. (2014). Allostatic load in parents of children with developmental disorders: Modering influence of positive affect. *Journal of Health Psychology*, *19*(2), 262–272. doi:10.1177/1359105312468193

Taanila, A., Järvelin, M., & Kokkonen, J. (1998). Parental guidance and counselling by doctors and nursing staff: Parents' views of initial information and advice for families with disabled children. *Journal of Clinical Nursing*, *7*, 505–511. doi:10.1046/j.1365-2702.1998.00190.x

Part II

Perspectives, Contributions, and Lived Experiences of Individuals with IDD and Their Families on the Journey

5 Understanding and Supporting Identity Formation and Meaning Making

Kami L. Gallus, PhD and Jennifer L. Jones, PhD

Introduction

Garrett: "Mom, can I play football?"
Mom: "No. Playing football is not safe because of your feeding tube and your disability."
Garrett: "What is my disability?"

This conversation in our minivan with my then 12-year-old son marked the first time I (JLJ) used the word *disability* when talking with Garrett. My husband and I had not intentionally avoided disability terms, we just had not explicitly used them. I had carefully prepared Garrett for every surgical procedure—sewing tracheostomies and feeding tubes into stuffed animals, explaining why another surgery was necessary and what to expect when he awoke from the anesthesia. We worked hard to create opportunities for him to exercise real choice and genuine control. We encouraged him to be proud of his body and helped him to show off his "tummy tube" for first grade show-and-tell. In elementary school, he played basketball, baseball, soccer, and hockey with his friends who did not have intellectual or physical disabilities, while simultaneously competing in Special Olympics (2017).

Looking back, I can see the evolution of my acceptance with Garrett having an intellectual disability (ID). As a new mom, I fought for him to not be labeled by medical and educational professionals—often requesting his records and asking for unsubstantiated diagnoses to be removed (e.g., mental retardation at the age of three—arguing that IQ was not stable until age eight). By the time Garrett was six, I had a new perspective. I was grateful Garrett had survived many life-threatening surgeries and was less concerned with the labels placed on him by others. By the time Garrett was nine, I was comfortable with the MR label and even explained to his third-grade teacher why retaining him was not in his best interest, "He's not going to catch up, Sharon. He has MR. He also has a very supportive group of friends who include him in the classroom, on the playground, and outside of school. He needs to stay with his peers."

You see, I was a "good" mom, a progressive mom. Not only was I unashamed that my son had an intellectual disability, I celebrated his disability as diversity that enriched our lives. I was successfully navigating my own journey of acceptance and had laid claim to my identity as a mom of a child with an intellectual disability. Why then had I waited until he was 12 years old to introduce the word *disability*? Had I somehow missed giving my son the language he needed to navigate his own identity journey?

Language that Influences Identity

Language is part of what makes us human. Since the 1960s, researchers in the field of linguistic anthropology have explored how language serves as our primary tool for communication and helps to organize our beliefs and worldviews (Duranti, 2003). Perhaps most important has been the increased understanding of how language shapes our identity. While the term *identity* derives from the Latin word *identitas* meaning sameness—being the same with something described—*identity formation* paradoxically encompasses uniqueness as well as affiliation (Erikson, 1968). Ultimately, identity helps individuals make sense of different and distinct parts of themselves. Disability is a unique identity context that distinguishes one as both unique and as part of a group (Oyserman, Elmore, & Smith, 2012).

Similar to other traits that contribute to identity (e.g., race, gender), intellectual and developmental disability (IDD) operates as a unique identity context that distinguishes an individual within society. In the social constructivist view, identities have meaning only within a complex web of social relations and shared activity (Gergen, 1990). Socially, individuals with IDD are given labels, defined primarily by their disability, and diagnosed because their intellectual functioning differs from what has been socially defined as "normal" (Manion & Bersani, 1987). The clinical terminology used to refer to individuals with IDD has evolved significantly over the past century with shifts from the traditional medical model to a social-ecological model of disability. As Schalock (2013) noted, the language of thought and one's mental model influence the terms that are used to refer to individuals with IDD.

Our goal for this chapter is to sensitize helping professionals to the important role language and communication play in individual and family meaning making and identity development, to inform professionals of the unique challenges faced, and to offer recommendations to promote communication among individuals and families regarding their meaning making and identity journey. Specifically, in this chapter we will explain the evolution of terminology used to refer to individuals with IDD and how shifts in terminology reflect changes in the conceptualization of individuals with IDD in society. Next, we will explore what is known about how individuals with IDD and their families acquire the language associated with intellectual and developmental disability and family members' comfort with using the professionally and socially ascribed terminology. We will explore how families' communication regarding intellectual and developmental disability and comfort with language and labels potentially impacts meaning and identity formation among both individuals and family members. Finally, we will provide recommendations for professionals to promote communication among individuals and families regarding their meaning making and identity journey.

The Language of Intellectual Disability

Intellectual disability (ID) is the most common developmental disorder, with an estimated prevalence rate of approximately 1% (American Psychiatric Association [APA], 2013). The term *intellectual disability* does not refer to a singular disease; rather, ID is a diagnosis with thousands of genetic (e.g., Down syndrome) and environmental causes (e.g., Fetal Alcohol Syndrome). Yet, for 30–50% of individuals with ID and their families, there is no known etiology to account for cognitive impairment (see Percy, 2007).

The American Association on Intellectual and Developmental Disabilities (AAIDD, 2017) defines intellectual disability as a disability originating before the age of 18 and characterized by significant limitations both in ***intellectual functioning*** (reasoning, learning, problem-solving) and in ***adaptive behavior***, which covers a range of everyday social and practical skills (Schalock *et al.*, 2010). Many individuals with ID also have developmental disabilities. *Developmental disability* is an umbrella term that includes intellectual disability as well as other disabilities manifested before the age of 22 and likely continue throughout the life span (AAIDD, 2017). Developmental disabilities are severe chronic disabilities that can be physical (e.g., epilepsy) or cognitive (e.g., dyslexia) or both (e.g., Down syndrome). Since intellectual and other developmental disabilities often co-occur, professionals often work with people who have both types of disabilities (AAIDD, 2017).

Changes in Disability Terminology

Individuals with IDD and their families are not alone in their struggle to find terminology and labels that fit their experiences and understanding of ID. Even within the field of intellectual disability, there have been significant shifts in the frameworks used to understand disability and in the terminology used to describe the phenomenon now known as intellectual disability. Throughout the twentieth century, language shifted from *feeble-minded* to *mental retardation* with institutional classification systems of *idiot, moron*, or *imbecile* and educational categories of *educable* or *trainable* (Wehmeyer, 2013a). At the turn of the century, in an effort led by and with self-advocates (i.e., individuals with IDD advocating for their own interests, desires, needs, and rights), the term *intellectual disability* replaced the term *mental retardation* (Schalock *et al.*, 2010). This change in terminology is much more than an attempt at political correctness. The change in terminology reflects an understanding of disability that has evolved from a person-centered trait (i.e., deficit) to a human phenomenon resulting from organic and social factors (Schalock, 2013). The movement from a medical model to a social-ecological model of disability (Schalock *et al.*, 2010) redefines disability as the interaction between personal competencies and contextual demands and recognizes the critical role of formal and informal supports as well as building on the strengths and capacities of persons with IDD (Wehmeyer, 2013b).

The Three Waves of the ID Movement: Professionals, Parents, and Self-Advocates

The changes in ID terminology are illustrated across the waves of the disability movement identified by Wehmeyer and other leaders in the field of IDD (see Wehmeyer, 2013a; Wehmeyer, Bersani, & Gagne, 2000). Three significant waves have brought about changes not only in terminology but in understanding the unique societal contributions of individuals with IDD: professionals, parents, and self-advocacy and self-determination.

1. **Professionals in the ID movement.** For the first half of the 1900s, professionals were viewed as the ultimate experts. Individuals with IDD were segregated from their families and society by being placed in large state-run institutions where sterilization was practiced to control the spread of feeble-mindedness (Wehmeyer *et al.*, 2000). Leaders and decision makers in the field of IDD were often physicians who served as superintendents of the state institutions. Parents and society assumed these professionals knew best and individuals with IDD had no basic civil rights, including access or rights to an education (Wehmeyer *et al.*, 2000).

2. **Parents in the ID movement.** With the return of many veterans with disabilities from World War II, a shift began in the disability movement, and the parent movement emerged in the early 1950s. People with disabilities were viewed as "objects to be fixed, cured, or rehabilitated, and simultaneously pitied" (Wehmeyer *et al.*, 2000, p. 107). As parents began to advocate publicly for their children with disabilities, the poster child became a primary strategy in fund-raising. Poster children promoted an understanding of individuals with IDD as innocent, eternal children. In contrast to the professional movement when individuals with IDD were feared and individuals and families experienced social shame and blame, the parent movement promoted an understanding of individuals with disabilities as needing societal care, protection, and pity. Many of today's leading disability organizations (e.g., The Arc, 2016; Special Olympics, 2017) were born out of a parent or family member's advocacy during this time. Professionals slowly joined parents in developing services and lobbying for legislation to ensure basic civil rights for individuals with disabilities (Wehmeyer *et al.*, 2000).

3. **Self-advocacy and self-determination.** With the foundation laid for individuals with IDD to begin speaking for themselves, the third wave, self-advocacy and self-determination, emerged during the 1970s and 1980s (Wehmeyer *et al.*, 2000). Self-advocacy and self-determination were fueled by the normalization principle (creating conditions where individuals with disability experience the normal respect extended to human beings leading to consideration of individual choices, desires, and aspirations) and the deinstitutionalization movement

(changes in primary residence of individuals with IDD from institutions to living in the community with residential supports; Wehmeyer *et al.*, 2000). Self-advocates have spent the past 40 years fighting for the right to choose where they live and work and with whom they interact. Self-determination reflects the belief that all individuals have the right to make choices and direct their own lives and is a key dimension of individual quality of life (Schalock *et al.*, 2005; Shogren, 2016).

Professional Communication About IDD

In our experience, the three waves of the disability movement illustrate how most individuals and families are introduced to the language of IDD and the associated challenge for parents and individuals of developing a personal meaning and cultural identity around IDD. While the professional wave "ended" nearly 70 years ago, most parents begin their journey seeking answers from professionals (Nelson Goff *et al.*, 2013). Medical professionals often provide the first IDD diagnosis, introducing parents to a new language. In interviews with 23 parents and siblings of adults with IDD, every parent specifically recalled the first time the language of disability was used to define their child (Richardson, 2016). Parents recall with emotion and detail the life-altering conversations they had with a physician and the language used to describe their child (Nelson Goff *et al.*, 2013; Richardson, 2016). Given the powerful impact of professionals' words and tone in delivering the news of IDD, much research is needed to understand and develop best practices in not only delivering the diagnosis, but helping families move forward in making meaning.

Family Communication About IDD

Once parents are given the initial diagnosis and language by a professional, they shift into a new and important role of giving meaning to the language, influencing their own and their child's identity. Research indicates that children often seek information concerning their disability from their parents (Connors & Stalker, 2007), but may encounter parents who are ill-prepared or unwilling to engage in the discussion (Jones, Oseland, Morris, & Larzelere, 2014; Shearn & Todd, 1997).

Parents' discomfort with engaging their children with IDD in conversations about disability appears to span the life course. Following a two-year study with 26 children with IDD aged seven to 15, Connors and Stalker (2007) concluded that a significant contributing factor to children's identity and meaning making struggle is a lack of positive language that can be used to discuss difference. They reported children with IDD were often discouraged from discussing their disability at home or school and that parental avoidance extended to siblings as well, as one 13-year-old brother reported his mother had forbidden him to discuss his sister's impairment, saying, "keep it in between the family" (Connors & Stalker, 2007, p. 24).

In research examining communication about disability between parents and adolescents with IDD, parents appear to struggle with the timing, context, and content of such conversations (Jones *et al.*, 2014). Overall, the majority of parents (62%) reported talking to their adolescent about differences between the child and his or her peers, and slightly less than half (44%) of the parents reported having a conversation about the child's disability. When parents did engage in conversations, it was often reactive rather than proactive, with many parents reporting first engaging in conversations about disability when their child had been bullied or as an explanation regarding exclusion from an age-normed activity such as driving, dating, or attending college. Among the parents who reported attempts to actively engage their adolescent in conversations about disability or difference, many stated these conversations were met by sadness or confusion from their child. Parents of adolescents for whom the etiology of the child's intellectual and developmental disability was unknown were most reluctant to engage in conversations. These parents may remain caught in a more ambiguous state and have fewer resources than families who have a tangible cause for a child's intellectual and developmental disability.

Finally, parents of adults with IDD may choose to avoid conversations about disability out of concern that such conversations could lead to emotional distress. Shearn and Todd (1997) found parents use specific strategies of avoidance, which include withholding disability-related information from their son or daughter, providing anxiety-dampening excuses when s/he is unable to accomplish a task due to his/her disability, concealing the social meaning of disability, and abstaining from the use of disability terminology in front of their son or daughter.

The Double Bind of Language for Individuals with IDD

Narratives from my (second author's) research and reflection on the conversations around my own dinner table remind me of the difficulty in choosing to engage individuals with IDD in conversations about their disability. After our initial conversation about why it was not safe for Garrett to play football, we began to use the language of disability and the term *intellectual disability* in many conversations. Garrett adopted this language readily and often used intellectual disability to describe himself; however, the struggle toward identity formation and meaning making have been ongoing and at times painful for all of us. One evening at dinner when Garrett was 16, he informed us that he was going to ask for a wishing rock for his birthday. I flippantly asked why he would want a wishing rock. His response left me breathless "Because I will close my eyes and wish that I do not have a disability anymore. Will that really work, Mom?" My eyes filled with tears and later that night I wrote, "There are no words to describe the flood of emotions that erupted in me—sadness, guilt, anger. Maybe I have done it all wrong in 'telling him' […] maybe it would have been better […] however, he *knows* he is different. He knows the limitations he experiences. Where is the handbook for this?" (J. L. Jones, personal communication, April 17, 2010).

Due to the difficult nature of these conversations, it is understandable why many professionals and family members choose to avoid discussing disability with individuals with IDD. That night at dinner, I questioned if giving Garrett the language of intellectual disability had created a double bind for him. He had adopted the terminology readily, but once he began to understand how the label had excluded him from opportunities (e.g., the social construction of intellectual disability), he wanted to wish it away. However, avoidance of such conversations does not negate the lived experience and stigma that individuals with IDD encounter throughout their lives (Cunningham & Glenn, 2004; Cunningham, Glenn, & Fitzpatrick, 2000; Davies & Jenkins, 1997).

Research indicates (see Shogren, 2016) and we believe there is everything to be gained by empowering individuals with IDD to know and understand themselves fully, including knowledge of their disability. Too often families and professionals avoid conversations regarding the details and ramifications of disability with individuals with IDD. Yet, in order to be the primary causal agent in one's life, individuals need to know themselves and understand how their disability might impact their relationships, employment, participation, and need for supports (Shogren, 2013).

Principles for Practice

Beart, Hardy, and Buchan (2005) offered that for individuals without ID, understanding of intellectual disability lies at the level of discourse rather than that of experience. They challenged researchers to acknowledge their limited perspective and to "try to understand at the level of experience by listening carefully to the people who live this identity every day" (Beart *et al.*, 2005, p. 55). We pose this is not only a challenge for the researcher, but for all professionals who work alongside individuals with IDD and their families. We also want to acknowledge the meaning making and identity formation journey for individuals with IDD who experience more profound limitations in cognition or communication may look very different than that of Garrett and others represented in the IDD literature. It may well be a journey that others can never truly understand because, for them, "dialogue" is all about other people trying to decipher the meaning of their behaviors that communicate (often in broad strokes, without a lot of precision) their emotions (e.g., happy, sad, frustrated; K. Roberson, personal communication, June 16, 2016).

Even when professionals in human service fields have personal experience or advanced training, most still feel ill-equipped to work with individuals with IDD and their families (see Werner & Stawski, 2012). It is clearly demonstrated within the literature that many individuals with IDD and their families are struggling with the meaning making and identity process (e.g., Davies & Jenkins, 1997; Jones, 2012; Shearn & Todd, 1997). Just as helping professionals are challenged to develop cultural competence in working with diverse populations, individuals with IDD and their families represent an underserved and vulnerable population that helping professionals must seek to better understand and effectively support.

The following principles reflect the values we believe professionals must ascribe to when working alongside individuals with IDD and their families as they navigate identity development and meaning making across the life span.

We are keenly aware there is no simple five-step approach that will guarantee success. We also recognize that not all individuals with IDD will be able to engage in meaningful dialogue. However, we hope by outlining these five broad principles helping professionals will be empowered to engage many individuals and families in navigating their own journeys.

Understand Your Values

Recognizing that the mental model helping professionals carry into their work with individuals and families greatly impacts the helping process, it is important for professionals to identify and acknowledge their personal values and beliefs regarding disability. As professionals, we each have a working mental model of disability that serves to define our understanding of disability, determines the terminology we use, and ultimately provides the basis upon which we devise strategies for providing supports and services. All professionals must be aware of the mental model they bring to the helping relationship and how their own working model impacts meaning and identity processes. Professionals must check their biases, including believing the common myth that having a family member with a disability is a liability to marriage and family relationships. To the contrary, research suggests that while families face unique stressors, having a family member with IDD can positively impact relationships and individual and family quality of life (see Blacher, Baker, & Berkovits, 2013). Strategies applied when working with families of individuals with IDD must include recognition of the unique strengths, gifts, and resources of each family member, including the individual with ID.

Embrace the Language of IDD

When working with individuals with IDD and their families, professionals must also acknowledge their own comfort level or lack thereof with the language of disability. Individuals and families may need assistance with learning or becoming more comfortable with using disability terminology that is specific and empowers them to access the services and supports needed. It is not uncommon for individuals, families, and professionals to use broad imprecise terms (e.g., special needs) or incorrect terms that do not accurately identify the individual's current condition (e.g., using the term developmental delay for children or adults over the age of eight or learning disability for an individual with an ID). Professionals who are not adequately equipped with the appropriate terms and language as specified within the intellectual and developmental disability field cannot comfortably introduce the appropriate clinical language to individuals and families with whom they work. Professionals should educate themselves on the most current and specific terminology within the IDD field in order to avoid mislabeling individuals and misinforming families. Organizations such as the American Association on Intellectual and Developmental Disabilities (AAIDD, 2017), National Down Syndrome Congress (NDSC, 2014), National Down Syndrome Society

(NDSS, 2012), and The Arc (2016) provide excellent resources. While it is important for professionals to introduce language, not all individuals and family members will readily adopt disability terminology. It is important to respect their choices and give them time as they navigate their identity and meaning making as individuals and as a family system.

Encourage Individuals with IDD and Their Families to Tell Their Unique Narratives

It is crucial for professionals to remember that while individuals with IDD may share a diagnosis or language, each individual's and family's experience is unique. Professionals are often knowledgeable and aware of the unique challenges encountered by individuals and their families, but may forget that individuals and their family members are our best teachers and the experts on their own lives. As professionals, we must help individuals and their family members find the voice and space to share their stories. In return, we must listen, modeling for individuals and families the importance of hearing one another's perspectives and experiences. As a parent (JLJ) of an individual with IDD for 20 years, I am often reminded that my perspective as a parent is just that—the perspective of one mom. I do not know what it feels like to be Garrett—the only person with IDD in a family, in a classroom, or in a workplace, nor do I understand my other children's perspectives of having lived their entire lives with a brother with IDD. Professionals who model a "listening to understand" stance broaden family members' perspectives and foster a greater appreciation for the unique meaning making and identity development of each individual in the family system.

Identity Development and Meaning Making as Dynamic Processes

In the United States, family members are expected to be lifelong caregivers. The overwhelming majority of individuals with IDD of all ages live in the home of a family member (Braddock *et al.*, 2015; Larson *et al.*, 2015). As professionals, we must strive to understand the family system we are collaborating with today within the context of their long history of meaning making and identity development. Parents of individuals with IDD face one marathon after another in the quest to get a diagnosis, accept the label, and assimilate the meaning and experience of IDD into their own personal and social identity. So too, siblings of individuals with IDD often comprise the primary social network for their brother or sister with IDD and are called upon to be the primary caregiver or overseer when parents are no longer able to do so (see Seltzer, Orsmond, Greenberg, & Lounds, 2005; also see Chapter 16 in this text). Recognizing that individuals with IDD often sustain a high level of involvement with their family throughout the life span, the family system plays a uniquely important role in meaning making and identity formation. Therefore, professionals working alongside individuals with IDD and their families would benefit from an understanding of general system theory (Satir, 1967; von Bertalanffy, 1968) and family quality of life (Zuna, Summers, Turnbull, Hu, & Xu, 2010). Professionals who adhere to these systemic approaches exhibit a richer understanding of families as systems whose parts are interdependent and open to change.

Navigating a Bicultural Identity: Merging Two Worlds

In our experience, individuals and their family members are often asked to navigate two cultures: the mainstream culture of typical development and the subculture of intellectual disability. These two cultures can at times feel in opposition to one another; however, individuals and families should not have to choose philosophically or logistically between access to full community inclusion (e.g., living and working in the community) and services and supports designed specifically to meet the needs of persons with IDD (e.g., employment supports) and their family members (e.g., parent support groups). We believe the value of community inclusion is not negated by programs or services designed specifically for individuals with ID.

As we identify with a group, we begin to make meaning of our belonging. Individuals with IDD report that connecting with others in the disability community is a powerful experience (Caldwell, 2010, 2011). Studies also show that after receiving a diagnosis for their child's disability, families begin to adopt new vocabularies, roles, rules, structures, and expectations that influence family functioning and overall coping (Bingham, Correa, & Huber, 2012; Bostrom, Broberg, & Hwang, 2010; Graungaard & Skov, 2007). Likewise, a large body of research supports the benefits of community inclusion for individuals with and without disabilities (see Hewitt, Nord, Bogenschutz, & Reinke, 2013). As professionals who work toward best practices of including individuals with IDD in our schools, religious institutions, neighborhoods, and workplaces, we often struggle to encourage the value of maintaining a place in both cultures. Professionals should acknowledge the challenge and reward of both cultures and encourage individuals and families in developing what we define as *bicultural identity*.

"Mom, There are Some Good Things About Having a Disability"

It has been 10 years since I (JLJ) introduced disability terminology to Garrett. Having terminology and language allows him to ask questions (e.g., "Is my intellectual disability because I was really sick when I was a baby?") and grow in his knowledge of how his disability impacts his life (e.g., "Is it a bad idea for me to have kids because of my disability?"). Our conversations about the meaning of intellectual disability and the implications of his diagnosis on his daily life and future are ongoing and at times exhausting. However, through continual dialogue and guided reflection with us and helping professionals, Garrett has navigated his own journey of identity formation and meaning making around intellectual disability.

It is not uncommon for Garrett to say he is frustrated by his disability or by the lack of opportunities available to him as compared to his peers and siblings without disabilities. However, at the age of 22, Garrett began to embrace some positive attributes of his disability, beginning conversations with "Mom, you know, there are some good things about having a disability." Each time I hear him reframe his disability in a positive light, my heart swells as he engages in the hard work of identity formation. Listening to him work to make meaning of intellectual disability and acknowledge both the very real challenges and rewards of a diagnosis he did not choose, but is learning to accept, validates that while the conversations are difficult, they are worth having for the individual with IDD and others.

For Garrett and me as individuals and for our family system, as we acquired language and assimilated that language comfortably into our lives, we have engaged in conversations that helped us make our own meaning of intellectual and developmental disability and solidify our identities as individuals and as a family unit. For us the dynamic processes of identity formation and meaning making led to an outcome of bicultural identity for each individual family member and our family unit. We value our relationships in the mainstream of community and support and embrace the unique attributes each member brings to the family system (e.g., all of my children, both with and without IDD, participate as athletes in Special Olympics, 2017). Garrett brought the unique attribute of IDD into our family system. Through and with him, we are able to acknowledge the very real challenges experienced by individuals with IDD and their family members without negating the unique joys and benefits that come with intellectual disability.

Conclusion

Making meaning of intellectual disability is challenging for professionals, for family members, and for the individual with IDD. Our goal for this chapter was to sensitize helping professionals to the important role that language and communication play in individual and family meaning making and identity development, to inform professionals of the unique challenges faced, and to offer recommendations to promote communication among individuals and families regarding their meaning making and identity journey.

We approached this chapter with caution. We in no way intended to portray that identity formation and meaning making at the individual or family level is simple or easy—there is no handbook or simple five-step approach. And we by no means believe that the outcomes of the difficult conversations will always be positive. We do, however, believe that if we are to make progress as a society and as helping professionals, we can no longer be afraid of the journey or let fear hold us back from engaging in the conversations and struggles of making meaning and forming identity around intellectual and developmental disability.

Key Messages from This Chapter

- **For individuals with IDD and their families**: Families' communication regarding intellectual disability and comfort with language and labels impacts meaning and identity formation among both individuals and family members. Thus, parents need to be encouraged and open to engaging in conversations about intellectual disability and identity.

- **For professionals**: Helping professionals play an important role in promoting communication among individuals and families regarding their meaning making and identity journey. Therefore, it is critical that professionals know and understand the language of intellectual and developmental disability, and appreciate the paradox of sameness amidst difference that exists within the identity of IDD.
- **For policy makers**: The professional and social terminology used to refer to individuals with IDD has evolved over the years. Shifts in terminology reflect changes in the conceptualization of how individuals with IDD belong in society. As we move from a medical model to a social-ecological model of disability, policies are needed that support and address the psychosocial needs of individuals with IDD and their families.

References

American Association on Intellectual and Developmental Disabilities. (2017). *Frequently asked questions on intellectual disability.* Retrieved from http://aaidd.org/intellectual-disability/definition/faqs-on-intellectual-disability

American Psychiatric Association. (2013). *Diagnostic and statistical manual of mental disorders* (5th ed.). Washington, DC: Author.

Beart, S., Hardy, G., & Buchan, L. (2005). How people with intellectual disabilities view their social identities: A review of the literature. *Journal of Applied Research in Intellectual Disabilities, 18*, 47–56. doi:10.1111/j.1468-3148.2004.00218.x

Bingham, A., Correa, V. I., & Huber, J. J. (2012). Mothers' voices: Coping with their children's initial disability diagnosis. *Infant Mental Health Journal, 33*, 372–385. doi:10.1002/imhj.21341

Blacher, J., Baker, B. L., & Berkovits, L. D. (2013). Family perspectives on child intellectual disability: Views from the sunny side of the street. In M. L. Wehmeyer (Ed.), *Oxford handbook of positive psychology and disability* (pp. 166–181). New York, NY: Oxford University Press.

Bostrom, P. K., Broberg, M., & Hwang, P. (2010). Parents' descriptions and experiences of young children recently diagnosed with intellectual disability. *Child: Care, Health, and Development, 36*, 93–100. doi:10.1111/j.1365-2214.2009.01036.x

Braddock, D., Hemp, R., Rizzolo, M. C., Tanis, E. S., Haffer, L., & Wu, J. (2015). *The state of states in intellectual and developmental disabilities: Emerging from the great recession.* Washington, DC: American Association on Intellectual and Developmental Disabilities.

Caldwell, J. (2010). Leadership development of individuals with developmental disabilities in the self-advocacy movement. *Journal of Intellectual Disability Research, 54*(11), 1004–1014. doi:10.1111/j.1365-2788.2010.01326.x.

Caldwell, J. (2011). Disability identity of leaders in the self-advocacy movement. *Intellectual and Developmental Disabilities, 49*(5), 315–326. doi:10.1352/1934-9556-49.5.315

Connors, C., & Stalker, K. (2007). Children's experiences of disability: Pointers to a social model of childhood disability. *Disability and Society, 22*, 19–33. doi:10.1080/09687590601056162

Cunningham, C., & Glenn, S. (2004). Self-awareness in young adults with Down syndrome: I. Awareness of Down syndrome and disability. *International Journal of Disability, Development, and Education*, *51*, 335–361. doi:10.1080/1034912042000295017

Cunningham, C. C., Glenn, S., & Fitzpatrick, H. (2000). Parents telling their offspring about Down syndrome and disability. *Journal of Applied Research in Intellectual Disabilities*, *13*, 47–61. doi:10.1046/j.1468-3148.2000.00012.x

Davies, C., & Jenkins, R. (1997). She has different fits to me: How people with learning difficulties see themselves. *Disability and Society*, *12*, 95–109. doi:10.1080/09687599727498

Duranti, A. (2003). Language as culture in U. S. anthropology: Three paradigms. *Current Anthropology*, *44*(3), 323–348. doi:10.1086/368118

Erikson, E. H. (1968). *Identity: Youth and crisis*. New York, NY: Norton.

Gergen, K. J. (1990). Social understanding and the inscription of self. In J. W. Sigler, R. A. Shweder, & G. Herdt (Eds.), *Cultural psychology: Essays on comparative human development* (pp. 569–606). New York, NY: Cambridge University Press.

Graungaard, A. H., & Skov, L. (2007). Why do we need a diagnosis? A qualitative study of parents' experiences, coping and needs, when the newborn child is severely disabled. *Child: Care, Health and Development*, *33*, 296–307. doi:10.1111/j.1365-2214.2006.00666.x

Hewitt, A. S., Nord, D., Bogenschutz, M., & Reinke, J. (2013). Community living. *Inclusion*, *1*, 17–28. doi:10.1352/2326-6988-1.1.017

Jones, J. L. (2012). Factors associated with self-concept: Adolescents with intellectual and developmental disabilities share their perspectives. *Intellectual and Developmental Disabilities*, *50*, 31–40. doi:10.1352/1934-9556-50.1.31

Jones, J. L., Oseland, L. M., Morris, K., & Larzelere, R. (2014). Parent report of conversations with their adolescents with intellectual disabilities. *Journal of Applied Research in Intellectual Disabilities*, *27*, 521–530. doi:10.1111/jar.12090

Larson, S. A., Hallas-Muchow, L., Aiken, F., Hewitt, A., Pettingell, S., Anderson, L. L., Moseley, C., Sowers, M., Lee Fay, M., Agosta, J., Smith, D., & Kardell, Y. (2015). *In-home and residential long-term support and services for persons with intellectual or developmental disabilities: Status and trends through 2013.* Minneapolis, MN: University of Minnesota, Institute on Community Integration, Research and Training Center on Community Living.

Manion, M., & Bersani, H. (1987). Mental retardation as a western sociological construct: A cross-cultural analysis. *Disability, Handicap & Society*, *2*, 231–245. doi:10.1080/02674648766780301

National Down Syndrome Congress. (2014). *Down syndrome informational brochure*. Retrieved from http://www.ndsccenter.org/

National Down Syndrome Society. (2012). *About NDSS*. Retrieved from http://www.ndss.org/About-NDSS/

Nelson Goff, B. S., Springer, N., Foote, L. C., Frantz, C., Peak, M., Tracy, C., Veh, T., Bentley, G.E., & Cross, K. A. (2013). Receiving the initial Down syndrome diagnosis: A comparison of prenatal and postnatal parent group experiences. *Intellectual and Developmental Disabilities*, *51*, 446–457. doi:10.1352/1934-9556-51.6.446

Oyserman, D., Elmore, K., & Smith, G. (2012). Self, self-concept, and identity. In M. R. Leary & J. P. Tangney (Eds.), *Handbook of self and identity* (2nd ed., pp. 69–104). New York, NY: Guilford.

Percy, M. (2007). Factors that cause or contribute to intellectual and developmental disabilities. In I. Brown, & M. Percy (Eds.), *A comprehensive guide to intellectual and developmental disabilities* (pp. 125–148). Baltimore, MD: Paul H. Brookes.

Richardson, N. (2016). *A lifetime of ambiguity: Understanding the experiences of families impacted by intellectual disability.* (Unpublished master's thesis). Oklahoma State University, Stillwater, OK.

Satir, V. (1967). *Conjoint family therapy* (2nd ed.). Palo Alto, CA: Science and Behavior Books.

Schalock, R. L. (2013). Introduction to the intellectual disability construct. In M. L. Wehmeyer (Ed.), *The story of intellectual disability* (pp. 1–15). Baltimore, MD: Paul H. Brookes.

Schalock, R. L., Borthwick-Duffy, S. A., Bradley, V. J., Buntinx, W. H. E., Coulter, D. L., Craig, E. M., Gomez, S. C., Lachapelle, Y., Luckasson, R., Reeve, A., Shogren, K. A., Snell, M. E., Spreat, S., Tassé, M. J., Thompson, J. R., Verdugo-Alonso, M. A., Wehmeyer, M. L., & Yeager, M. H. (2010). *Intellectual disability: Definition, classification, and systems of support* (11 ed.). Washington, DC: American Association on Intellectual and Developmental Disabilities.

Schalock, R. L., Verdugo, M. A., Jenaro, C., Wang, M., Wehmeyer, M., Jiancheng, X., & Lachapelle, Y. (2005). Cross-cultural study of quality of life indicators. *American Journal on Mental Retardation, 110*(4), 298–311. doi:10.1352/0895-8017(2005)110[298: CSOQOL]2.0.CO;2

Seltzer, M. M., Orsmond, J. S., Greenberg, G. I., & Lounds, J. L. (2005). Life course studies of siblings of individuals with developmental disabilities. *Mental Retardation, 43*, 354–359. doi:10.1352/0047-6765(2005)43[354: LCSOSO]2.0.CO;2

Shearn, J., & Todd, S. (1997). Parental work: An account of day-to-day activities of parents of adults with learning disabilities. *Journal of Intellectual Disability Research, 41*, 285–301. doi:10.1111/j.1365-2788.1997.tb00712.x

Shogren, K. A. (2013). *Self-determination and transition planning.* Baltimore, MD: Paul H. Brookes.

Shogren, K. A. (2016). Self-determination and self-advocacy. In American Association on Intellectual and Developmental Disabilities, *Critical issues in intellectual and developmental disabilities: Contemporary research, practice, and policy* (pp. 1–18). Washington, DC: American Association on Intellectual and Developmental Disabilities.

Special Olympics. (2017). *History.* Retrieved from http://www.specialolympics.org/Sections/What_We_Do/History_of_Special_Olympics.aspx

The Arc. (2016). *Who we are.* Retrieved from http://www.thearc.org/who-we-are

von Bertalanffy, L. (1968). *General system theory: Foundations, developments, applications.* New York, NY: George Braziller.

Wehmeyer, M. L. (Ed.). (2013a). *The story of intellectual disability.* Baltimore, MD: Paul H. Brookes.

Wehmeyer, M. L. (Ed.). (2013b). *The Oxford handbook of positive psychology and disability.* New York, NY: Oxford University Press.

Wehmeyer, M., Bersani, H. J., & Gagne, R. (2000). Riding the third wave: Self-determination and self-advocacy in the 21st century. *Focus on Autism and Other Developmental Disabilities, 15*, 106–115. doi:10.1177/108835760001500206

Werner, S., & Stawski, M. (2012). Mental health: Knowledge, attitudes and training of professionals on dual diagnosis of intellectual disability and psychiatric disorder. *Journal of Intellectual Disability Research*, *56*, 291–304. doi:10.1111/j.1365-2788.2011.01429.x

Zuna, N., Summers, J. A., Turnbull, A. P., Hu, X., & Xu, S. (2010). Theorizing about family quality of life. In R. Kober (Ed.), *Enhancing the quality of life of people with intellectual disabilities: From theory to practice* (pp. 241–278). Amsterdam, The Netherlands: Springer Netherlands.

6 Perspectives from Mothers

Recognizing Their Strengths and Contributions beyond Caregiving

Jessica D. Cless, MS and Christyne Stephenson, MS

Introduction

Mothers of children with a disability often have a unique perspective of what it means to be a parent. Parents of children with intellectual and developmental disabilities (IDD) often face more challenges than those with typically developing children (Glidden, Billings, & Jobe, 2006). Mothers share a special part in this story, as their perspective is shaped not only by what it is like to raise a child with a disability, but also uniquely what it means to bring the child into the world through pregnancy and birth. This chapter addresses what is known about the experiences of mothers of children with IDD, including those mothers who are primary caregivers and represent single-parent families. Recommendations for professionals working with mothers of children with IDD are offered in consideration of the unique experiences and attributes of this population.

Mothers as Primary Caregivers

Caring for children has traditionally been viewed as the primary responsibility of mothers (Traustadottir, 1991). Previous literature on mothers of children with IDD has reported that they tend to be the main caregivers for their child (Marcenko & Myers, 1991), a traditional role that may continue in various settings even with the blurring of traditional gender roles in modern American culture. Even recent research examining the effects of parenting a child with IDD on primary caregivers uses data that is primarily descriptive of mothers (see Feldman *et al.*, 2007). This role of primary caregiver may be in part due to traditional gender roles, but may also be related to mothers' feelings regarding who is best to care for their child with a disability. In one study, mothers expressed feeling either hesitant or fearful of giving up their role as primary caregiver of their child with IDD, as they perceived themselves to be the most fit to understand and meet the complex and unique needs of the child (Hubert, 2011). While it may sometimes be the case that mothers of children with IDD prefer to be the primary caregivers for their children, some mothers, specifically single mothers, may not have a choice.

Single Mothers

Today's families come in all shapes and sizes, including single-parent households, which represent the environment for around 28% of children in the United States (Vespa, Lewis, & Kreider, 2013). Additionally, less than half of children with IDD reside with both biological parents, with 25% in single mother households, 5% in single father households, and another subset residing in various other households, such as grandparents, foster homes, or residential treatment facilities (Marshak, 2015). Whether single-parent homes are the result of divorce, death, deployment, adoption, or other means, single-parent homes may experience additional complexities compared to those faced by two-parent homes, which can be both a source of difficulty as well as a source of strength for mothers.

Single mothers of children with a disability may be more vulnerable to mental health disorders, including depression, compared to their married counterparts (Olsson & Hwang, 2001). In addition to the psychological adjustments necessary to cope with their child's disability, single mothers may also be required to adjust to divorce, death of a spouse, military deployment, or loneliness that may coincide with going solo while raising a child with IDD. Additionally, single mothers may experience increased isolation, emotional and physical stress, and limited relief from caregiving, which may prevent them from maintaining their mental health (Lloyd & Rosman, 2005). Solo parents may also face additional stressors of dating, limited social support, and increased isolation and potential for burnout (Marshak, 2015).

Single mothers also may face economic hardships. In dual-parent homes, there may be multiple avenues of income, which allows for some mothers to be full-time caretakers for their child. However, in single-parent homes, the responsibility often lies completely on the solo parent to financially provide for the family. Parish, Rose, Swaine, Dababnah, and Mayra (2012) found that single mothers of children with a developmental disability were worse off financially than both married mothers of developmentally disabled children as well as single mothers of typically developing children. Regarding placement in residential care facilities, single, older mothers may be more likely to consider placement, whereas families who possess enough economic resources and stability may be less likely to consider this as an option (Green, 2004). Additionally, single mothers of children with IDD have markedly fewer resources for retirement yet continue their caretaking role, at times leading them to depend entirely on other income such as social security.

Despite the potential challenges faced by single mothers of children with IDD, most still demonstrate resilience. Mothers may facilitate resilience through intentional actions meant to strengthen their relationship with their children and view them as a source of happiness, which leads to increased well-being (Levine, 2009). Themes emerging from research by Levine (2009) included shifting stigma to being a "chosen mother," viewing disability as normal, drawing upon resources both current and possible, and possessing an empowered expert stance regarding their children. Mothers have also demonstrated the ability to reframe their single status to an advantage in being able to make unanimous decisions for their child, having increased opportunities to develop special bonds with their children, and having opportunity to be completely devoted to their well-being (Marshak, 2015).

Caregiver Stress

While normative daily stressors affect all parents, much of the unique stress that mothers of children with IDD experience may be described as caregiving stress (Murphy, Christian, Caplin, & Young, 2007). Caregiving stress may be related not only to everyday stressors of caring for a child with IDD, such as meeting with professionals, coordinating educational needs, and providing basic care, but also to medical and financial concerns, as well as to future planning for the child and family. Mothers of children with IDD have related their stress to a lack of control and worry about the future, while some have regarded the role of continuous advocate as particularly stressful (Murphy, 2007; Ogston, Mackintosh, & Myers, 2011). Aside from emotional experiences, mothers must often dedicate a significant amount of time and money to provide care for a child with IDD, as well as carry the responsibility of helping the individual manage symptoms and build skills to serve him/her later in life (Norton & Drew, 1994). Sometimes, this responsibility may be more burdensome on the caregiver, especially when the child is not able to maintain safety or communicate his/her needs.

Employment Among Mothers of Children with Special Needs

Traditional gender roles have prescribed that women should fulfill their role as caretakers for children and, to a certain extent, have left the task of pursuing full-time careers to men. However, as women have increased their participation in the work force, societal views have grown more accepting of working mothers (Bolzendahl & Myers, 2004). Even in the midst of a changing social climate, the expectation of domestic responsibility may be especially heightened when mothers have a child with IDD, who often need more care and support. Parents of children with IDD specifically face the difficulty of balancing the demands of both parenting and employment (DeRigne & Porterfield, 2010). Working mothers may struggle to find a balance between providing care for their children, including regular and frequent service appointments, extra care needs that childcare providers may be unable to fulfill, and extensive costs that mothers of typically developing children may not experience. Mothers report having to make decisions regarding employment based on an abundance of care demands, lack of flexibility in the workforce, limited social supports, and social pressures that women should sacrifice for the family (Scott, 2010). Mothers whose careers are interrupted may experience emotional distress and frustration for an inability to manage care for their child and their career, leading to isolation and feelings of incompetency and inadequacy, as well as feeling they have lost a part of themselves (Scott, 2010). Furthermore, mothers of children with more severe

IDD may be more likely to report financial problems (Looman, O'Conner-Von, Ferski, & Hildenbrand, 2009), heightening the need for reliable income as well as for support and care from their parents.

Psychological Well-Being and Coping

Traditionally, much of the literature on parenting children with IDD has focused on the effects of stressors on parents, but specifically mothers in primary caretaking roles. Understanding coping and psychological well-being in mothers of children with IDD may provide a window into the effects of having a child with IDD on the parent, as well as highlight avenues toward possible support and intervention to remediate these effects. Seligman and Darling have applied concepts from *systems theory* (von Bertalanffy, 1968) to families with children with IDD, in which the family is "operating as an interactive unit, in which what affects one member affects all members" (Seligman & Darling, 2009, p. 17). Family systems theory provides a lens through which to consider the importance of maternal well-being and coping and their effects on the child and the rest of the family, shifting the focus of intervention and prevention from primarily child-centered efforts to include whole family and/or parent care. Professionals should recognize the importance of maternal well-being, as whole-family wellness begins with the parents. As professionals provide services for mothers of children with various aims to affect family outcomes, understanding psychological well-being in mothers can be considered a first step in providing care toward positive systemic change.

Variations in Coping: Reported Negative Effects on Mothers

How mothers experience the relationship with their child is affected by both the child's diagnosis and the demands of care for the child. These factors have therefore been studied in terms of mother's psychological well-being as a health outcome. Some studies have shown that parent levels of stress and well-being has tended to vary based on the disability of the child (Abbeduto *et al.*, 2004; Stoneman, 2007). Variations in child behavior, level of care needed, certainty and timing of diagnosis, as well as community support may all contribute to differing effects on mothers' psychological well-being (Abbeduto *et al.*, 2004; Horton & Wallander, 2001; Lenhard, Breitenbach, Ebert, Schindelhauer-Deutscher, & Henn, 2005).

Mothers' reactions to the child's IDD diagnosis have the potential to evoke such feelings as denial, anger, fear, disappointment, and self-blame (Bernier, Mao, & Yen, 2010), which can notably impact mothers' well-being. Parents also may experience ambiguous loss which is defined as an incongruence between the psychological and physical family (Boss, 1999, 2002). Particularly upon learning of their child's diagnosis, mothers may experience this ambiguity in which their child is physically present however psychologically distant to varying degrees of the disability's effect on the child's social, emotional, and intellectual development.

When ambiguous loss occurs, mothers may have difficulty making decisions or defining roles and relationship boundaries (Boss & Couden, 2002). Grieving an ambiguous loss of this nature can be unique for mothers, as grief may exist alongside other contrasting emotions, such as joy. In one study, mothers of children with a developmental disability expressed feeling unjustified in their feelings of grief due to their simultaneous love and responsibility to care for their child (Kearney & Griffin, 2001). Mothers may also experience cyclical grief from time to time, especially around milestones (Marshak, 2015). The future trajectory of mothers of children with IDD may be different than previously planned, which may affect mothers' own future goals which are no longer possible with the additional responsibilities and constraints (Marshak, 2015).

Effects of Stigma

Another issue that impacts mothers of children of IDD is the effect of stigma surrounding a disability diagnosis. Although the 1990 Americans with Disabilities Act set the foundation for a shift in attitudes and policy to decrease discriminatory acts against persons with a disability (Scheid, 2005), U.S. culture continues to favor ability over impairment. While individuals living with disability are surely affected by social stigmas, mothers of children with IDD have described the effect of this stressor on their own experiences.

Stigma, whether actual or perceived, can contribute to mothers' depression, feelings of shame, and social isolation (Green, 2003). The effects of stigma tend to be cyclical, as certain negative experiences may crystallize in the memory of mothers and instill more widespread perceptions of stigma. In this way, maternal stress is increased by mothers' perceptions of stigma against their child, which may lead to less interaction with other mothers, and, at times, barring them from peer support (Green, 2003). Mothers of children with IDD who are more severely stigmatized in society also are more likely to consider placing their children in a residential care facility due to feelings of burden or perceived discomfort from others in the community related to interactions with the child, especially children under the age of five (Green, 2004). Just as the experiences of mothers vary by disability, so may the experiences of stigma and discrimination. The child's disability may not be as obvious to others such as children with autism when compared with a child with Down syndrome (DS), which may decrease the amount of stigma experienced. On the other hand, mothers may also experience stigma when their child acts out due to others not realizing it to be a function of the disability, as behavioral indicators of mental illness and other disorders are often stigmatized (Hinshaw, 2005). Since mothers' experiences of stigma may vary depending on the diagnosis and specific behaviors exhibited by the child, varying responses and coping with stigma in mothers of children with IDD is to be expected.

Cultural context also is important to consider in understanding the effects of stigma on mothers. For example, mothers of children with DS in China have described the difficulty of having a child with IDD in relation to the competitive and achievement-focused nature of their culture (Lam & Mackenzie, 2002). Group marginalization or oppression should be considered, as experiences of discrimination based on race or ethnicity may overlap with disability-based discrimination in mothers possessing a minority status. In one study, Mexican-American mothers described experiences of discrimination related to having a child with IDD that intersected with race-related discrimination, such as being treated poorly by service providers because of their race or dealing with stereotypes that their own behaviors, such as drug use, was the likely cause of their child's condition (McHatton & Correa, 2005). For these groups, discrimination and stigma that were already experienced due to minority status may be compounded when a child with IDD becomes a part of the family system.

Because the experiences of mothers of children with IDD vary depending on the child's diagnosis and care requirements, mothers' own levels of stress and support, as well as variables such as stigma and culture, a mother's coping and well-being may vary greatly from person to person. While there has been a significant amount of research that has focused on the negative effects of having a child with IDD, it should not be assumed that these reported negative effects and challenges are the defining components of mothers' personal stories.

Positive Effects on Mothers of Children with IDD

Research tends to focus on the negative effects related to the presence of a child with IDD in the family. This greater presence of negative rather than positive research on impacts and outcomes has been formally recognized, although studies that investigate and highlight positive experiences of parents and families with a child with IDD continue to be sparse (Helf & Glidden, 1998). While extra stressors and unique challenges do exist within this population, it should be noted that mothers also describe rewarding experiences of fulfillment and joy, although these may be less publicized. Some reported positive effects of having a child with IDD on mothers include the personal experience of growth and joy, family benefits, and gaining new meaning and perspective (Springer, McCallum, Pounds, & Nelson Goff, 2011).

Joy, happiness, and personal growth. Various studies have shown that mothers of children with a child with IDD often experience joy and happiness when interacting with and parenting their child (Pillay, Girdler, Collins, & Leonard, 2012; Stainton & Besser, 1998). In a study of parents of children with DS, mothers described that the child's personality itself was a source of joy in daily life (Cless, Cless, Farkas, & Nelson Goff, 2017). In addition to joyful experiences, mothers' personal growth has also been identified as a theme in the literature on the positive effects of parenting (Hastings & Taunt, 2002; Pillay *et al.*, 2012; Springer *et al.*, 2011). Some specific elements of personal growth and transformation have been described as having an increased sense of tolerance and patience, and taking on new roles, such as advocate or a leader of parent groups (Scorgie & Sobsey, 2000).

Another point of joy that mothers describe is the experience of witnessing and celebrating their child's accomplishments and milestones. In a study by Green (2007), the majority of mothers strongly agreed that witnessing their child's accomplishments made all the work and challenges worth it, and reported that they would never trade their child for a child without a disability. Mothers of children with DS have also described how joyous experiences related to parenting a child with an IDD diagnosis, such as being able to celebrate the child's milestones and experiencing the uniqueness of the child's personality, have had a positive effect on their life (Cless *et al.*, 2017). These points of personal growth through the joyous experience of parenting a child with IDD are just a few examples of the various positive effects on mothers.

Relational benefits. The presence of a child with IDD brings with it positive experiences not only for mothers individually, but also in the context of mothers' relationships. An overall sense of increased family unity has been reported by some families with children with IDD (Hastings & Taunt, 2002; Stainton & Besser, 1998). Although some couples with a child with IDD experience relationship strain, many mothers may experience a strengthened relationship with their partner (Risdal & Singer, 2004). Specifically, Scorgie and Sobsey (2000) found that parents of children with IDD described that the hardships they experienced related to times of stress and crisis made their relationship stronger. Mothers may also find that the experience of having a child with IDD promotes acceptance of diversity in their typically developing children (Scorgie & Sobsey, 2000) and that a positive sibling relationship may result from both mutual understanding and acceptance between children (Moyson & Roeyers, 2012). Finally, mothers of children with IDD may find their relationships outside the family transforming, as they engage in new friendships and partnerships in the IDD community and through advocacy activities (Scorgie & Sobsey, 2000). Examining mothers' positive relational contexts may highlight how having a child with IDD can transform women's lives, often for the better (Springer *et al.*, 2011).

Meaning making. The process of meaning making is described in the literature as crucial for mothers of children with IDD. Focusing on positive aspects of parenting a child with IDD may promote optimism, which is a protective factor against stress (Marshak, 2015). Making meaning and finding the benefits in the parent role is associated with adaptive and positive coping (Pakenham, Sofronoff, & Samios, 2004). Furthermore, a parent's perception of the child having a positive impact on his or her life has been found to moderate the relationship between child behavioral problems and parent stress (Blacher & Baker, 2007), highlighting the potential positive impact of a parent's own personal meaning of the child's presence in the family.

Establishing meaning in the role of parenting a child with IDD seems to arise through consideration of positive experiences. Mothers have reported finding meaning through having the opportunity to overcome adversity to sacrifice for the benefit of another (Marshak, 2015). Meaning may come for mothers through spiritual growth (Pillay *et al.*, 2012), and a transformation of perspective, in which mothers reconsider their values, priorities, and appreciate life in new ways (Scorgie & Sobsey, 2000). Whatever way mothers make meaning out of their experience, it should be noted that this process often brings to the forefront the positive aspects of raising a child with IDD, as well as each mothers' unique strengths and qualities.

Principles for Practice

A variety of professionals may interact with mothers of children with IDD, including, but not limited to mental health clinicians, healthcare providers, educational professionals, disability and social service agency staff members, and support group facilitators. Regardless of their role, professionals can help mothers by providing services that are sensitive and understanding in light of mothers' experiences, as outlined in this chapter. In recognition of the role that mothers fill in relation to the child with IDD as well as the family as a whole, professionals should be ready to provide additional supports and resources to mothers within the scope of their practice in order to help families grow together toward their goals.

Working with Mothers in the Primary Caregiver Role

Regardless of the family structure, when mothers are the primary caregivers for their child, the role of support becomes incredibly important. One study found that both single and married mothers reported significantly low levels of help with daily aspects of caregiving, such as household chores or child care (Marcenko & Myers, 1991). Daily life stressors may begin to compound with stressors related to the IDD diagnosis, calling for an increased need for support or respite for mothers. Primary caregivers for children with IDD versus typically developing children may experience more daily stress and higher levels of depression and anxiety (Ones, Yilmaz, Cetinkaya, & Caglar, 2005). As is true for any child, the health and well-being of the child with IDD in the family is affected by the health of their parents. However, mothers who are primary caregivers may experience poorer health than those spending less time providing care (Murphy *et al.*, 2007), leading to additional and unique needs for these mothers.

Recognizing Mothers' Unique Challenges and Strengths

Despite the research literature that aims to compare the experiences of mothers of children with IDD, practitioners should take care to consider each family's strengths and goals to draw upon the abilities present rather than focusing solely on challenges related to the disability. Professionals can help by acknowledging that parenting a child with an IDD diagnosis is not only limited to times of stress and hardship, but also includes times of happiness and wonder, celebrations of milestones, and positive lessons learned. Professionals who also share in these experiences may help mothers to shift the narrative of negative parenting experiences to also include positive elements combined with some challenges and times of stress.

Considering the unique challenges and needs that each family faces can assist professionals in tailoring services according to the needs of the family, rather than the assumed needs of the diagnosis. Since the parent's and child's needs will vary, professionals should get to know the situation of the family in order to gain empathy and to be able to make specialized recommendations. Individualized services may also help mothers gain trust in the professional. In one study, mothers of children with IDD were more likely to trust school personnel when they perceived that the staff member authentically cared for their child's well-being by implementing individualized approaches and demonstrating acceptance of the child, which helped mothers believe that the professionals understood the child's unique characteristics (Angell, Stoner, & Shelden, 2009). Infrequent communication, inadequate follow up, and delayed communication inhibited trust by mothers (Angell *et al.*, 2009).

When working with mothers in this role, professionals should assess for both personal and professional support available to and being utilized by the mother, as well as provide recommendations for additional resources, when necessary. Professionals may wish to frame the use of outside supports in terms of resourcefulness, courage, and strength. By highlighting both mothers' personal unique strengths as well as the strengths and individuality of the child with IDD, mothers may feel more hope and acceptance even amidst times of stress and challenges.

Ameliorating Stress and Stigma

Some mothers of children with IDD may experience stress and challenges that require seeking help or resources from outside professionals. Professionals may benefit from approaching this work from a biopsychosocial perspective, in order to understand mothers' experiences through consideration of biogenetic, somatic, psychological, social, and cultural risk factors (Schotte, Van Den Bossche, De Doncker, Claes, & Cosyns, 2006). Some interventions have been identified to target caregiving stress specifically, or in the context of an IDD diagnosis. One study found that mindfulness training was helpful to mothers in reducing stress and anxiety related to caregiving (Benn, Akiva, Arel, & Roeser, 2012). Other studies have suggested that cognitive behavioral interventions, both individually and in group settings, are helpful for parents of children with IDD (Hastings & Beck, 2004). As research continues to examine and identify interventions aimed at remediation of caregiver stress, professionals should be informed of new and effective practices that may be useful in work with mothers of children with IDD.

The responsibility of combatting stigma is often led by parents of children with IDD, but should be seen as the responsibility of society as a whole. Parents can be helped by understanding that acceptance of a disability is "refusing to be devalued or seen as 'less than' others" (Marshak, 2015, p. 16). Helping professionals should work not only to combat stigma and discrimination in their own lives and practice, but also in communities as well. Practicing inclusion has been described as one way to reduce stigma (Carter, Satcher, & Coelho, 2013), and should become part of the professional's perspective and approach when working with mothers of children with IDD. Modeling inclusion may not only affect positive change within the mother and family system, but also in others who may come into contact with persons with IDD.

Professional organizations also may provide recommendations for working with individuals with IDD and their family members. The American Psychological Association (2016) provides guidelines for assessment and interventions with persons with disabilities. Such resources can help professionals become better informed and aware of the experiences and perspectives of mothers of children with IDD.

Conclusion

This chapter provided an overview of the literature that addresses mothers of children with IDD, as this group is often the focus of much of the research available addressing this population. Mothers of children with IDD may encounter challenges, with single and working mothers often more at-risk for stress than their full-time parent counterparts; however, moments of stress and difficulty do not define this population, as mothers also describe the positive impact that parenting a child with IDD has had on their life. For persons with IDD, recognition that mothers often balance challenging experiences with feelings of joy is important to note as conversations in this field of study shift away from mostly negative to a more positive and balanced framing of what it means to have an IDD diagnosis. Professionals working with mothers should consider utilizing a more rounded and holistic perspective, taking into account both positive and negative experiences that mothers may hold as a part of their story, and respond according to the needs of each unique mother. Finally, policy-makers may wish to consider how mothers' experiences of raising and caring for children with IDD are unique in comparison to mothers of typically developing children, and shape laws and policies according to the needs of a diverse community.

Key Messages from This Chapter

- **For individuals with IDD and their families**: As mothers still often provide primary caregiving for their children with IDD, it is important to more deeply understand the experiences of these mothers, who may encounter both challenges and unique joys. Mothers who must balance caring for their children and employment, as well as single mothers, may find they need extra support in order to best care for themselves as they care for their children.
- **For professionals**: Professionals working with mothers of children with IDD may wish to assess for both positive and negative effects on mothers in order to understand how to assist each mother in her unique needs. Providers should be sensitive to mothers' needs, which may include processing grief or stress and stigma, connecting mothers to support resources, and providing mothers a space to reflect on their specific parenting role.

- **For policy makers**: For those who have the power to influence policy, mothers' experiences of raising children with IDD should be noted. Especially for mothers who are primary caregivers and are either single and/or working parents, relevant policies in the workplace should address the needs of these mothers. Mothers of children with IDD often have expenses that typically developing children may not require, making work even more essential for single-income families. Policies should enable parents to be fully present both in the workplace and for their children.

References

Abbeduto, L., Seltzer, M. M., Shattuck, P., Krauss, M. W., Orsmund, G., & Murphy, M. M. (2004). Psychological well-being and coping in mothers of youths with autism, Down syndrome, or Fragile X syndrome. *American Journal on Mental Retardation, 109*(3), 237–254. doi:10.1352/0895-8017(2004)109%3C237:PWACIM%3E2.0.CO;2

American Psychological Association. (2016). *Guidelines for assessment of and intervention with persons with disabilities.* Retrieved from http://www.apa.org/pi/disability/resources/assessment-disabilities.aspx

Angell, M. E., Stoner, J. B., & Shelden, D. L. (2009). Trust in education professionals: Perspectives of mothers of children with disabilities. *Remedial and Special Education, 30*(3), 160–176. doi:10.1177/0741932508315648

Benn, R., Akiva, T., Arel, S., & Roeser, R. W. (2012). Mindfulness training effects for parents and educators of children with special needs. *Developmental Psychology, 48*(5), 1–12. doi:10.1037/a0027537

Bernier, R., Mao, A., & Yen, J. (2010). Psychopathology, families, and culture: Autism. *Child and Adolescent Psychiatric Clinics of North America, 19*(4), 855–867. doi:10.1016/j.chc.2010.07.005

Blacher, J., & Baker, B. L. (2007). Positive impact of intellectual disability on families. *American Journal on Mental Retardation, 112*(5), 330–348. doi:10.1352/0895-8017(2007)112[0330: PIOIDO]2.0.CO;2

Bolzendahl, C. I., & Myers, D. J. (2004). Feminist attitudes and support for gender equality: Opinion change in women and men, 1974-1998. *Social Forces, 83*(2), 759–789. doi:10.1353sof.2005.0005

Boss, P. (1999). *Ambiguous loss: Learning to live with unresolved grief.* Cambridge, MA: Harvard University Press.

Boss, P. (2002). *Family stress management: A contextual approach.* Thousand Oaks, CA: Sage.

Boss, P., & Couden, B. (2002). Ambiguous loss from chronic physical illness: Clinical interventions with individuals, couples and families. *Journal of Clinical Psychology, 58*(11), 1351–1360. doi:10.1002/jclp.10083

Carter, R., Satcher, D., & Coelho, T. (2013). Addressing stigma through social inclusion. *American Journal of Public Health, 103*(5), 773. doi:10.2105/AJPH.2012.301167

Cless, J. D., Cless, A. W., Farkas, L., & Nelson Goff, B. S. (2017). *Positive and negative experiences of parents of children with Down syndrome.* Manuscript submitted for publication.

DeRigne, L., & Porterfield, S. (2010). Employment change and the role of the medical home for married and single-mother families with children with special health care needs. *Social Science & Medicine*, *70*(4), 631–641. doi:10.1016/j.socscimed.2009.10.054

Feldman, M., McDonald, L., Serbin, L., Stack, D., Secco, M. L., & Yu, C. T. (2007). Predictors of depressive symptoms in primary caregivers of young children with or at risk for developmental delay. *Journal of Intellectual Disability Research*, *51*(8), 606–619. doi:10.1111/j.1365-2788.2006.00941.x

Glidden, L. M., Billings, F. J., & Jobe, B. M. (2006). Personality, coping style and well-being of parents rearing children with developmental disabilities. J*ournal of Intellectual Disability Research*, *50*(12), 949–962. doi:10.1111/j.1365-2788.2006.00929.x

Green, S. E. (2003). "What do you mean 'What's wrong with her?'": Stigma and the lives of families of children with disabilities. *Social Science & Medicine*, *57*, 1361–1374. doi:10.1016/S0277-9536(02)00511-7

Green, S. E. (2004). The impact of stigma on maternal attitudes toward placement of children with disabilities in residential care facilities. *Social Science & Medicine*, *59*, 799–812. doi:10.1016/j.socscimed.2003.11.023

Green, S. E. (2007). "We're tired, not sad": Benefits and burdens of mothering a child with a disability. *Social Science & Medicine*, *64*(1), 150–163. doi:10.1016/j.socscimed.2006.08.025

Hastings, R. P., & Beck, A. (2004). Practitioner review: Stress intervention for parents of children with intellectual disabilities. *Journal of Child Psychology and Psychiatry*, *45*(8), 1338–1349. doi:10.1111/j.1469-7610.2004.00357.x

Hastings, R. P., & Taunt, H. M. (2002). Positive perceptions in families of children with developmental disabilities. *American Journal of Mental Retardation, 107*(2), 116–127. doi:10.1352/0895-8017(2002)107 0116:PPIFOC 2.0.CO;2

Helf, C. M., & Glidden, L. M. (1998). More positive or less negative? Trends in research on adjustment of families rearing children with developmental disabilities. *Mental Retardation*, *36*, 457–464. doi:10.1352/00476765(1998)036%3C0457:MPOLNT%3E2.0.CO;2

Hinshaw, S. P. (2005). The stigmatization of mental illness in children and parents: Developmental issues, family concerns, and research needs. *Journal of Child Psychlology and Psychiatry*, *46*(7), 714–734. doi:10.1111/j.1469-7610.2005.01456.x

Horton, T. V., & Wallander, J. L. (2001). Hope and social support as resilience factors against psychological distress of mothers who care for children with chronic physical conditions. *Rehabilitation Psychology*, *46*(4), 382–399. doi:10.1037//0090-5550.46.4.382

Hubert, J. (2011). "My heart is always where he is". Perspectives of mothers of young people with severe intellectual disabilities and challenging behaviour living at home. *British Journal of Learning Disabilities*, *39*, 216–224. doi:10.1111/j.1468-3156.2010.00658.x

Kearney, P. M., & Griffin, T. (2001). Between joy and sorrow: Being a parent of a child with developmental disability. *Journal of Advanced Nursing*, *34*(5), 582–592. doi:10.1046/j.1365-2648.2001.01787.x

Lam, L., & Mackenzie, A. E. (2002). Coping with a child with Down syndrome: The experiences of mothers in Hong Kong. *Qualitative Health Research*, *12*(2), 223–237. doi:10.1177/104973202129119856

Lenhard, W., Breitenbach, E., Ebert, H., Schidenlhauer-Deutscher, H. J., & Henn, W. (2005). Psychological benefit of diagnostic certainty for mothers of children with disabilities: Lessons from Down syndrome. *American Journal of Medical Genetics, 133A*, 170–175. doi:10.1002/ajmg.a.30571

Levine, K. A. (2009). Against all odds: Resilience in single mothers of children with disabilities. *Social Work in Health Care, 48*, 402–419. doi:10.1080/00981380802605781

Lloyd, C. M., & Rosman, E. (2005). Exploring mental health outcomes for low-income mothers of children with special needs: Implications for policy and practice. *Infants & Young Children, 18*(3) 186–199. doi:10.1097/00001163-200507000-00003

Looman, W. S., O'Conner-Von, S. K., Ferski, G. J., & Hildenbrand, D. A. (2009). Financial and employment problems in families of children with special health care needs: Implications for research and practice. *Journal of Pediatric Health Care, 23*(2), 117–125. doi:10.1016/j.pedhc.2008.03.001

McHatton, P. A., & Correa, V. (2005). Stigma and discrimination: Perspectives from Mexican and Puerto Rican mothers of children with special needs. *Topics in Early Childhood Special Education, 25*(3), 131–142. doi:10.1177/02711214050250030101

Marcenko, M. O., & Myers, J. C. (1991). Mothers of children with developmental disabilities: Who shares the burden? *Family Relations, 40*(2), 186–190. doi:10.2307/585481

Marshak, L. E. (2015). *Going solo while raising children with disabilities*. Bethesda, MD: Woodbine House.

Moyson, T., & Roeyers, H. (2012). 'The overall quality of my life as a sibling is all right, but of course, it could always be better'. Quality of life of siblings of children with intellectual disability: The siblings' perspectives. *Journal of Intellectual Disability Research, 56*(1), 87–101. doi:10.1111/j.1365-2788.2011.01393.x

Murphy, N., Christian, B. J., Caplin, D., & Young, P. (2007). The health of caregivers for children with disabilities: Caregiver perspectives. *Child Health and Development, 33*(2), 180–187. doi:10.1111/j.1365-2214.2006.00644.x

Norton, P., & Drew, C. (1994). Autism and potential family stressors. *American Journal of Family Therapy, 22*(1), 67–76. doi:10.1080/01926189408251298

Ogston, P. L., Mackintosh, V. H., & Myers, B. J. (2011). Hope and worry in mothers of children with an autism spectrum disorder or Down syndrome. *Research in Autism Spectrum Disorders, 5*, 1378–1384. doi:10.1016/j.rasd.2011.01.020

Olsson, M. B., & Hwang, C. P. (2001). Depression in mothers and fathers of children with intellectual disability. *Journal of Intellectual Disability Research, 45*(6), 535–543. doi:10.1046/j.1365-2788.2001.00372.x

Ones, K., Yilmaz, E., Cetinkaya, B., & Caglar, N. (2005). Assessment of the quality of mothers of children with Cerebral palsy (primary caregivers). *Neurorehabilitation & Neural Repair, 19*(3), 232–237. doi:10.1177/1545968305278857

Pakenham, K., Sofronoff, K., & Samios, C. (2004). Finding meaning in parenting a child with Asperger Syndrome: Correlates of sense making and benefit finding. *Research in Developmental Disabilities, 25*(3), 245–264. doi:10.1016/j.ridd.2003.06.003

Parish, S. L., Rose, R. A., Swaine, J. G., Dababnah, S., & Mayra, E. T. (2012). Financial well-being of single, working-age mothers of children with developmental disabilities. *American Journal on Intellectual and Developmental Disabilities, 117*(5), 400–412. doi:10.1352/1944-7558-117.5.400

Pillay, D., Girdler, S., Collins, M., & Leonard, H. (2012). "It's not what you were expecting, but it's still a beautiful journey": The experience of mothers of children with Down syndrome. *Disability & Rehabilitation*, *34*(18), 1501–1510. doi:10.3109/09638288.2011.650313

Risdal, D., & Singer, G. H. (2004). Marital adjustment in parents of children with disabilities: A historical review and meta-analysis. *Research and Practice for Persons with Severe Disabilities*, *29*(2), 95–103. doi:10.2511/rpsd.29.2.95

Scheid, T. L. (2005). Stigma as a barrier to employment: Mental disability and the Americans with disabilities act. *International Journal of Law and Psychiatry*, *28*(6), 670–690. doi:10.1016/j.ijlp.2005.04.003

Schotte, C. K. W., Van Den Bossche, B., De Doncker, D., Claes, S., & Cosyns, P. (2006). A biopsychosocial model as a guide for psychoeducation and treatment of depression. *Depression and Anxiety*, *23*, 312–324. doi:10.1002/da.20177

Scorgie, K., & Sobsey, D. (2000). Transformational outcomes associated with parenting children who have disabilities. *Mental Retardation, 38*(3), 195–206. doi:10.1352/0047-6765(2000)038Z 0195:TOAWPC 2.0.CO;2

Scott, E. K. (2010). "I feel as if I am the one who is disabled": The emotional impact of changed employment trajectories of mothers caring for children with disabilities. *Gender & Society*, *24*(5), 672–696. doi:10.1177/0891243210382531

Seligman, M., & Darling, R. B. (2009). *Ordinary families, special children: A systems approach to childhood disability.* New York, NY: Guilford.

Springer, N., McCallum, S., Pounds, M., & Nelson Goff, B. (2011, March). *Resilience and hope: Embracing life with Down syndrome.* Poster presented at the Texas Association of Marriage and Family Therapy Annual Conference, San Antonio, TX.

Stainton, T., & Besser, H. (1998). The positive impact of children with an intellectual disability on the family. *Journal of Intellectual & Developmental Disability*, *23*(1), 57–70. doi:10.1080/13668259800033581

Stoneman, Z. (2007). Examining the Down syndrome advantage: Mothers and fathers of young children with disabilities. *Journal of Intellectual Disability Research*, *51*(12), 1006–1017. doi:10.1111/j.1365-2788.2007.01012.x

Traustadottir, R. (1991). Mothers who care: Gender, disability, and family life. *Journal of Family Issues*, *12*, 211–228. doi:10.1177/019251391012002005

Vespa, J., Lewis, J. M., & Kreider, R. M. (2013). America's families and living arrangements: 2012. *Current Population Characteristics, 20*, 570–604. Retrieved from https://www.census.gov/prod/2013pubs/p20-570.pdf

von Bertalanffy, L. (1968). *General system theory: Developments, foundations, applications.* New York, NY: George Braziller.

7 Perspectives from Fathers

Recognizing Their Strengths and Contributions beyond Breadwinning

Gail E. Bentley, PhD, Matthew D. Brown, PhD, and Jason B. Whiting, PhD

Introduction

Two of the most influential people in everyone's lives are their parents. This chapter will summarize the current literature on fathers of children with disabilities. Fathers often experience life with disability from the periphery, which may be by choice, but often fathers have a critical perspective that is overlooked in the research and by professionals. The chapter reviews available research from two studies that specifically included fathers of children with Down syndrome (DS) and autism spectrum disorder (ASD). The chapter provides information for professionals on working to ensure fathers are included as important contributors to the family system.

Fathering

Although fathers may be a major part of most people's narratives regarding their development, for the last 100 years, research and theories of child development have focused more on the mother-child relationship. In the latter half of the twentieth century, there were calls for research including the contributions of fathers and their role in their child's development. As systemic research has developed, it has become easier, and indeed necessary, to acknowledge the father role in the context of child development (Fitzgerald & Bradley, 2012; Fitzgerald, Mann, & Barratt, 1999; Lamb, 1975, 1987). Fathers who are willing and able to choose paternal involvement contribute to a more positive family environment. Involved fathers who feel good about their family relationships contribute to a family context that is supportive of positive developmental outcomes for children (Hodapp, 2007; Lamb, 1987).

Modern society has increased the expectations of father involvement, yet fathers often have traditional concepts of their role. The constraints of work, especially for those in low paying jobs, prevent many fathers from feeling as if they can spend time with their families (Harrison, Henderson, & Leonard, 2007). In addition, many fathers lack confidence in their capacity to care for their child (Zvara, Schoppe-Sullivan, & Dush, 2013). This is an unfortunate scenario, as fathers make a unique and important contribution to their families and their children's well-being. Studies have shown that school-aged children with involved fathers tend to have higher grades, improved emotional development, and lower risk-taking behaviors (Allen & Daly, 2007; Bronte-Tinkew, Moore, & Carrano, 2006; Rosenberg & Wilcox, 2006). They also have higher levels of cognitive competence, greater empathy, a stronger internal locus of control, and less stereotypical concepts of gender roles.

Fathering and IDD

The special needs of a child can be a primary influence on the context of fathering. Although it is known that the acceptance, or rejection, of a child with special needs by their father is impactful, there is limited information about fathers of children with special needs or IDD (Brotherson & Dollahite, 1997; Hodapp, 2007; Hornby, 1994). Father involvement and emotional availability with children who have special needs often is similar to father involvement with typically developing children (de Falco, Venuti, Esposito, & Bornstein, 2009; Fenning, Baker, Baker, & Crnic, 2014).

Although still limited, research on fathers may be helpful to parents of children with IDD, as well as the professionals working with this population. This chapter will explore some of the specific factors research has found, related to fathers, which can contribute to positive adjustment and resilience in their families. Two recent studies have identified some of the positive influence of fathers in families with a child with IDD. Brown (2012) looked at how couples cope when they have a child with ASD and the role of the marital relationship as a primary source of parenting support. Bentley, Zvonkovic, McCarty, and Springer (2015) took a non-deficit approach to examining the hope and satisfaction factors for fathers of a child with Down syndrome (DS). The samples for both studies were limited in their generalizability, as they used small samples of well-educated men, yet they provide some insight that can be valuable to practitioners. Still, fathers of children with IDD have unique concerns, including feelings of self-blame, denial, guilt, and uncertainty about the future. Fathers also report concerns about their marriage and the constant strain of caregiving (Bentley *et al.*, 2015; Hornby, 1992). Current research suggests that fathers address these issues in different ways than mothers, which will be described next.

Recent Research Parameters

Ambiguous Loss

The theory of ambiguous loss (Boss, 1999, 2006) addresses situations of loss that are neither typical nor clear. For example, when a loved one dies, the loss is grieved in culturally sanctioned ways. However, when a loved one is missing, or affected by a disability, there is a loss, but it can be difficult to know how to feel or deal with it. The cultural parameters do not exist for a grieving process. Parents of a child with IDD face unique circumstances in that they have a child with challenges, and it is not the path they expected. For example, fathers of children with IDD report guilt about having negative feelings about their child, and the restrictions on their family life. They sometimes cope by being in denial about the extent of their child's disability (Hornby, 1992). Yet, most of them move forward with their life and family (Bentley *et al.*, 2015; Brown, 2012). It does not mean they forget or abandon the child they thought they would have; instead, they focus on the child that is born to them. Still, the unknown about the level of functioning their child will have, as well as the changes that will occur in the daily life of their family, are now ambiguous. An ambiguous loss denies closure and can be both painful and ongoing (Boss, 1999).

In a study of parents of children with ASD, one mother illustrated this when asked about coping with autism: "You have in your mind the type of parent you want to be when you're expecting a child, but you don't think that your child won't be typical when you envision those things for your relationship. Now it feels like everyone else gets to enjoy normal joys and challenges and we don't" (Brown, 2012, p. 109). A father in the same study said: "I feel like I am on pins and needles with daycares and school because he is frequently expelled" (p. 109).

In a study of fathers of children with DS, three different ways of managing this ambiguous loss were identified (Bentley, 2011; Bentley *et al.*, 2015): *mastering*, *connecting*, and *thriving*. The *mastering* group expressed what is identified as a *mastery mindset*, which is a point of view that hard work will bring the reward of a positive conclusion (Boss, 1999, 2006). This acceptance, often with resignation, is seen in this father's comment:

> Although I wouldn't change any decision I've made, and I love him as much as a parent loves any child, there are days where I hate that he has Down syndrome, that he has to struggle every day, that he didn't get the same chances that most kids get. That his future is extremely challenging, and I feel pretty helpless, because there's little I can do to change it. I love how he's 13 but still just a child, but I'm also saddened because he'll never be a "normal" teenager or adult. He'll always be a little kid … I wonder sometimes how different our lives would be if he was healthy. I had a much more positive attitude for years, but I'm feeling a lot older and tired. It wears on you, the daily struggle.
>
> (Bentley, 2011, p. 66)

For the *connecting* group, the sense of ambiguous loss was evident as they expressed a certain mourning for the life they expected, but would not have. Along with family and friends, they attempted to determine how to cope with this new, unexpected life experience, as the following quote describes:

> My wife was in shock and then in depression for some time [upon learning their child's diagnosis]. I, on the other hand, went into anger and denial for a short period of time. When we were first married, we were having trouble getting pregnant and carrying the baby to full term. So, we began to think about adoption … However, once we had our first child, I had pushed that

> to the back of my head. So, when we had the second child, your hopes and dreams take a beating at first, until you realize all will be ok. For my wife, people were sending condolence cards instead of congratulations and that paired with post-partum depression really took its toll.
>
> (Bentley, 2011, p. 71)

The fathers in the *thriving* group embraced the ambiguity of their new life, which led these fathers to find importance simply in the experience of fathering. Boss (1999, 2007) described this type of behavior as meaning making, and one father summed up the reaction of this group by referencing the essay "Welcome to Holland" (Kingsley, 1987):

> You make all these plans and dreams for a lifetime trip to Italy. On the way, your plane is rerouted to Holland. Now you can spend a lifetime complaining about how you were rerouted and didn't get to see Italy ... or you can make the effort to open your eyes and see the wonderful things about Holland.
>
> (Bentley, 2011, p. 74)

Satisfaction and the Couple Relationship

Hornby (1992) identified a list of key issues experienced by fathers of children with disabilities that included the strains of caregiving, negative experiences of service provision, and negative reactions from the community. Similarly, Harrison and colleagues (2007) described common barriers that fathers report, including feelings of exclusion and conflicting demands. Satisfaction is a personal evaluation of quality of life that would take all of those concerns into account (Diener, Emmons, Larsen, & Griffin, 1985). Studies of marital satisfaction have led to a better understanding of how couples respond to challenges and the ways that response can lead to resilience (Bradbury, Fincham & Beach, 2000). Despite many life stressors, parents of children with special needs report that they are satisfied with their life, they see their lives as both challenging and satisfying (Asberg, Vogel, & Bowers, 2007; Bentley *et al.*, 2015; Brown, 2012). Studies provide support for the conclusion that addressing marital satisfaction can increase parental satisfaction and decrease levels of parenting stress.

The context in which fathers influence the family and the ways fathers engage with their children also influences their experiences as fathers. The couple relationship contributes to children's well-being by providing a foundation that provides social, emotional, and economic support in which children can grow and develop (Amato, 1998; Brotherson & Dollahite, 1997; Doherty, 1997; Hawkins & Palkovitz, 1999). Hornby (1992) found that the effect on marriage was a key issue for fathers of children with IDD. When parents of children with disabilities perceive that the burden of parenting is shared, they report higher parenting satisfaction (Adbo & Fischer, 2003). Likewise, when there is a discrepancy between actual and expected levels of spouse or partner support, parenting quality suffers

(Bristol, Gallagher, & Schopler, 1988). Parents of children with ASD also report lower relationship satisfaction than parents of neurotypical children (Brobst, Clopton, & Hendrick, 2009; Brown, 2012). Hornby (1994) found that marital satisfaction was not significantly different in groups with and without children with DS. Fathers of children with DS reported high levels of hope and satisfaction about their marriages and about life in general (Bentley *et al.*, 2015). Thus, the quality of the couple's relationship, and the support of fathers' involvement by mothers, may influence both father involvement and fathering activities (Fox, Nordquist, Billen, & Savoca, 2015).

Brown (2012) found that the couple relationship and positive coping strategies were resources in alleviating parenting stress in parents of children with ASD. The study also found that fathers reported lower parenting stress than mothers, while the mothers in the study described parenting as a growth experience more often than the fathers. Still, it was fathers who expressed that the experience of parenting had brought the couple closer together (Brown, 2012). In the Bentley *et al.* (2015) study, all three groups of fathers of children with DS identified levels of satisfaction with their marriage that were above average levels. Overall, an increase in relationship satisfaction is connected to a decrease in parenting stress (Brown, 2012; Floyd & Zmich, 1991). Marital quality may also affect a father's level of involvement with his children, as marital satisfaction has been related to better coping (Bentley *et al.*, 2015; Bowman, 1990; Brown, 2012; Cowan & Cowan, 2000; Mehall, Spinrad, Eisenberg, & Gaertner, 2009).

Stress and Coping

Raising a child with IDD brings a variety of challenges related to development, medical needs, social interactions, and education. Thus, locating resources to address those needs are common stressors articulated by parents (Flaherty & Masters Glidden, 2000; Glidden, Billings, & Jobe, 2006). Planned, positive strategies for coping lead to a greater sense of mastery and more positive outcomes. The types of coping strategies activated often reflect available resources (Folkman & Lazarus, 1988; Minnes, Graffi, Nolte, Carlson, & Harrick, 2000). Activation of social support networks, reframing, and meaning making are strategies that help families adapt to these stressors (McCubbin & Thompson, 1991; Twoy, Connolly, & Novak, 2007).

Bentley *et al.* (2015) found three different types of coping behaviors in their sample of fathers. The mastery group coped by attempting to gain control of situations:

> We both expect him to behave and contribute to our family. We want him to achieve as much academic success as possible. We want him to communicate better, so we can truly understand his cognitive level.
>
> (p. 71)

The difficulty with their mastery mindset is that hard work does not always change the outcome, and it may reduce the resilience for this group of fathers. In comparison, the connecting group of fathers focused on using engagement strategies for coping. Boss (1999) described this tactic as an inability to control the ambiguity, with a willingness to take responsibility for daily life. Connecting fathers shared examples of reframing, a strategy used to put difficulties in a more positive perspective (McCubbin & Thompson, 1991), describing their involvement in community organizations that provided support for families of individuals with IDD:

> The biggest impact for me personally has been a "resetting" of my life priorities. I was a career-focused person prior to [my son] being born, always looking at what job is next and in what location. Having him as part of my life shifted my focus and provided a greater balance between my home and work life. I no longer focus, as much, on what my title is at work or what job I am in next. I see my job as a means to an end. A necessity to support my family and their needs. This shift in focus has allowed me to get involved in the DS community in our area and see all of the opportunities that still need to be opened up to my son and others with disabilities. It is these things where I want to spend my energy and time. All of this has given me a much different perspective on life … and provided a passion that I lacked prior to having [my son].
>
> (p. 67)

Finally, the thriving group demonstrated harmony with their life. The level of personal acceptance is seen in one father's response when asked about his attitude toward his son's diagnosis: "What's your attitude about your son having brown eyes?" Statements from the thriving group indicated that they used reframing, or meaning making, as a coping skill, as demonstrated by the following quote:

> We are very fortunate to have a well-adjusted, fun, inquisitive stubborn fourth grader who happens to have Down syndrome. Can she be difficult? Yes. Can she be obnoxious? Yes. Can she be disruptive? Yes, but so can our other two children. I would say that [my daughter] more often displays these negative behaviors but she is also much more caring, sympathetic and responsive to the needs of others. You have to take the good with the bad and in our case, [my daughter] has much more good than bad.
>
> (p. 69)

This ability to create meaning in the midst of ambiguity illustrates positive coping strategies and behaviors, which lead to resilience and strength (Boss, 1999, 2013). These studies demonstrate how the special needs context influenced these fathers as they chose their responses to their responsibilities as parents. That context appears to influence how parents developed the relationships in their lives, both within and outside of their families, as one of the fathers in the Brown study stated:

> It has helped me to grow more as an individual. I am constantly trying to be a better father and be more patient … If anything, I am a better person because of my child with ASD.
>
> (p. 116)

Principles for Practice

Ambiguous loss theory (Boss, 1999, 2006) provides an approach for identifying both the unexpected pleasures, as well as the challenges often found in raising a child with IDD. It also provides some therapeutic implications for those working with this population of fathers. For many professionals working with families of individuals with IDD, there may be a gap in their understanding of how to engage fathers in services. Fletcher (2008) called for using multicultural training when interacting with fathers and to be sensitive to fathers' expectations. Fathers' needs and concerns are often different from those of mothers. Fathers' concerns focus more on the big picture for their family, financial needs, as well as characteristics that may contribute to their child being excluded from society (Hodapp, 2007). Most family services are provided by female professionals and often geared toward mothers. To reach fathers effectively, some programs have hired more men and have sought different avenues to engage father's participation, particularly in recognizing the unique contributions fathers bring to parenting.

Recognizing Fathers' Unique Challenges and Strengths

Research has shown that fathers may process their child's diagnosis of a disability differently than mothers. Hobart (2008) found that parents identified four stages of reaction to a diagnosis: shock (numbness, disbelief, or denial), recoil (anger, confusion, blaming, guilt, and bargaining), depression/anxiety, and reorganization (acceptance and recovery). Fathers reported moving more slowly through these steps, particularly the shock stage. This could perhaps be due to the general lack of information and interaction with helping professionals as reported by fathers. Perhaps a better understanding of the responses of fathers to the birth of their child with IDD can assist professionals in adjusting their interactions.

Clinicians and helping professionals should create more parity in their interactions with fathers and mothers. This process can begin in the hospital. For instance, with the support of perinatal nurses, fathers can develop competence and thus subsequent confidence in caring for their newborn child. It is important for healthcare professionals to be aware of their own stereotypes of fathers, as they are in a unique position to support fathers in developing nurturing behaviors that will influence their relationship with their child.

Fathers tend to connect or bond differently with their children than mothers. Mothers have been shown to prefer quiet activities to promote emotional bonds, fathers favor exciting activities that generally involve physical play, risk taking, and exploration (Paquette, 2004; Yogman, 1994). Similarly, while the mother-child attachment relationship serves to calm the child, the father-child activation relationship (Paquette, 2004) serves the child's need to be stimulated. When IDD creates situations where these types of bonding activities are inhibited, fathers may be less likely to develop those bonds or more cautious about how to interact with their child with IDD. This can perpetuate the cycle of the mother being more aligned with their child and providing the primary caregiving responsibilities, which may disconnect the father from developing his parenting skills or accessing professional resources.

It is important for professionals to help parents understand the unique contributions and challenges fathers experience in bonding with their child with IDD. Education regarding the positive child outcomes associated with strong father-child bonds may help parents shift out of patterns that could diminish this relationship. Professionals should encourage fathers to take an active role in parenting and find creative ways to play with their children. Helping normalize some of the concerns that mothers may express regarding the limitations the child may have (e.g., the child may be medically fragile or easily overwhelmed), while promoting fathers' pursuit of new ways to connect could also facilitate flexibility in father involvement. It is important for professionals to be careful not to replicate patterns of stepping in and correcting fathers in these interactions, but encouraging and reinforcing their attempts to connect and assume a more active role in parenting.

Support Within the Couple or Co-Parenting Relationship

Due to the nature of caring for children with IDD, parents may adopt a "divide and conquer" strategy, and sadly, in some cases, never strike that balance and end up completely divided (Marshak & Prezant, 2007). A functional division of labor can serve an important role in relieving stress and providing support; however, parents may find themselves with an arrangement that further promotes fathers being distant from the resources they need to be more directly involved with their children (Seligman & Darling, 2007) and mothers may fall into micromanaging the relationship between fathers and children (Zvara *et al.*, 2013). Many researchers have only included mothers in research on children with IDD, asking them to report on the well-being and functioning of other family members (Hornby, 1994), which perpetuates the potentially problematic pattern of mothers absorbing the stress of the family (Seligman & Darling, 2007). Mothers may also be experiencing the dual stress of being a caregiver and intervention provider (Tehee, Honan, & Hevey, 2009).

Fathers sometimes emotionally detach or become neutral toward their child as a way of coping and they also report that they are hesitant to share their concerns when mothers are present (Kersh, Hedvat, Hauser-Cram, & Warfield, 2006; King & Coleman, 2007; Krauss, 1993). Perhaps as a result, they also report having no one to confide in. In addition to helping parents utilize their couple relationship as a resource for stress-related coping, it is important for professionals to help improve communication and support, which can strengthen the couple relationship or partnership as co-parents.

Fathers should be encouraged to understand the impact that their involvement in parenting has on their couple relationship. Engaging fathers in the responsibilities of caregiving may help reduce stress for mothers, while also increasing the quality of the couple relationship (Ireland, Sanders, & Markie-Dodds, 2003). King and Coleman (2007) found that fathers reported feeling both powerless to "fix" their child's disability and, therefore, useless in their contributions. Due to the tendency fathers may have to disengage when they see little chance of success (e.g., emotional distancing when bonding with their child seems difficult), helping fathers see that their involvement can lead to positive outcomes both for the child and their spouse/partner may increase engagement. Research suggests that couples who work together to address the stressors they face, and use their relationship as a resource, adapt better to stressors (Adbo & Fischer, 2003). Consequently, professionals working with this population should consider the health, strength, and satisfaction of the couple relationship in their interventions, as this may be the most meaningful resource for fathers (Bentley *et al.*, 2015; Brown, 2012). Ensuring that fathers are included as contributors to the family system is an important task for all professionals working with individuals with IDD and their families.

Areas of Specific Social Support and Coping for Fathers

While fathers of children with DS in the Bentley *et al.* (2015) study all scored above the mean on the measure of coping strategies, each group demonstrated different coping behaviors. Understanding these existing coping styles may provide practitioners deeper insight on ways to reach fathers more effectively. Fathers of children with DS all scored above the mean on the coping scale (Bentley *et al.*, 2015). Yet, each group demonstrated different coping behaviors. Understanding these existing coping styles may provide practitioners deeper insight with regards to ways to reach fathers more effectively.

Some of the common barriers to services and programs for fathers include a loss of previous friends and confidants with whom to share their feelings and concerns about their children, their family, and themselves (Harrison *et al.*, 2007). The concept of *universality* (i.e., a common experience shared by a group of people) can help fathers who may be isolated not only from their child's services, but also from other adults who are experiencing the same situation and challenges. Normalizing their experience could increase their involvement in their children's lives (Beatty & King, 2008; Bentley *et al.*, 2015; Harrison *et al.*, 2007).

There are a number of specialized programs for fathers that address these issues in father-friendly ways. For example, a program entitled *Hey, Dad! For Fathers Who Have a Child with a Disability* (Beatty & King, 2008; King & Coleman, 2007), implements sessions that focus on many of the concerns addressed in this chapter. This program, from the Fatherhood Institute in the United Kingdom, as well as the Australian Department of Social Services, provides a wealth of detailed information related to reaching fathers with services (Fatherhood Institute, 2007). In the Down syndrome area, Dads Appreciating Down Syndrome (DADS, 2014) is a fathering initiative with chapters in the United States, Canada, Australia, and United Kingdom. Fathers often seek information to deal with their circumstances and may engage with organizations that provide information and support (Bentley *et al.*, 2015). Developing father-friendly programs available through IDD organizations is likely to be appreciated by fathers, resulting in more engaged, active, and confident fathers.

Conclusion

This chapter provided an overview of the available literature on fathers of children with IDD. Although the current research literature that specifically focuses on fathers or targets fathers as direct participants is limited, the increasing attention and move toward fathers becoming more engaged and involved in their families is also important in families with a child with IDD. Fathers play an important role in the development of their children and they should be viewed as providing important contributions to their family system. When facing an IDD diagnosis, parents may respond differently to the information, as their knowledge, stress, responsibilities, coping strategies, and resources may vary. In the past, fathers were often viewed as peripheral or disengaged from their families, including those with children with IDD. Fathers may have felt unappreciated or misunderstood by professionals, who may have felt challenged or defensive when fathers attempted to participate in services for their child's care.

We hope that the information in this chapter will be useful for families and professionals. Two of the authors (MDB and JBW) are fathers of children with special needs, so we have an investment in improving the lives of children with IDD. We hope that the information and principles for practice in this chapter will help professionals value father involvement and take steps to encourage and support their inclusion and to engage with their child with IDD.

Key Messages from This Chapter

- **For individuals with IDD and their families**: Raising a child with IDD has its challenges, but it is also a satisfying experience. Fathers are valuable contributors, beyond their typical financial role, and the relationship between mothers and fathers is important for fathering but also in helping to create a balance in caregiving demands.
- **For professionals**: Fathers respond to their child's diagnosis in unique ways, coping styles can vary from mastery-oriented efforts to community engagement to meaning making. Professionals should invite and reinforce father involvement in parenting their child with IDD.
- **For policy makers**: Paternity/medical/sick leave for fathers should be available to support early bonding and increased caregiving involvement, and employers can be supportive by allowing for flexible work schedules. Father-focused programs need to collect program effectiveness data to better inform future programming efforts.

References

Adbo, A., & Fischer, J. M. (2003). Factors relevant to parental alliance for parents of children with disabilities. *Journal of Applied Rehabilitation Counseling*, *34*(3), 10–15.

Allen, S., & Daly, K. (2007). *The effects of father involvement: An updated research summary of the evidence inventory*. Guelph, Ontario, Canada: Centre for Families, Work & Well-Being, University of Guelph. Retrieved from http://www.fira.ca/cms/documents/29/Effec

Amato, P. R. (1998). More than money? Men's contributions to their children's lives. In A. Booth, & A. C. Crouter (Eds.), *Men in families: When do they get involved? What difference does it make?* (pp. 241–278). Mahwah, NJ: Lawrence Erlbaum.

Asberg, K. K., Vogel, J. J., & Bowers, C. A. (2007). Exploring correlates and predictors of stress in parents of children who are deaf: Implications of perceived social support and mode of communication. *Journal of Child and Family Studies, 17*, 486–499. doi:10.1007/s10826-007-9169-7

Beatty, D., & King, A. (2008). Supporting fathers who have a child with a disability: The development of a new parenting program. *Groupwork, 18*(3), 69–87. doi:10.1921/gpwk.v18i3.659

Bentley, G. E. (2011). *The up side of Down syndrome and fathering: An exploration of hope, satisfaction, and coping.* (Unpublished doctoral dissertation). Texas Tech University, Lubbock, TX.

Bentley, G. E., Zvonkovic, A. M., McCarty, M., & Springer, N. (2015). Down syndrome and fathering: An exploration of ambiguous loss. *Fathering, 13*(1), 1–17. doi:10.3149/fth.1301.1

Boss, P. (1999). *Ambiguous loss: Learning to live with unresolved grief.* Cambridge, MA: Harvard Press.

Boss, P. (2006). *Loss, trauma, and resilience: Therapeutic work with ambiguous loss.* New York, NY: W. W. Norton.

Boss, P. (2007). Ambiguous loss theory: Challenges for scholars and practitioners. *Family Relations, 56*(2), 105–111. doi:10.1111/j.1741-3729.2007.00444.x

Boss, P. (2013, November). *Myth of closure: What is normal grief after loss, clear or ambiguous?* Paper presented at the annual conference of the National Council on Family Relations, San Antonio, TX.

Bowman, M. L. (1990). Coping efforts and marital satisfaction: Measuring marital coping and its correlates. *Journal of Marriage and the Family, 52*(2), 463–474. doi:10.2307/353040

Bradbury, T. N., Fincham, F. D., & Beach, S. R. H. (2000). Research on the nature and determinants of marital satisfaction: A decade in review. *Journal of Marriage and Family Therapy, 62*(4), 964–980. doi:10.1111/j.1741-3737.2000.00964.x

Bristol, M. M., Gallagher, J. J., & Schopler, E. (1988). Mothers and fathers of young developmentally disabled and nondisabled boys: Adaptation and spousal support. *Developmental Psychology, 24*, 441–451. doi:10.1037/0012-1649.24.3.441

Brobst, J. B., Clopton, J. R., & Hendrick, S. S. (2009). Parenting children with autism spectrum disorders: The couple's relationship. *Focus on Autism and Other Developmental Disabilities, 24*(1), 38–49. doi:10.1177/1088357608323699

Bronte-Tinkew, J., Moore, K. A., & Carrano, J. (2006). The father-child relationship, parenting styles, and adolescent risk behaviors in intact families. *Journal of Family Issues, 27*(6), 850–881. doi:10.1177/0192513x05285296

Brotherson, S. E., & Dollahite, D. C. (1997). Generative ingenuity in father work with young children with special needs. In A. J. Hawkins & D. C. Dollahite (Eds.), *Generative fathering: Beyond deficit perspectives* (pp. 89–104). Thousand Oaks, CA: Sage.

Brown, M. (2012). *Dyadic coping, relationship satisfaction, and parenting stress among parents of children with an autism spectrum disorder: The role of couple relationship.* (Unpublished doctoral dissertation). Texas Tech University, Lubbock, TX.

Cowan, C. P., & Cowan, P A. (2000). *When partners become parents: The big life change for couples.* Mahwah, NJ: Lawrence Erlbaum.

Dads Appreciating Down Syndrome. (2014). *About us.* Retrieved from www.Dadsnational.org

de Falco, S., Venuti, P., Esposito, G., & Bornstein, M. H. (2009). Mother-child and father-child emotional availability in families of children with Down syndrome. *Parenting: Science and Practice, 9*(3–4), 198–215. doi:10.1080/15295190902844381

Diener, E., Emmons, R.A., Larsen, R.J., & Griffin, S. (1985). The Satisfaction with Life Scale. *Journal of Personality Assessment, 49*(1), 71–75. doi:10.1207/s15327752jpa4901_13

Doherty, W. J. (1997). The best of times and the worst of times: Fathering as a contested arena of academic discourse. In A. J. Hawkins & D. C. Dollahite (Eds.), *Generative fathering: Beyond deficit perspectives* (pp. 217–227). Thousand Oaks, CA: Sage.

Fatherhood Institute. (2007). *Hey, dad! For fathers who have a child with a disability.* Retrieved from www.fatherhoodinstitute.org/2007/hey-dad-for-fathers-of-children-with-disabilities/

Fenning, R. M., Baker, J. K., Baker, B. L., & Crnic, K. A. (2014). Parent-child interaction over time in families of young children with borderline intellectual functioning. *Journal of Family Psychology, 28*, 326–335. doi:10.1037/a0036537

Fitzgerald, H. E., & Bradley, R. (2012). Paternal family relationships, child risk, and child outcomes. *Family Science, 3*(3–4), 141–144. doi:10.1080/19424620.2012.779421

Fitzgerald, H. E., Mann, T., & Barratt, M. (1999). Fathers and infants. *Infant Mental Health Journal, 20*(3), 213–221. doi:10.1002/(SICI)1097-0355(199923)20:3 213::AID-IMHJ1 3.0.CO;2-G

Flaherty, E., & Masters Glidden, L. (2000). Positive adjustment in parents rearing children with Down syndrome. *Early Education and Development, 11*(4), 407–422. doi:10.1207/s15566935eed1104_3

Fletcher, R. (2008). *Father-inclusive practice and associated professional competencies.* Melbourne, Australia: Australian Institute of Family Studies.

Floyd, F. J., & Zmich, D. E. (1991). Marriage and the parenting partnership: Perceptions and interactions of parents with mentally retarded and typically developing children. *Child Development, 62*(6), 1434–1448. doi:10.2307/1130817

Folkman, S., & Lazarus, R. (1988). Coping as a mediator of emotion. *Journal of Personality and Social Psychology, 54*(3), 466–475. doi:10.1037/0022-3514.54.3.466

Fox, G. L., Nordquist, V. M., Billen, R. M., & Savoca, E. F. (2015). Father involvement and early intervention: Effects of empowerment and father role identity. *Family Relations, 64*(4), 461–475. doi:10.1111/fare.12156

Glidden, L. M., Billings, F. J., & Jobe, B. M. (2006). Personality, coping style and well-being of parents rearing children with developmental disabilities. *Journal of Intellectual Disability Research, 50*(12), 949–962. doi:10.1111/j.1365-2788.2006.00929.x

Harrison, J., Henderson, M., & Leonard, R. (2007). *Different dads: Fathers' stories of parenting disabled children.* London, UK: Jessica Kingsley.

Hawkins, A. J., & Palkovitz, R. (1999). Beyond ticks and clicks: The need for more diverse and broader conceptualizations and measures of father involvement. *The Journal of Men's Studies, 8*(1), 11–32. doi:10.3149/jms.0801.11

Hobart, H. M. (2008). Autism and family in the People's Republic of China: Learning from parents' perspectives. *Research and Practice for Persons with Severe Disabilities, 33*(1/2), 37–47. doi:10.2511/rpsd.33.1-2.37

Hodapp, R. M. (2007). Families with persons with Down syndrome: New perspectives and findings, and research and service needs. *Mental Retardation and Developmental Disabilities Research and Reviews*, *13*, 279–287. doi:10.1002/mrdd

Hornby, G. (1992). A review of fathers' accounts of their experiences of parenting children with disabilities. *Disability, Handicap & Society*, *7*(4), 363–374. doi:10.1080/02674649266780431

Hornby, G. (1994). Effects of children with disabilities on fathers: A review and analysis of the literature. *International Journal of Disability, Development and Education*, *41*(3), 171–184. doi:10.1080/0156655940410302

Ireland, J. L., Sanders, M. R., & Markie-Dodds, C. (2003). The impact of parent training on marital functioning: A comparison of two group versions of the Triple-P Positive Parenting Program for parents of children with early-onset conduct problems. *Behavioural and Cognitive Psychotherapy*, *31*, 127–142. doi:10.1017/S1352465803002017

Kersh, J., Hedvat, T. T., Hauser-Cram, P., & Warfield, M. E. (2006). The contribution of marital quality to the well-being of parents of children with developmental disabilities. *Journal of Intellectual Disability Research*, *50*, 883–893. doi:10.1111/j.1365-2788.2006.00906.x

King, A., & Coleman, A. (2007). *Hey, dad! For fathers who have a child with a disability. A parenting program for men*. Sydney, Australia: UnitingCare Burnside and Centacare Broken Bay. Retrieved from http://trove.nla.gov.au/work/34782123?q&versionId=43105527

Kingsley, E. P. (1987). *Welcome to Holland*. Retrieved from http://firefliesofhope.typepad.com

Krauss, M. W. (1993). Child-related and parenting stress: Similarities and differences between mothers and fathers of children with disabilities. *American Journal of Mental Retardation*, *97*, 393–404. Retrieved from http://psycnet.apa.org/psycinfo/1993-21637-001

Lamb, M. E. (1975). Fathers: Forgotten contributors to child development. *Human Development*, *18*, 245–266. doi:10.1159/000271493

Lamb, M. E. (Ed.) (1987). *The father's role: Cross-cultural perspectives*. Hillsdale, NJ: Lawrence Erlbaum.

McCubbin, H. I., & Thompson, A. I. (Eds.) (1991). *Family assessment inventories for research and practice*. Madison, WI: University of Wisconsin.

Marshak, L. E., & Prezant, F. P. (2007). *Married with special-needs children: A couple's guide to keeping connected*. Bethesda, MD: Woodbine House.

Mehall, K. G., Spinrad, T. L., Eisenberg, N., & Gaertner, B. M. (2009). Examining the relations of infant temperament and couples' marital satisfaction to mother and father involvement: A longitudinal study. *Fathering*, *7*(1), 23. doi:10.3149/fth.0701.23

Minnes, P., Graffi, S., Nolte, M.L., Carlson, P., & Harrick, L. (2000). Coping and stress in Canadian family caregivers of persons with traumatic brain injuries. *Brain Injury*, *14*(8), 737–748. doi:10.1080/026990500413768

Paquette, D. (2004). Theorizing the father-child relationship: Mechanisms and developmental outcomes. *Human Development*, *47*(4), 193–219. doi:10.1159/000078723

Rosenberg, J., & Wilcox, W.B. (2006). *The importance of fathers in the healthy development of children*. U. S. Department of Health and Human Services Administration for Children and Families, Administration on Children, Youth and

Families, Children's Bureau, Office on Child Abuse and Neglect. Retrieved from http://nccanch.acf.hhs.gov/profess/toolspusermanual.cfm

Seligman, M., & Darling, R. B. (2007). *Ordinary families, special children* (3rd ed.), New York, NY: Guilford.

Tehee, E., Honan, R., & Hevey, D. (2009). Factors contributing to stress in parents of individuals with autistic spectrum disorders. *Journal of Applied Research in Intellectual Disabilities*, *22*, 34–42. doi:10.1111/j.1468-3148.2008.00437.x

Twoy, R., Connolly, P. M., & Novak, J. M. (2007). Coping strategies used by parents of children with autism. *Journal of the American Academy of Nurse Practitioner*, *19*, 251–260. doi:10.1111/j.1745-7599.2007.00222.x

Yogman, M. W. (1994). Observations on the father-infant relationship. In S. H. Cath, A. R. Gurwitt, & J. M. Ross (Eds.), *Father and child: Developmental and clinical perspectives* (pp. 101–122). Hillsdale, NJ: The Analytic Press.

Zvara, B. J., Schoppe-Sullivan, S. J., & Dush, C. K. (2013). Fathers' involvement in child health care: Associations with prenatal involvement, parents' beliefs, and maternal gatekeeping. *Family Relations*, *62*(4), 649–661. doi:10.1111/fare.12023

8 The Sibling Experience
More than My Brother's Keeper

Carolyn Shivers, PhD

Introduction

> "Ben" and "Brandon" are 16-year-old twins. Their parents were recently divorced, and their 19-year-old sister, Amy, has been diagnosed with autism spectrum disorder (ASD). While Amy is high-functioning, she has struggled in school, and her mother has described "a lot of conflict" in trying to find Amy an appropriate educational setting. When asked about her sons, their mom expressed optimism and hope that they could have their own lives, while still recognizing the gifts and benefits of having a sister, regardless of her diagnosis. In contrast, Ben and Brandon often focus on the ways having a sister with ASD makes their lives different. Ben stated, "The way our family functions is more tailored to her. We have to act differently toward her and, even though I'm not the oldest, I have to take more responsibility." When asked if there were any benefits of having a sister with a disability, Brandon replied, "I don't think there are many really clear benefits, but there's probably something there."

Although Ben and Brandon's perceptions are not unusual, they cannot be classified as "typical" of the sibling experience either. Individual differences in age, gender, family composition, and the nature of a sibling's disability can all influence sibling outcomes (Giallo & Gavidia-Payne, 2006; Hodapp & Urbano, 2007; Rossiter & Sharpe, 2001). Since the 1950s, research on siblings of individuals with IDD has focused on understanding how siblings of individuals with IDD differ from those with typically developing siblings and which factors impact these differences. This chapter will summarize results from existing sibling research, including individual, demographic, and family factors, as well as specific outcomes for the siblings of individuals with IDD. Although some researchers have focused on siblings of individuals with IDD as a group (i.e., siblings of individuals with any type of IDD), other researchers have addressed siblings of individuals with a particular diagnosis, such as autism spectrum disorder (ASD) or Down syndrome (DS), which are noted throughout the chapter.

Overview of Research on Sibling Outcomes

Many sibling studies have sought to quantify the sibling experience, focusing on specific outcomes that are likely when one has a sibling with IDD, and how those outcomes may be different from outcomes for siblings of individuals without disabilities. Much of the early research focused on psychosocial adjustment of siblings, often describing the impact on siblings as primarily negative or that siblings were inherently more at risk for problems. These early studies indicated more behavior problems, cognitive problems, and poorer psychosocial adjustment in siblings (Breslau, 1982, 1983; Lobato, 1983; San Martino & Newman, 1974). These outcomes were attributed primarily to the extra demands on parents caring for a child with a disability. For example, it was purported that siblings had more problems because parents had less time to devote to the typically developing siblings, due to the extra demands of having a child with IDD. Another explanation was that the siblings took on more responsibilities and "parentified" roles (i.e., they had to take on extra chores and caregiving activities at home), turning them into additional parental figures rather than siblings, which resulted in poorer outcomes for the typically developing siblings (Lamorey, 1999). Like Ben, who described having more responsibilities than he would have otherwise, because he was not the oldest child, early work by researchers and clinicians suggested that such heightened expectations for responsibility were both common and detrimental to siblings of individuals with IDD (see San Martino & Newman, 1974). While these results suggest problems in siblings were more prevalent in early studies, recent studies have also suggested that siblings of individuals with IDD may be at greater risk for individual problems and impaired family relationships (c.f., Fisman, Wolf, Ellison, & Freeman, 2000; Hastings, 2003; Hodapp & Urbano, 2007; Shivers, Deisenroth, & Taylor, 2013; Williams *et al.*, 2010). Later, these studies will be described in more detail and related to specific characteristics and factors that have been examined in the research.

Not all research on siblings of individuals with IDD suggests negative outcomes. In contrast, some research has indicated positive outcomes and benefits from having a sibling with IDD, including individual effects (e.g., personal growth, pride, empathy and other psychological or intrapersonal outcomes), as well as positive family relationships (e.g., closeness, reduced conflict; Floyd, Purcell, Richardson, & Kupersmidt, 2009; Meyer & Holl, 2014). Although some research indicates either positive or negative outcomes for siblings of individuals with IDD, other researchers have found no differences between siblings of individuals with and without IDD, specifically on measures of behavior problems, self-efficacy, social skills, and mental health symptoms, including anxiety and depression (see Gau *et al.*, 2010; Grissom & Borkowski, 2002; Hastings & Petalas, 2014; Kaminsky & Dewey, 2002; Neely-Barnes & Graff, 2011; Quintero & McIntyre, 2010; Rodgers *et al.*, 2016) or mixed outcomes, suggesting both positive and negative effects (see Graff *et al.*, 2012; Petalas, Hastings, Nash, Reilly, & Dowey, 2012; Williams *et al.*, 2003). In an effort to synthesize these mixed results, Rossiter and Sharpe (2001) conducted a meta-analysis of 25 sibling studies published between 1972–1999. Their results indicated a small negative effect on siblings of individuals with IDD; however, they also noted the importance of accounting for individual differences in personal and family situations to understand the experiences of siblings of individuals with IDD. These unique factors that may be at work and impact whether a sibling experiences negative effects or more positive outcomes will be described next.

Research on Specific Factors Related to Sibling Outcomes

In addition to studies that have found either negative or positive outcomes for siblings, a common theme in early research was the belief that siblings of individuals with IDD "comprise [of] one important identifiable group" (San Martino & Newman, 1974 p. 168). The nature of the brother or sister's disability was unimportant, as the sibling experience was seen to be the same across different disability diagnoses. For example, siblings of children with hearing impairments were thought to have similar experiences as siblings of children with DS. While this convention shaped sibling research for many years, recent research is now far more likely to examine the specific differences within and among families that predict varying outcomes for typically developing siblings. These factors include demographic variables, such as age and gender of the sibling and/or child with IDD, birth order of the sibling, and specific characteristics of the sibling with IDD, as well as other individual and family factors, which will be described next.

Demographic Characteristics

Some of the earliest variables studied in relation to sibling outcomes were the gender and birth order of the sibling, as well as demographic factors and family-related variables, such as family structure, problem-solving, or parental stress. Female siblings, as well as sole siblings (individuals who have no other typically developing brothers or sisters) are more likely to plan for greater levels of future involvement in caring for their brother/sister with IDD in adulthood (Burke, Taylor, Urbano, & Hodapp, 2012). Additionally, the combination of genders may have an impact on sibling outcomes, with same-gender dyads (e.g., brother-brother or sister-sister pairs) exhibiting more warmth in the sibling relationship than opposite-gender dyads (Begum & Blacher, 2011). Therefore, Ben and Brandon may struggle more to relate to their sister with ASD than they would to a brother with IDD. Among siblings of children with ASD, researchers have also found differences based on the gender of the sibling, particularly for male siblings. Shivers *et al.* (2013) found that male siblings were more likely to exhibit sub-clinical anxiety symptoms than female siblings, while Hastings (2003) reported that male siblings engaged in fewer prosocial behaviors than female siblings. Similarly, male siblings may show lower levels of social competence, psychosocial adjustment, and emotional symptoms (Kaminsky & Dewey, 2002; Macks & Reeve, 2007).

In contrast to the research on male siblings, some studies have found that female siblings of individuals with ASD seem to be doing well and are well-adjusted. As previously noted, female siblings have been found to exhibit more prosocial behavior and better social competence and are at lower risk for adjustment problems than male siblings (Hastings, 2003; Kaminsky & Dewey, 2002). Additionally, Verté, Roeyers, and Buysse (2003) found that female siblings between the ages of 12 and 16 had better social skills and more positive self-concept than siblings of individuals without disabilities. This may suggest that female siblings report benefits not only in comparison to male siblings of individuals with IDD, but also in comparison to their typically developing peers in the general population.

In addition to gender, sibling age as well as the relative birth order of the sibling (i.e., older or younger than the child with IDD) may be related to sibling outcomes. While younger siblings of individuals with ASD have been found to exhibit fewer prosocial behaviors (Hastings, 2003), older siblings have reported more problems with psychosocial and behavioral adjustment (Macks & Reeve, 2007). Compared to adult siblings, adolescent siblings have reported more shared activities with their sibling with ASD and more perceived support from family and friends, but lower levels of problem-focused (i.e., adaptive) coping and higher levels of emotion-focused (i.e., maladaptive) coping (Orsmond, Kuo, & Seltzer, 2009). Siblings of children with ASD may experience more internalizing and externalizing behaviors, as well as more anxious behaviors and adjustment problems than child siblings of individuals without IDD (Fisman *et al.*, 2000; Shivers *et al.*, 2013; Verté *et al.*, 2003). However, other researchers (Dempsey, Llorens, Brewton, Mulchandani, & Goin-Kochel, 2012; Kaminsky & Dewey, 2002) did not find greater emotional or behavioral problems in child siblings of individuals with ASD. Additionally, Floyd, Costigan, and Richardson (2016) reported that the sibling relationship improved over time, with conflict decreasing and emotional closeness increasing from adolescence to adulthood. Similarly, Skotko, Levine, and Goldstein (2011) found that the majority of adolescent siblings of individuals with DS reported liking and being proud of their sibling and indicated that their sibling relationship was positive. Based on a sample of siblings of those with DS, researchers indicated that sibling participants reported both positive and negative factors but also shared that they "would not change anything about their experience" (Graff *et al.*, 2012, p. 187). In general, female siblings appear to have better outcomes than male siblings; however, the research on differences across various age groups of siblings is mixed.

Characteristics of Siblings with IDD

Two factors specific to the sibling with IDD that have been addressed in research include comparisons across types of IDD diagnoses (e.g., siblings of individuals with ASD compared to DS, siblings of individuals with IDD compared to siblings of individuals without IDD) and severity of behavior problems in the sibling with IDD. Specifically, research comparing different sibling groups has been quite extensive and will be described next.

Comparing different sibling groups. When studying outcomes among siblings of individuals with IDD, some researchers have found negative results, both in comparison to siblings of children without disabilities and siblings of children with another IDD diagnosis. As with other areas, these comparison studies have resulted in mixed results. Fisman *et al.* (2000) found that siblings of individuals with pervasive developmental disorder (a diagnosis on the autism spectrum) demonstrated more problems with adjustment than both siblings of individuals without disabilities and siblings of individuals with DS. Similarly, Hastings (2003) reported that siblings of children with autism were at greater risk for poorer psychological adjustment compared to other children. Gau and colleagues (2010) found that siblings exhibited higher rates of delinquent behavior and withdrawal compared to siblings of children without ASD in a Taiwanese sample. Recent studies have shown that siblings of individuals with IDD or ASD reported more anxiety symptoms than control samples (e.g., O'Neill & Murray, 2016; Shivers *et al.*, 2013). However, other researchers have found no differences in psychosocial adjustment between ASD, DS, and typically developing sibling groups (Dempsey *et al.*, 2012). Floyd *et al.* (2009) even suggested that siblings of individuals with IDD exhibited more warmth and less conflict with their sibling than did siblings of typically developing individuals.

Although the literature on adult siblings of individuals with IDD is scarce, one study found significant differences between adult siblings of individuals with ASD compared to adult siblings of individuals with DS (Hodapp & Urbano, 2007). Siblings of individuals with ASD reported significantly poorer outcomes on nearly every measure: greater self-reported health problems and depressive symptoms, as well as less closeness and a more negative overall appraisal of the relationship with their sibling (Hodapp & Urbano, 2007). In both groups (ASD siblings and DS siblings), sibling relationship quality was positively related to the ability to make and maintain friendships in the sibling with ASD or DS and negatively related to emotional/behavioral problems in the sibling with ASD or DS. This research on the impact of behavior problems in the individual with IDD will be described in the next section.

Behavior problems of siblings with IDD. One of the most consistent predictors of negative outcomes among typically developing siblings is the presence of behavior problems in the sibling with IDD. In one study, parents of siblings of young children with IDD reported more problems in the target child than parents of siblings of typically developing children, but those differences disappeared when target child behavior problems were controlled for in the analyses (Neece, Blacher, & Baker, 2010). That is, children's behavior problems had an adverse impact on siblings, regardless of whether the child was diagnosed with IDD. Similarly, in a longitudinal study, sibling behavior problems measured at one time point predicted higher levels of sibling behavior problems measured two years later, even when controlling for initial levels of sibling behavior problems (Hastings, 2007).

Similar to siblings of children with other types of IDD, outcomes for siblings of children with ASD seem to be more impacted by the presence of behavior problems in the child with IDD. Tomeny, Barry, and Bader (2012) found that internalizing behavior problems in the child with IDD predicted internalizing behavior problems in the sibling, regardless of whether or not the target child had a disability. Benson and Karlof (2008) reported that increased severity of behavior problems, frequently seen in individuals with ASD, significantly predicted lower levels of prosocial behavior and higher levels of behavioral mental health problems among siblings. Likewise, Orsmond *et al.* (2009) reported that sibling behavior problems predicted significantly lower levels of positive affect in the sibling relationship among adolescents. Smith, Elder, Storch, and Rowe (2015) found that behavior problems in the child with IDD had a negative impact on the siblings' ability to manage stress. While behavior problems of the child with IDD seem to have a consistent, negative impact on typically developing siblings, the actual presence of an IDD diagnosis may not matter as much as the severity of the behavior problems of siblings with IDD.

Family and Personal Factors

Although the behavior and characteristics of the child with IDD is important, variables related to parental behavior and the family structure, in general, may also play a role in sibling outcomes. Understandably, siblings, particularly in childhood and adolescence, cannot always change the behavior of their family members. However, like studies of parents and caregivers, some sibling research has identified personal factors and behaviors, as well as family characteristics that may impact sibling outcomes. Collectively, research indicates that family stability and coping predict better sibling outcomes (Giallo & Gavidia-Payne, 2006; Smith *et al.*, 2015), while parental stress and depressive symptoms predicted more sibling problems (Meyer, Ingersoll, & Hambrick, 2011; Rivers & Stoneman, 2003; Shivers *et al.*, 2013; Tomeny, Baker, Barry, Eldred, & Rankin, 2016). In one study, parents' greater levels of perceived stress predicted more problems in siblings, while better family problem-solving, family stability, and time spent together specifically predicted fewer sibling difficulties (Giallo & Gavidia-Payne, 2006). In a study of siblings of individuals with ASD, Smith *et al.* (2015) found that siblings with more coping strategies showed little to no change in stress management when they had more stressors in life, while siblings who had few coping strategies reported a significant decrease in their ability to maintain health when more stressors were present. While it is clear that more research is needed, it is important to consider family and individual factors when working to maximize positive outcomes for siblings. Cuskelly and Gunn (2006) suggested that *within family* processes were likely more important in understanding sibling adjustment and risks, than an IDD diagnosis in and of itself. Their design is one of only a few studies that included a matched comparison group of typically developing siblings and collected responses on adjustment-related measures from both parents and siblings.

In summary, several factors related to sibling outcomes have been studied: age and gender of the siblings, type of IDD diagnosis, severity of behavior problems in the sibling with IDD, and family characteristics. Much of the research shows mixed results, with some studies indicating differences in these factors and others indicating no differences between groups. Specifically, gender of the sibling, behavior problems of the individual with IDD, and family-related qualities are the factors with the clearest outcomes, or in which there are not studies with mixed results. While these are not the only important factors to consider in understanding the siblings of individuals with IDD, it does provide a picture of what may be most needed in programs available to siblings and families, as well as further research on these and other factors. Specifically, further understanding and awareness of the risk and protective factors for siblings of individuals with IDD is needed.

Principles for Practice

The current consensus among researchers is that many siblings of individuals with IDD are doing well—having a sibling with IDD is not the risk factor professionals once believed. However, certain factors, such as increased behavior problems in the sibling with IDD and parental stress and depression, may contribute to negative outcomes for the siblings. It is important for parents to keep their expectations developmentally appropriate and not place too much adult responsibility on siblings of individuals with IDD. Additionally, communication is important. Studies show that parents and siblings often have different opinions on how the siblings are doing (e.g., Guite, Lobato, Kao, & Plante, 2004; Senner & Fish, 2010). Open communication can help parents better understand whether or not siblings are struggling and how to best address specific concerns.

Areas for Future Research

It is important to recognize that siblings, parents, and others (e.g., teachers) all have different perspectives on the sibling experiences. Many sibling studies rely solely on parent reports of adjustment, impact, and behavior of the sibling. Because parents typically serve as sources of information for the individual with IDD, having parents also answer questions about the sibling can save time and ensure full participation. However, studies have shown that parents and siblings do not always agree on the impact of having a sibling with IDD (Diener, Anderson, Wright, & Dunn, 2015; Guite *et al.*, 2004; Rossiter & Sharpe, 2001; Senner & Fish, 2010). Parents and siblings may develop different cognitive frameworks of the sibling interactions, which indicates that including multiple perspectives and direct input from siblings is necessary in research studies, support programs, and policies for individuals with IDD.

There are a number of limitations in the current research on siblings of individuals with IDD. Very few studies exist on siblings in adulthood, although anecdotal evidence suggests that many adult siblings become responsible for caring for their brother or sister when the parents are no longer able (see Chapter 16). More research is needed to identify the individual and family factors that promote healthy sibling outcomes, including positive relationships between siblings, as well as specific areas of change in the sibling relationship at different ages and across the life span (see Hodapp & Urbano, 2007). Further research is also needed with larger samples across different comparison groups. In addition, to date, only one meta-analysis study (Rossiter & Sharpe, 2001) has been conducted on the available research on siblings of individuals with IDD.

Much of the early research, which focused on the negative effects on siblings, may have asked the wrong questions. Instead of asking *how* siblings are affected, assuming either positive or negative effects, perhaps the questions to be asked are *which* siblings are most negatively impacted, and what factors contribute to both positive and negative outcomes, as well as resilience in other siblings? Recent studies have revealed sub-threshold levels of symptoms among certain siblings, particularly with regards to anxiety (e.g., O'Neill & Murray, 2016). Professionals, including school personnel, mental health professionals, healthcare professionals, and others, need to be aware that not all sibling outcomes manifest into full, clinical disorders, nor do siblings exhibit negative outcomes or impairment due to simply having a sibling with IDD (Cuskelly & Gunn, 2006). By considering family risk factors, including behavior problems of siblings with IDD and parent stress and mental health, professionals who interact with siblings can recognize individuals and families who may be more susceptible to negative outcomes. With this knowledge, professionals can also identify more subtle symptoms and specific risk factors that may indicate potential sibling problems and direct them to support programs and services.

Developing Programs for Siblings of Individuals with IDD

Although research on siblings of individuals with IDD still has a long way to go in identifying siblings most at-risk for negative outcomes, there are several programs designed to support siblings of individuals with IDD (Sibling Support Project, 2017; The Arc, 2016). In addition, the National Down Syndrome Congress (NDSC, 2014) offers a sibling-specific activity track at their annual convention, with specific programming for siblings. Brian Skotko, a physician and sibling of a sister with DS, along with Susan Levine (2009), published a book which serves as an informative guide for understanding the facts about DS, managing peers, handling frustrating or uncomfortable situations, and addressing family challenges. The book was their effort to identify and address common questions raised by siblings of individuals with DS, during brother and sister meetings for teens (some held during the Brothers & Sisters Conference held at the NDSC Annual Convention; see NDSC, 2014). This resource is specifically valuable for the DS community, but similar resources could benefit siblings with other IDDs, like ASD.

Sibling programs comprise of various support activities, including introducing siblings to peers, teaching problem-solving methods, expressing feelings and seeking feedback and validation, and developing strategies for coping with stress (e.g., Roberts *et al.*, 2015). Anecdotal feedback for such programs is largely positive; unfortunately, few empirical studies have analyzed whether participating in these programs had any effect on sibling outcomes. Of the studies that have been conducted, most showed some positive outcomes for siblings, including increased knowledge of their siblings with IDD (Williams *et al.*, 2003), fewer behavior problems (Lobato & Kao, 2002), improved emotional and behavioral functioning (Roberts *et al.*, 2015), improvements in attitude and self-esteem (Williams *et al.*, 2003), and improvements in the sibling relationship (Phillips, 1999). Small sample studies also suggest that the majority of siblings enjoy these programs and would recommend them to other siblings (D'Arcy, Flynn, McCarthy, O'Connor, & Tierney, 2005).

Conclusion

Sibling research has expanded significantly since the first exploratory studies during the 1950s–1960s. Overall, researchers have determined that most siblings are doing well, with little to no risk for significant psychological or mental health issues. However, certain siblings may be at risk for sub-threshold levels of individual symptoms; in particular, several studies have shown increased rates of anxiety in siblings of individuals with IDD as compared to normative groups (e.g., Shivers *et al.*, 2013). More importantly, researchers have identified several predictors of sibling outcomes, furthering the notion that simply having a brother or sister with IDD does not automatically imply difficulties for typically developing siblings (Cuskelly & Gunn, 2006). The most consistently analyzed of these factors is by far the presence of behavior problems in the sibling with IDD. Ultimately, more research is needed to determine the mechanisms driving both risk and resilience factors for sibling outcomes, and, most crucially, how to best support siblings who face more challenging situations. Sibling relationships are among the longest-lasting that humans will experience; thus, it is essential to minimize the challenges and maximize the benefits of these relationships for all.

Key Messages from This Chapter

- **For individuals with IDD and their families**: Having a sibling with IDD is not the risk factor professionals once believed. Although some studies show overall differences in emotional and behavioral outcomes between siblings of individuals with and without IDD, family-level differences, and behavior problems of the child with IDD, seem to have a greater impact on the sibling than the presence of a disability itself.
- **For professionals**: Certain factors, such as increased behavior problems in the sibling with IDD and parental stress, may contribute to negative outcomes for siblings. Professionals who interact with individuals with IDD and their families need to recognize those who may be most susceptible to negative outcomes, specifically symptoms and problems that indicate potential sibling difficulties.
- **For policy makers**: Lack of services is consistently identified as a source of stress for families; therefore, policy makers should work to make lifelong

services available for individuals with IDD. Simpler and more comprehensive access to such services across the life span would make the lives of siblings easier, both in childhood, as peers to their brothers and sisters with IDD, and in adulthood, as potential future caregivers.

References

Begum, G., & Blacher, J. (2011). The siblings relationship of adolescents with and without intellectual disabilities. *Research in Developmental Disabilities*, *32*, 1580–1588. doi:10.1016/j.ridd.2011.01.056

Benson, P. R., & Karlof, K. L. (2008). Child, parent, and family predictors of latter adjustment in siblings of children with autism. *Research in Autism Spectrum Disorder*, *2*, 583–600. doi:10.1016/j.rasd.2007.12.002

Breslau, N. (1982). Siblings of disabled children: Birth order and age-spacing effects. *Journal of Abnormal Child Psychology*, *10*(1), 85–96. doi:10.1007/BF00915953

Breslau, N. (1983). The psychological study of chronically ill and disabled children: Are healthy siblings appropriate controls? *Journal of Abnormal Child Psychology*, *11*(3), 379–391. doi:10.1007/bf00914246

Burke, M. M., Taylor, J. L., Urbano, R., & Hodapp, R. M. (2012). Predictors of future caregiving by adult siblings of individuals with intellectual and developmental disabilities. *American Journal on Intellectual and Developmental Disabilities*, *117*(1), 33–47. doi:10.1352/1944-7558-117.1.33

Cuskelly, M., & Gunn, P. (2006). Adjustment of children who have a sibling with Down syndrome: Perspectives of mothers, fathers and children. *Journal of Intellectual Disability Research*, *50*(12), 917–925. doi:10.1111/j.1365-2788.2006.00922.x

D'Arcy, F., Flynn, J., McCarthy, Y., O'Connor, C., & Tierney, E. (2005). Sibshops: An evaluation of an interagency model. *Journal of Intellectual Disabilities*, *9*(1), 43–57. doi:10.1177/1744629505049729

Dempsey, A. G., Llorens, A., Brewton, C., Mulchandani, S., & Goin-Kochel, R. P. (2012). Emotional and behavioral adjustment in typically developing siblings of children with autism spectrum disorders. *Journal of Autism and Developmental Disorders*, *42*(7), 1393–1402. doi:10.1007/s10803-011-1368-9

Diener, M. L., Anderson, L., Wright, C. A., & Dunn, M. L. (2015). Sibling relationships of children with autism spectrum disorder in the context of everyday life and a strength-based program. *Journal of Child and Family Studies*, *24*(4), 1060–1072. doi:10.1007/s10826-014-9915-6

Fisman, S., Wolf, L., Ellison, D., & Freeman, T. (2000). A longitudinal study of siblings of children with chronic disabilities. *Canadian Journal of Psychiatry-Revue Canadienne De Psychiatrie*, *45*(4), 369–375. doi:10.1177/070674370004500406

Floyd, F. J., Costigan, C. L., & Richardson, S. S. (2016). Sibling relationships in adolescence and early adulthood with people who have intellectual disability. *American Journal on Intellectual and Developmental Disabilities*, *121*(5), 383–397. doi:10.1352/1944-7558-121.5.383

Floyd, F. J., Purcell, S. E., Richardson, S. S., & Kupersmidt, J. B. (2009). Sibling relationship quality and social functioning of children and adolescents with intellectual disability. *American Journal on Intellectual and Developmental Disability*, *114*(2), 110–127. doi:10.1352/2009.114.110-127

Gau, S., Chou, M., Lee, J., Wong, C., Chou, W., Chen, M., Soong W. T., & Wu, Y. (2010). Behavioral problems and parenting style among Taiwanese children with autism and their siblings. *Psychiatry and Clinical Neurosciences*, *64*(1), 70–78. doi:10.1111/j.1440-1819.2009.02034.x

Giallo, R., & Gavidia-Payne, S. (2006). Child, parent and family factors as predictors of adjustment for siblings of children with a disability. *Journal of Intellectual Disability Research*, *50*, 937–948. doi:10.1111/j.1365-2788.2006.00928.x

Graff, C., Mandleco, B., Dyches, T. T., Coverston, C. R., Roper, S. O., & Freeborn, D. (2012). Perspectives of adolescent siblings of children with Down syndrome who have multiple health problems. *Journal of Family Nursing*, *18*(2), 175–199. doi:10.1177/1074840712439797

Grissom, M. O., & Borkowski, J. G. (2002). Self-efficacy in adolescents who have siblings with or without disabilities. *American Journal on Mental Retardation*, *107*(2), 79–90. doi:10.1352/0895-8017

Guite, J., Lobato, D., Kao, B., & Plante, W. (2004). Discordance between sibling and parent reports of the impact of chronic illness and disability on siblings. *Children's Health Care*, *33*(1), 77–92. doi:10.1207/s15326888chc3301_5

Hastings, R. P. (2003). Brief report: Behavioral adjustment of siblings of children with autism. *Journal of Autism and Developmental Disorders*, *33*(1), 99–104. doi: 10.1023/A:1022290723442

Hastings, R. P. (2007). Longitudinal relationships between sibling behavioral adjustment and behavior problems of children with developmental disabilities. *Journal of Autism and Developmental Disorders*, *37*, 1485–1492. doi:10.1007/s10803-006-0230-y

Hastings, R., & Petalas, M. (2014). Self-reported behaviour problems and sibling relationship quality by siblings of children with autism spectrum disorder. *Journal of Applied Research in Intellectual Disabilities*, *27*(4), 363–363. doi:10.1111/cch.12131

Hodapp, R. M., & Urbano, R. C. (2007). Adult siblings of individuals with Down syndrome versus with autism: Findings from a large-scale U. S. survey. *Journal of Intellectual Disability Research*, *51*, 1018–1029. doi:10.1111/j.1365-2788.2007.00994.x

Kaminsky, L., & Dewey, D. (2002). Psychosocial adjustment in siblings of children with autism. *Journal of Child Psychology and Psychiatry*, *43*(2), 225–232. doi:10.1111/1469-7610.00015

Lamorey, S. (1999). Parentification of siblings of children with disability or chronic disease. In N. D. Chase (Ed.), *Burdened children: Theory, research, and treatment of parentification* (pp. 75–91). Thousand Oaks, CA: Sage.

Lobato, D. (1983). Siblings of handicapped children: A review. *Journal of autism and developmental disorders*, *13*(4), 347–364. doi:10.1007/BF01531585

Lobato, D. J., & Kao, B. T. (2002). Integrated sibling-parent group intervention to improve sibling knowledge and adjustment to chronic illness and disability. *Journal of Pediatric Psychology*, *27*, 711–716. doi:10.1093/jpepsy/27.8.711

Macks, R. J., & Reeve, R. E. (2007). The adjustment of non-disabled siblings of children with autism. *Journal of Autism and Developmental Disorders*, *37*(6), 1060–1067. doi:10.1007/s10803-006-0249-0

Meyer, D., & Holl, E. (2014). *The sibling survival guide: Indispensable information for brothers and sisters of adults with disabilities.* Bethesda, MD: Woodbine House.

Meyer, K. A., Ingersoll, B., & Hambrick, D. Z. (2011). Factors influencing adjustment in siblings of children with autism spectrum disorders. *Research in Autism Spectrum Disorders*, *5*, 1413–1420. doi:10.1016/j.rasd.2011.01.027

National Down Syndrome Congress. (2014). *Brothers & Sisters Conference*. Retrieved from https://www.ndsccenter.org/brothers-sisters-conference/

Neece, C., Blacher, J., & Baker, B. (2010). Impact on siblings of children with intellectual disability: The role of child behavior problems. *American Journal on Intellectual and Developmental Disabilities*, *115*(4), 291–306. doi:10.1352/1944-7558-115.4.291

Neely-Barnes, S. L., & Graff, J. C. (2011). Are there adverse consequences to being a sibling of a person with a disability? A propensity score analysis. *Family Relations*, *60*(3), 331–341. doi:10.1111/j.1741-3729.2011.00652.x

O'Neill, L. P., & Murray, L. E. (2016). Anxiety and depression symptomatology in adult siblings of individuals with different developmental disability diagnoses. *Research in Developmental Disabilities*, *51*, 116–125. doi:10.1016/j.ridd.2015.12.017

Orsmond, G. I., Kuo, H., & Seltzer, M. M. (2009). Siblings of individuals with an autism spectrum disorder: Sibling relationships and wellbeing in adolescence and adulthood. *Autism*, *13*(1), 59–80. doi:10.1177/1362361308097119

Petalas, M. A., Hastings, R. P., Nash, S., Reilly, D., & Dowey, A. (2012). The perceptions and experiences of adolescent siblings who have a brother with autism spectrum disorder. *Journal of Intellectual and Developmental Disability*, *37*(4), 303–314. doi:10.3109/13668250.2012.734603

Phillips, R. (1999). Intervention with siblings of children with developmental disabilities from economically disadvantaged families. *Families in Society*, *80*(6), 569–577. doi:10.1606/1044-3894.1781

Quintero, N., & McIntyre, L. L. (2010). Sibling adjustment and maternal well-being: An examination of families with and without a child with an autism spectrum disorder. *Focus on Autism and Other Developmental Disabilities*, *25*(1), 37–46. doi:10.1177/1088357609350367

Rivers, J. W., & Stoneman, Z. (2003). Sibling relationships when a child has autism: Marital stress and support coping. *Journal of Autism and Developmental Disorders*, *33*(4), 383–394. doi:10.1023/A:1025006727395

Roberts, R. M., Ejova, A., Giallo, R., Strohm, K., Lillie, M., & Fuss, B. (2015). A controlled trial of the SibworkS group program for siblings of children with special needs. *Research in Developmental Disabilities*, *43–44*, 21–31. doi:10.1016/j.ridd.2015.06.002

Rodgers, J. D., Warhol, A., Fox, J. D., McDonald, C. A., Thomeer, M. L., Lopata, C., Darrow, A. M., Szyszkowski, A. L., Biscotto, A. A., & Sheffield, T. (2016). Minimal risk of internalizing problems in typically-developing siblings of children with high-functioning autism spectrum disorder. *Journal of Child and Family Studies*, *25*(8), 2554–2561. doi:10.1007/s10826-016-0407-8

Rossiter, L., & Sharpe, D. (2001). The siblings of individuals with mental retardation: A quantitative integration of the literature. *Journal of Child and Family Studies*, *10*(1), 65–84. doi:10.1023/A:1016629500708

San Martino, S., & Newman, M. B. (1974). Siblings of retarded children: A population at risk. *Child Psychiatry and Human Development*, *4*(3), 168–177. doi:10.1007/BF01436025

Senner, J. E., & Fish, T. (2010). Comparison of child self-report and parent report on the sibling need and involvement profile. *Remedial and Special Education*, *33*(2), 103–109. doi:10.1177/0741932510364547

Shivers, C. M., Deisenroth, L. K., & Taylor, J. L. (2013). Patterns and predictors of anxiety among siblings of children with autism spectrum disorders. *Journal of Autism and Developmental Disorders*, *43*(6), 1136–1346. doi:10.1007/s10803-012-1685-7

Sibling Support Project. (2017). *The sibling support project*. Retrieved from www.siblingsupport.org

Skotko, B. G., & Levine, S. P. (2009). *Fasten your seatbelt: A crash course on Down syndrome for brothers and sisters*. Bethesda, MD: Woodbine House.

Skotko, B. G., Levine, S. P., & Goldstein, R. (2011). Having a brother or sister with Down syndrome: Perspectives from siblings. *American Journal of Medical Genetics Part A*, *155*(10), 2348–2359. doi:10.1002/ajmg.a.34228

Smith, L. O., Elder, J. H., Storch, E. A., & Rowe, M. A. (2015). Predictors of sense of coherence in typically developing adolescent siblings of individuals with autism spectrum disorder. *Journal of Intellectual Disability Research*, *59*, 26–38. doi:10.1111/jir.12124

The Arc. (2016). *I am a sibling*. Retrieved from www.thearc.org/siblings

Tomeny, T. S., Baker, L. K., Barry, T. D., Eldred, S. W., & Rankin, J. A. (2016). Emotional and behavioral functioning of typically-developing sisters of children with autism spectrum disorder: The roles of ASD severity, parental stress, and marital status. *Research in Autism Spectrum Disorders*, *32*, 130–142. doi:10.1016/j.rasd.2016.09.008

Tomeny, T. S., Barry, T. D., & Bader, S. H. (2012). Are typically-developing siblings of children with an autism spectrum disorder at risk for behavioral, emotional, and social maladjustment? *Research in Autism Spectrum Disorders*, *6*, 508–518. doi:10.1016/j.rasd.2011.07.012

Verté, S., Roeyers, H., & Buysse, A. (2003). Behavioural problems, social competence and self-concept in siblings of children with autism. *Child: Care, Health and Development*, *29*(3), 193–205. doi:10.1046/j.1365-2214.2003.00331.x

Williams, P. D., Piamjariyakul, U., Graff, J. C., Stanton, A., Guthrie, A. C., Hafeman, C., & Williams, A. R. (2010). Developmental disabilities: Effects on well siblings. *Issues in Comprehensive Pediatric Nursing*, *33*(1), 39–55. doi:10.3109/01460860903486515

Williams, P. D., Williams, A. R., Graff, C., Hanson, S., Stanton, A., Hafeman, C., Liebergen, A., Leuenberg, K., Setter, R. K., Ridder, L., Curry, H., Barnard, M., & Sanders, S. (2003). A community-based intervention for siblings and parents of children with chronic illness or disability: The ISEE study. *Journal of Pediatrics*, *143*, 386–393. doi:10.1067/S0022-3476(03)00391-3

9 Grandparents

Meaningful Contributors to a Changing Family Landscape

Sandra Woodbridge, PhD and Laurie Buys, PhD

Introduction

Professionals working with families do so in an environment that bears little resemblance to society 50 years ago. Significant changes to family and social structures have occurred over time. In modern society, single parent families; same sex families; blended families as well as the more traditional family structure (nuclear family) of mother, father, and children, are well accepted and integrated in many societies across the world (Tomlin, 1998). Throughout history, grandparents have been featured as part of the family, but changes to "traditional" family structures in recent times have resulted in the changing roles of grandparents (Uhlenberg & Kirby, 1998). These changes have increased the likelihood that extended family members, including grandparents, play a critical role in the challenges faced by parents and their children, particularly when children in the family are diagnosed with an intellectual or developmental disability (IDD) (Organisation for Economic Cooperation and Development, 2011). Whether the diagnosis occurs at or around the birth of the child or later as a result of illness or an accident, grandparents are confronted with many issues that will challenge their expectations, their identities, their roles, and their relationships. While some grandparents may be overwhelmed by the prospect, others will adapt their roles and contribute to the overall well-being of the family.

The purpose of this chapter is to provide insight into the experiences of grandparents who have a grandchild with IDD. This insight will explore the demographic factors that have resulted in the growing numbers of grandparents in this situation and the impact that having a child with IDD can have on family relationships across generations. The chapter will describe the roles grandparents adopt with their grandchildren and the emotional responses they may have at the time of diagnosis. As there has been limited research attention given to the impact of having a grandchild with IDD, this chapter also makes an important contribution to the knowledge of professionals who seek to ensure that the family has the best support available by providing recommendations for consideration.

Becoming a Grandparent

Leopold and Skopek (2015) described the event of becoming a grandparent as "a counter-transition—not self-initiated" (p. 803), with the timing being completely out of the grandparents' control. Despite this lack of direct involvement, the birth of a grandchild significantly changes the lives of grandparents on many levels and will be experienced in a variety of ways. Some grandparents will fully embrace this new role and everything that comes with it, while others may be more circumspect and unsure about how their lives may be affected. This differing response is also seen in grandparents who are processing the news when their grandchild is diagnosed with an IDD (Miller, Buys, & Woodbridge, 2012). Becoming a grandparent is a significant life event, often described in terms of the enjoyment and pleasure that it brings, as well as the sense of purpose and meaning that having a grandchild often brings to the lives of the grandparent (Bengston, 1985; Lye, 1996; Margolis, 2016; Silverstein & Long, 1998). The realization that their grandchild has an IDD diagnosis often adds to the intensity of that experience (Margetts, Le Couteur, & Croom, 2006).

Family Relationships

While longer life expectancy extends the opportunities for becoming a grandparent, a growing number of grandchildren will experience multiple generations of grandparents (Uhlenberg, 2005). The phenomena of multi-generational families, while more a feature in Western societies, is a significant change from previous generations. It is not unusual for grandchildren to have multiple sets of grandparents (both biological and non-biological) as a result of the changing relationships of their parents. Negotiating these multiple relationships can present challenges for all involved. However, the relationships the grandchild has with each of these individual grandparents will often be quite unique with the relationship moderated by a number of factors, such as health status of the grandparents, availability (time), geographic mobility, marital status, expectations of all parties, and the nature of the relationships between the adults (Condon, Corkindale, Luscz, & Gamble, 2013).

For example, Condon and colleagues (2013) found that grandparents and first-time parents may have different expectations on the level of involvement they will have with their grandchild and often require a shared understanding of concepts such as "care" and "contact" in order to begin the conversations on the topic. Reaching a position where there is a shared understanding of the expectations of both parties is also critical in the circumstances where the grandchild has an IDD diagnosis. A number of studies have also identified that the relationship grandparents have with their grandchild may be influenced by the number and sets of grandchildren involved (Findler, 2014; Leopold & Skopek, 2015). However, Uhlenberg and Hammill (1998) found that the amount of time spent with grandchildren was not predicted by the number of grandchildren. As children of the baby boomer generation generally have smaller families (Uhlenberg, 2005), it could be expected that the number of grandchildren within families will be significantly less than that experienced by earlier generations. Therefore, it is important that professionals question assumptions about how individuals will respond to the IDD diagnosis of their grandchild, as it will often be a very individual experience for each person.

Roles of Grandparents

The role that grandparents play in the lives of their grandchild(ren) is influenced by a number of factors. Studies have identified that individuals will be influenced greatly by their own grandparenting experience, often deciding to be more involved with their grandchildren based on their limited engagement with their own grandparents (Kornhaber, 1996; Turnbull & Turnbull, 1990). For example, many current grandparents recalled having frail elderly grandparents who seemed aloof and withdrawn. As a result of this experience, older people have described the importance of developing a more positive relationship with their own grandchildren (Harwood & Lin, 2000; Woodbridge, 2010). On the other hand, some individuals may reflect on the wonderful experiences they had with their grandparents (or with some other significant older person in their lives) (Falk & Falk, 2002). In these cases, they will often identify that this is the type of role that they want to have with their grandchildren (Falk & Falk, 2002; Kornhaber, 1996). Grandparents are more likely to report better outcomes for the grandparent-grandchild relationship when they believe that they make contributions to their grandchildren's lives, enhancing their own feelings of self-worth and purpose, and providing an environment where they are able to share their wisdom and experiences (Erikson, Erikson, & Kivnick, 1986; Kornhaber, 1996; Reitzes & Mutran, 2004).

In general, grandparents will engage in a number of activities that can be categorized as either instrumental or symbolic roles (Fuller-Thomson & Minkler, 2001; Weibel-Orlando, 1990; Woodbridge, Buys, & Miller, 2011). Instrumental activities may include practical tasks such as childcare; assisting with the financial needs of the family (e.g., school fees, clothes, music, and sports lessons); meeting the housing needs of the family; attending school activities, such as a grandparent's day; and providing vacations and holiday excursions. There is also evidence that grandparents provide the majority of childcare for children, including children with a disability (Ferguson, Maughan, & Golding, 2008; Gonzales, Matz-Costa, & Morrow-Howell, 2015; Luo, La Pierre, Hughes, & Waite, 2012; Woodbridge *et al.*, 2011). Assistance can vary from providing full-time care for younger children and after-school care for older children but also holiday care, which makes a significant contribution to the well-being of families, especially given the cost of formal childcare and its limited availability in some communities.

Grandparents provide both emotional and practical help for their families. In the study by Woodbridge *et al.* (2011), grandparents identified that they had provided help and assistance to their children and grandchildren with IDD in several ways: learning sign language, making modifications to their house to accommodate wheelchair access and personal care needs, purchasing a wheelchair accessible car, taking early retirement to be more available, and providing holiday and respite care in order to provide the support needed to their child and grandchildren. In addition, grandparents involved themselves with their grandchildren's activities at school by attending reading groups, grandparent days, and athletic events, as well as ensuring that their grandchildren with IDD were not excluded from such events (Woodbridge *et al.*, 2011). According to Erikson *et al.* (1986), being a role model within the community, both the disability community and the broader social community, ensures older adults feel that they are contributing and leaving a legacy for future generations.

Gender Differences

Just as there have been significant changes to the roles grandparents have in contemporary families, there have been significant changes to the roles grandfathers and grandmothers may have as individuals, as well. Traditionally, mothers and grandmothers have often been seen as more likely to be involved with their children and families, in general, as fathers were somewhat distant or even absent from the daily activities within families. Mothers often saw their role very much as being responsible for building a cohesive and supportive family environment and were responsible to support the needs of the family (Mann, Khan, & Leeson, 2013; Margolis, 2016). In contrast, fathers were often more disengaged from the emotional and relationship needs of the family, deferring to their wife, mother, or grandmother to attend to these needs. Essentially, the role of fathers was viewed as going to work and providing financially for the family as their key responsibility (Thomas, 1994).

It is interesting that historically, grandfathers may have been more likely to adopt a distant style of grand-parenting, continuing to rely on their partner to take responsibility for the emotional and support needs of the family (Thomas, 1994). However, just as many fathers no longer view their role in the family as only that of "provider" and are more engaged in all aspects of family life, contemporary grandfathers are often more directly involved with their families and grandchildren. Grandfathers often report feeling that they missed out on so much by not being more involved as fathers with their children when they were younger (Lesperance, 2010; Woodbridge, 2008). They also report feeling more relaxed with their grandchildren than they did with their own children and speak fondly of the activities that they share, as well as the influence they are able to have on the relationships with their own children as a result (Ben Shlomo & Taubman-Ben-Ari, 2017; Stgeorge & Fletcher, 2014). Adult children are often surprised at just how engaged their father is with their grandchildren compared to their experience of him as a father (Lesperance, 2010; Woodbridge, 2010). Grandfathers who are engaged with their families in this way also appear to be able to make a very positive contribution to the overall well-being of their family when the grandchild has an IDD diagnosis (Mann *et al.*, 2013; Stgeorge & Fletcher, 2014). The experiences of having a grandchild with an IDD diagnosis will be described next.

Grandchildren with IDD: Grandparent Experiences

Whether a grandchild is diagnosed with a disability at birth or later in life, parents and grandparents alike are faced with significant challenges as they try to come to terms with the situation. In spite of these challenges, grandparents have an emotional connectedness with both their children and their grandchildren, and therefore, they have a vested interest in being available for both instrumental and symbolic support to their families. Grandparents often experience a variety of emotions when informed of the diagnosis and their responses may be quite varied based on a range of circumstances, including their own experience or knowledge of IDD, their prior and current roles and relationships within the family, and their own health and financial situation at the time of diagnosis (Findler, 2014; Hillman, 2007; Miller *et al.*, 2012; Woodbridge, 2010). Grandparents may experience a period of grief and mourning at the time of diagnosis, but at the same time, they may be aware of the emotional and instrumental needs of their own child and seek to find strategies to support the family, often drawing on their own personal strengths and coping strategies (Findler, 2014; Margetts *et al.*, 2006; Mirfin-Veitch, Bray, & Watson, 1997).

Diagnosis at Birth

Together with the expectant parents, prospective grandparents rarely consider that the birth of a grandchild will be anything but a joyous occasion. Rarely do they consider that the outcome of the pregnancy may present the family with potential challenges and new, sometimes difficult experiences. For some, the pregnancy may be problematic, and prenatal tests may clearly indicate that the child may be born with a disability. On the other hand, the pregnancy may be trouble-free or health assessments may not provide any warning that the birth will not result in the expected outcome of a "healthy child" (Hastings, 1997; Lee & Gardner, 2010; Mirfin-Veitch *et al.*, 1997; Woodbridge, 2010).

Parents and grandparents may experience conflicting emotions at the time of the diagnosis. While needing to come to terms with their own feelings and emotions, grandparents may want to ensure that they are there to support their child (the parent). This emotional conflict can be compounded by the current status of the relationship between the parents and the grandparents, physical distance between the parents and child with IDD and the grandparents, as well as other work and family responsibilities (Baranowski & Schilmoeller, 1999; Findler, 2014; Lee & Gardner, 2010; Mirfin-Veitch *et al.*, 1997).

Grandparents rely on their prior experiences to inform the specific grandparent roles they adopt within their families (Kornhaber, 1996). In the situation where a grandchild has been diagnosed with an IDD, grandparents often do not have any previous experiences to draw upon, which can add to the emotional turmoil they may feel. In the past, people with disabilities were often ostracized from society, attending "special schools" rather than mainstream schools, and as young adults, many spent their adulthood in institutions with little inclusion in society in general (Turnbull, Summers, & Brotherson, 1986). At the same time, grandparents may recall the negative, discriminative, and isolating language often used by other children and adults toward people with disabilities. These memories may be distressing for grandparents and limit their capacity to see a positive future for the child and their family. Despite grandparents reporting these initial concerns, in most cases, grandparents will adopt a positive attitude and seek to support the family, and in particular their own adult child, to negotiate the complex circumstances that often come with having a child with IDD (Woodbridge *et al.*, 2011; Woodbridge, 2010; Woodbridge & Clapton, 2012).

One of the particular challenges grandparents experience at the time of an IDD diagnosis is that they may not have access to the information needed to understand the diagnosis nor the prognosis for their grandchild. This can add to feelings of inadequacy in providing support for their child and has been reported by grandparents as a significant hindrance to the support they can provide to their family (Lee & Gardner, 2010). It does appear that non-judgemental emotional support provided by grandparents can be of great assistance to the family, even if they do not always have all of the information or knowledge that the parents may need. However, as a strategy for ensuring the parents of the child are well supported, there is value in keeping the grandparents well-informed, when possible (Woodbridge *et al.*, 2011).

Limited research is available on the grandparents' perspective on their role when a grandchild has a disability at birth, but what is available tends to report on the parents' perceptions of the role of grandparents at that time. For example, mothers of children with intellectual disability reported that they experienced less depression when they had significant emotional support from their own mother (Baranowski & Schilmoeller, 1999). Trute (2003) reported that in the case of parents of children with developmental disabilities, the emotional support provided by their parents resulted in better overall well-being than practical help did, reinforcing the important role grandparents can play. It has also been noted that emotional support provided to the parents by the grandparents can have a beneficial effect on the level of anxiety often observed in children and young adults with autism (Hillman, 2007).

Diagnosis in Later Life

In some circumstances, the grandchild may not present with any signs of a disability or a diagnosis at birth, or a disability may occur with no warning, such as acquiring a disability. In these cases, grandparents report that they experienced the same emotions as described with an early diagnosis, such as shock, sadness, or disbelief (Woodbridge, 2010). In addition, they often reported experiencing significant loss in relation to the changes that may occur for the child, as well as the anticipated changes with the relationship they have with their grandchild (Woodbridge, 2010). For example, grandparents who have been used to having their grandchild spend weekends and holidays with them may question whether they will still be able to manage this as the child's need for support changes

(Woodbridge, 2010). Grandparents also reported that the grief they felt for lost opportunities, for themselves, for their grandchild, and also for their own child, at times, overwhelmed them (Woodbridge, 2010).

Interestingly, grandparents reported that when an older grandchild is diagnosed with IDD, the diagnosis itself may come as a blessing (Woodbridge, 2010). They often reported a sense of relief that at least they know what they are dealing with (Woodbridge, Buys, & Miller, 2009), as a diagnosis may follow a significant period of concern that something "just does not seem right" or while seeking out specialists to provide answers to the many questions that may have arisen for the family along the way. With a clear diagnosis, plans for the future of the child and family can be made, as they may now know more about what they are facing. For some families, this feeling that "something is just not right" may continue for some time, even years (Woodbridge, 2010). Children may exhibit challenging behaviors, suffer from ongoing generalized illnesses, present with some features but not all facets of a diagnosis, and yet despite continuous investigations by multiple medical specialists and services, an actual diagnosis is not obtained. In this situation, grandparents may be called upon to provide emotional support to their families as they negotiate the complexity and uncertainty, while they continue to seek answers.

Grandparent Roles, Styles, and Identity Development

Despite the emotional impact of having a grandchild with IDD, grandparents still appear to adopt the specific grand-parenting roles (i.e., instrumental and symbolic) and styles (i.e., formal, fun-loving, distant, reservoirs of family wisdom, and surrogate parents) that have been identified in the literature on grandparenting (Kivinick, 1982; Neugarten & Weinstein, 1964; Weibel-Orlando, 1990; Westheimer & Kaplan, 1998). Likewise, grandparents with grandchildren who have IDD also identify with the concepts of *grandparent drive*, *latent grandparent identity*, and *functional grandparent identity* (Kornhaber, 1996), which have previously been applied to describe grandparents of typically developing grandchildren. Developing an identity or approach to being a grandparent is not something that grandparents do consciously but something that develops prior to becoming a grandparent.

Weibel-Orlando (1990) found that rather than being rigid in the adoption of these styles, grandparents often adapted the particular roles based on the individual grandchild's specific needs and circumstances. For families where the grandchild has an IDD diagnosis, grandparents may contribute by being available for school or medical appointments, which may reduce the demands on the parents (Gardner, Scherman, Mobley, Brown, & Schulter, 1994). Similarly, grandparents may contribute financially to the costs of specialized therapeutic services, adaptive technology, and medical aids, thus, also relieving some of the financial pressures on the parents. Parents have reported the importance of the support provided by grandparents in meeting the daily needs of the child with IDD (Baranowski & Schilmoeller, 1999; Findler, 2014; Mirfin-Veitch *et al.*, 1997; Woodbridge, 2010).

Family Relationships Following an IDD Diagnosis

Grandparents often find the circumstances surrounding an IDD diagnosis challenging, as the uncertainty may result in a tense situation for all family members. Grandparents may be called upon to defend the circumstances with other family members who may question the legitimacy of the situation and blame the child's behavior on other circumstances or not fully understand the IDD diagnosis (Hillman, 2007; Woodbridge, 2010). Grandparents sometimes must justify time spent supporting members of the family when a specific diagnosis of a disability has not been made (Woodbridge, 2010). Negotiating family relationships and advocating for the child with IDD can be an important role grandparents adopt and can contribute positively to the overall well-being of the family, including the grandparents (Hastings, 1997; Hillman, 2007).

While most families of children with IDD can be very supportive of each other and encourage the grandparents to be involved in the lives of all their grandchildren, in some families, the grandparents may find themselves caught in the middle of family conflict (Miller *et al.*, 2012). This conflict can be pre-existing but can intensify if one family member believes that the grandparents are providing more support in the case of the child with IDD than to their other typically developing grandchildren. Surprisingly, this tension and family conflict can be particularly challenging for the grandparent when the diagnosis of the disability is delayed (Findler, 2014; Hillman, 2007; Margetts *et al.*, 2006). Dealing with family conflict can be distressing for grandparents and can contribute to them taking on a mediator role within their family. Grandparents may choose to provide greater support to the family of the grandchild with IDD, deciding that their need is higher at that point in time. This may not be well received by their other adult children, and this decision can have long lasting repercussions for long-term relationships within the whole family. When conflict does arise, grandparents may experience disappointment and additional sadness and stress due to the fact that their family members are not able to support each other and may choose to have a more distant role in the life of their grandchild with IDD in order to "keep the peace" (Woodbridge, 2010).

Kahana *et al.* (2015) suggested that grandparents are ideally situated because of their unique relationships to ensure that communication with the broader family system is both timely and effective. However, many grandparents develop a great sense of pride at how supportive their families can be in the case of a child diagnosed with IDD (Hillman, 2007; Woodbridge *et al.*, 2009). This sense of pride reinforces their positive identity as parents and validates their desire to contribute positively to the overall well-being of the family (Erikson *et al.*, 1986; Woodbridge, 2008). As professionals, it is important to understand the complex family relationships that may exist for grandparents before placing expectations on them or questioning their commitment to be a support for the family.

Principles for Practice

While the numbers of children with disabilities is growing, parents are faced with ongoing challenges in order to ensure that their children are able to make their way in society. Drawing on the support of other family members and members of the IDD community, parents have the opportunity to benefit from the expertise of those around them to achieve their goals and aspirations. Grandparents are ideally placed in these situations as they not only have the expertise of their own life experiences but also their expert knowledge of their own families.

Grandparents as Resources

With multiple generations, professionals have a resource that they can draw on when seeking to support families, especially those who have children with IDD. Acknowledging the differences that can occur both within and among families, the multiple benefits gained by involving grandparents is unlimited both for the families and for the grandparents themselves.

As professionals who may be involved in supporting families of children with IDD, an important component of any assessment is to identify the level of support needed by the family and the availability and potential sources of that support. This chapter has identified how grandparents are able to contribute across a number of areas to the overall well-being of the family, both emotionally and instrumentally. Whether this is assisting the family financially, providing respite care, a listening ear, a place to cry, or a place to applaud their grandchild's achievements, grandparents can make a substantial difference to all involved. For most families, grandparents who are well-informed and encouraged through consultations and planning meetings may have the capacity to make an important contribution to the overall aspirations and achievements of the family and the child with IDD.

Grandparents bring important skills and knowledge from their own professional life to this situation and this should not be discounted. For example, many individuals who have worked in education and healthcare may have worked with children with the same diagnosis and are able to transfer these skills to the needs of their grandchild. Likewise, grandfathers who are/were builders, engineers, or mechanics could possibly design and build equipment and aids that would assist their grandchild to be more mobile and participate in community life. Grandparents have significant prior skills in accessing internet information, either through their work or as a personal interest, which can be used to identify possible resources for their grandchild. These are all invaluable skills to be able to access not only for their family but perhaps for other individuals with IDD.

Avoiding Professional Bias about Family Dynamics

It is important to understand the family dynamics that exist within each family. There may be complex situations that occurred in the past that will influence any possible strategies and initiatives suggested for the family. This can be sensitive and time consuming but is more likely to result in good outcomes for the family if discussed early in the professional relationship. Likewise, it is worth reviewing one's own attitude and experiences with older people and grandparents, as this may influence how professionals view the experience and possible support that grandparents may bring to the family. Ageist attitudes and stereotypes can limit the potential support grandparents could offer their family. It is also important to understand that not all grandparents will be retired or in declining health, as many continue working not only out of necessity but also out of choice (Margolis, 2016). It is important not to make assumptions about the time they may have available to support the family and their grandchild.

It is also necessary for professionals to ensure that all possible support initiatives are explored in order to achieve positive outcomes for the family and, in particular, the child. When it comes to understanding the possible roles grandparents may play, it is important to understand several key principles. Grandparents are not a homogeneous group of people. They will be diverse in age, life experiences, education levels, and financial status. Some may be in good health, while others may not be very active or have health impairments. It is therefore important for professionals to not assume their capacity or ability to contribute to the needs of the family. It is vital to develop a true picture of who they are and discuss their understanding of the situation before making decisions to include or not include them in any family discussions or planning for the child.

Conclusion

Just as the structure of families has changed, so has the nature of twenty-first century families. A number of factors such as the health and marital status of the grandparent, whether the grandparent is still working, the geographic location of family members, and importantly the nature of the relationship between the grandparent and their own child will impact the type of relationship grandparents have with their family and, in particular, their grandchildren (Uhlenberg, 2005). Grandparents can provide an integral part of family life, especially for families with a child with IDD. The role and relationship they have with their family is unique and will be experienced differently from one family to the next. In the past, limited life expectancy meant that many older adults were frail or died before meaningful relationships could be established. A benefit of the aging of the population is that many grandparents are now able to be involved with their families in a much more engaging and participatory way, providing support and contributing as an additional resource for a grandchild with IDD and their family.

Key Messages from this Chapter

- **For individuals with IDD and their families**: Grandparents can engage in many positive activities in their grandchildren's lives, ranging from occasional to more permanent arrangements. They can be there to support the wider family, especially their own child, and serve to connect the various services they receive and to advocate for their grandchild's needs and aspirations.
- **For professionals**: Grandparents can play an important role in achieving positive outcomes for their grandchild with IDD and the family. At the same

time, professionals must recognize that family relationships can be complex and have developed over many years, which may influence the ability or the desire of the grandparents to be involved and any judgements on the situation should be well-informed and evidence-based.

- **For policy makers:** It is important for policy makers to recognize the significant contribution grandparents make to the circumstances of people with IDD. This contribution, through the provision of a range of services from child care, education, transportation, and other areas considerably impacts the cost of government-provided services. At the same time, little recognition is given to grandparents for these financial savings. Policies that provide subsidies, such as transportation vouchers, access to therapeutic services, or housing modifications, would ensure that grandparents continue to make this important contribution not only to their families but also to society at large.

References

Baranowski, M. D., & Schilmoeller, G. L. (1999). Grandparents in the lives of grandchildren with disabilities: Mothers' perceptions. *Education and Treatment of Children, 22*(4), 427–446. Retrieved from http://www.jstor.org/stable/42899587

Ben Shlomo, S., & Taubman-Ben-Ari, O. (2017). What factors may assist social workers to promote life satisfaction and personal growth among first-time grandfathers? *Child and Family Social Work, 22*, 482–491. doi:10.1111/cfs.12267

Bengston, V. (1985). Diversity and symbolism in the grandparental role. In V. Bengston & J. V. Robertson (Eds.), *Grandparenthood* (pp. 11–26). Beverly Hills, CA: Sage.

Condon, J., Corkindale, C., Luscz, M., & Gamble, E. (2013). The Australian First-time Grandparents Study: Time spent with the grandchild and its predicators. *Australasian Journal on Ageing, 2*(1), 21–27. doi:10.1111/j.1741-6612.2011.00588.x

Erikson, E., Erikson, J. M., & Kivnick, H. Q. (1986). *Vital involvement in old age: The experience of old age in our time*. New York, NY: W. W. Norton.

Falk, U. A., & Falk, G. (2002). *Grandparents: A new look at the supporting generation*. Amherst, NY: Prometheus.

Ferguson, E. B., Maughan, B., & Golding, B. (2008). Which children receive grandparental care and what effect does it have? *Journal of Child Psychology and Psychiatry, 49* (2), 161–169. doi:10.1111/j.1469-7610.2007.01840.x

Findler, L. (2014). The experience of stress and personal growth among grandparents of children with and without intellectual disability. *Intellectual and Developmental Disabilities, 52*(1), 32–48. doi:10.1352/1934-9556-52.1.32

Fuller-Thomson, E., & Minkler, M. (2001). American grandparents providing extensive childcare to their grandchildren: Prevalence and profile. *The Gerontologist, 41*(2), 201–209. doi:10.1093/geront/41.2.201

Gardner, J. E., Scherman, A., Mobley, D., Brown, P. M., & Schulter, M. (1994). Grandparent's beliefs regarding their roles and relationships with special needs grandchildren. *Education & Treatment of Children, 17*, 185–196. Retrieved from http://www.jstor.org/stable/42899352

Gonzales, E., Matz-Costa, C., & Morrow-Howell, N. (2015). Increasing opportunities for the productive engagement of older adults. *The Gerontologist, 55*(2), 252–261. doi:10:1093/geront/gnv013

Harwood, J., & Lin, M. C. (2000). Affiliation, pride, exchange and distance in grandparents' accounts of relationships with their college-age grandchildren. *Journal of Communication*, *50*(3), 31–47. doi:10.1111/j.1460-2466.2000.tb02851.x

Hastings, R. P. (1997). Grandparents of children with disability: A review. *International Journal of Disability, Development and Education*, *44*, 329–340. doi:10.1080/0156655970440404

Hillman, J. (2007). Grandparents of children with autism: A review with recommendations for education, practice, and policy. *Educational Gerontology*, *33*(6), 514–527. doi:10.1080/036012701328425

Kahana, E., Lee, J. E., Kahana, J., Goler, T., Kahana, B., Burk, E., & Barnes, K. (2015). Childhood autism and proactive family coping: Intergenerational perspectives. *Journal of Intergenerational Relationships*, *13*(2), 150–166. doi:10.1080/15350770.2015.1026759

Kivinick, H. Q. (1982). Grandparenthood: An overview of meaning and mental health. *The Gerontologist*, *22*, 59–66. doi:10.1093/geront/22.1.59

Kornhaber, A. (1996). *Contemporary grandparenting*. Thousand Oaks, CA: Sage.

Lee, M., & Gardner, J. E. (2010). Grandparents' involvement and support of families with disabilities. *Educational Gerontology*, *36*, 467–499. doi:10.1080/03601270903212419

Leopold, T., & Skopek, J. (2015). The demography of grandparenthood: An international profile. *Social Forces*, *94*(2), 801–832. doi:10.1093/sf/sov066

Lesperance, D. (2010). Legacy, influence and keeping the distance: Two grandfathers, three stories. *The Journal of Men's Studies*, *18*(3), 199–217. doi:10.3149/jms.1803.199

Luo, Y., La Pierre, T. A., Hughes, M. E., & Waite, L. J. (2012). Grandparents providing care to grandchildren: A population based study of continuity and change. *Journal of Family Issues*, *33*(9), 1143–1167. doi:10.1177/0192513X12438685

Lye, D. N. (1996). Adult-child parent relationships. *Annual Review of Sociology*, *22*, 79–102. doi:10.1146/annurev.soc.22.1.79

Mann, R., Khan, H. T. A., & Leeson, G. W. (2013). Variations in grandchildren's perceptions of their grandfathers and grandmothers: Dynamics of age and gender. *Journal of Intergenerational Relationships*, *11*(4), 380–395. doi:10.1080/15350770.2013.839326

Margetts, J. K., Le Couteur, A., & Croom, S. (2006). Families in a state of flux: The experience of grandparents in autism spectrum disorder. *Child: Care, Health and Development*, *32*(5), 565–574. doi:10.1111/j.1365-2214.2006.00671.x

Margolis, R. (2016). The changing demography of grandparenthood. *Journal of Marriage and Family*, *78*, 610–622. doi:10.1111/jomf.12286

Miller, E., Buys, L., & Woodbridge, S. (2012). Impact of disability on family: Grandparents' perspectives. *Journal of Intellectual Disability Research*, *56*(1), 102–110. doi:10.1111/j.1365-2788.2011.01403.x

Mirfin-Veitch, B., Bray, A., & Watson, M. (1997). "We're just that sort of family": Intergenerational relationships in families including children with disabilities. *Family Relationships*, *46*, 305–311. doi:10.2307/585129

Neugarten, B. L., & Weinstein, K. (1964). The changing American grandparent. *Journal of Marriage and Family*, *26*(2), 199–204.

Organisation for Economic Cooperation and Development. (2011). *Doing better for families*. Retrieved from http://www.oecd.org/els/soc/doingbetterforfamilies.htm

Reitzes, D. C., & Mutran, E. J. (2004). Grandparent identity, intergenerational family identity, and well-being. *The Journals of Gerontology: Psychological Sciences and Social Sciences, 59*(4), S213–219. doi:10.1093/geronb/59.4.S213

Silverstein, M., & Long, J. D. (1998). Trajectories of grandparents' perceived solidarity with adult grandchildren: A growth curve analysis over 23 years. *Journal of Marriage and Family, 60*(4), 912–923. doi:10.2307/353634

Stgeorge, J. M., & Fletcher, R. J. (2014). Men's experience of grandfatherhood: A welcome surprise. *International Journal of Aging and Human Development, 78*(4), 351–378. doi:10.2190/AG.78.4.c

Thomas, J. (1994). Older men as fathers and grandfathers. In E. H. Thompson (Ed.), *Older men's lives* (pp. 197–218). Thousand Oaks, CA: Sage.

Tomlin, A. M. (1998). Grandparents' influence on grandchildren. In M. E. Szinovacz (Ed.), *Handbook on grandparenthood* (pp. 159–170). Westport, CT: Greenwood.

Trute, B. (2003). Grandparents of children with developmental disabilities: Intergenerational support and well-being. *Families in Society: The Journal of Contemporary Human Services, 84*(1), 119–126. doi:10.1606/1044-3894.87

Turnbull, A. P., Summers, J. A., & Brotherson, M. J. (1986). Family life cycle: Theoretical and empirical implications and future directions for families and mentally retarded members. In J. J. Gallagher & P. M. Vietz (Eds.), *Families of handicapped persons* (pp. 45–65). Baltimore, MD: Paul H. Brookes.

Turnbull, A. P., & Turnbull, H. R. (1990). *Families, professionals, and exceptionality* (2nd ed.). Columbus, OH: Merrill.

Uhlenberg, P. (2005). Historical forces shaping grandparent-grandchild relationships: Demography and beyond. *Annual Review of Gerontology and Geriatrics, 24*, 77–97. Retrieved from http://www.cpc.unc.edu/research/publications/2468

Uhlenberg, P., & Hammill, B.C. (1998). Frequency of grandparent contact with grandchild sets: Six factors that make a difference. *The Gerontologist, 38*(3), 276–285. doi:10.1093/geront/38.3.276

Uhlenberg, P., & Kirby, J. (1998). Grandparenting over time: Historical and demographic trends. In M. Szinovacz (Ed.), *Handbook on grandparenthood* (pp. 23–29). Westport, CT: Greenwood.

Weibel-Orlando, J. (1990). Grandparenting styles: Native American perspectives. In J. Sokolovsky (Ed.), *The cultural context of aging: Worldwide perspectives* (pp. 109–125). New York, NY: Bergin & Garvey.

Westheimer, R. K., & Kaplan, S. (1998). *Grandparenthood.* New York, NY: Bergin & Garvey.

Woodbridge, S. (2008). Sustaining families in the 21st century: The role of grandparents. *International Journal of Environmental, Cultural, Economic & Social Sustainability, 4*(2), 61–68. Retrieved from http://ijs.cgpublisher.com/product/pub.41/prod.404

Woodbridge, S. (2010). *Exploring the relationship between grandparents and their grandchild who has a disability.* (Unpublished doctoral thesis). Queensland University of Technology, Brisbane, Queensland, Australia. Retrieved from http://eprints.qut.edu.au/41020/1/Sandra_Woodbridge_Thesis.pdf

Woodbridge, S., Buys, L., & Miller, E. (2009). Grandparenting a child with a disability: An emotional rollercoaster. *Australasian Journal on Ageing, 28*(1), 37–40. doi:10.1111/j.1741-6612.2008.00344

Woodbridge, S., Buys, L., & Miller, E. (2011). My grandchild has a disability: Impact on grandparent identity, roles and responsibilities. *Journal of Aging Studies, 25*, 355–363. doi:10.1016/j.jaging.2011.01.002

Woodbridge, S., & Clapton, J. (2012). What should I do now? Exploring family roles and relationships when a child has a disability. The grandparent's perspective. *Journal of Intellectual Disability Research, 56*, 736. doi:10.1111/j.1365-2788.2012.01583_8.x

Part III

Navigating Professional Systems of Care

From Birth to Adolescence

10 The Medical Perspective Developing Health Literacy in Families

Karen Summar, MD, MS

Introduction

This chapter will include a brief overview of the movement away from the traditional medical model toward collaborative and integrated care, the various roles and interactions within the physician-patient-family relationship, as well as important aspects of interfacing with healthcare systems. Specifically, tips for developing good health literacy, including communication skills, effectively navigating hospitals and medical facilities, and understanding the utilization of insurance coverage are described. An application of how healthcare providers can influence health literacy in families, utilize person first language, invite advocacy-oriented patient-family communication, and foster self-agency in persons with IDD also will be provided. As a point of clarification, the terms *parent* and *caregiver* are used interchangeably in this chapter, as are the terms *patient* and *child*. In addition, individuals with IDD often have special healthcare needs and sometimes are used interchangeably here, as well.

From the Medical Model to Integrated Care

One of the most common frameworks many helping professionals are exposed to within their education and training experience is the medical model (Laing, 1971), which is largely focused on assessment, testing, diagnosis, and treatment of illness, with primary attention placed on the patient at the biological and/or physical level. However, a common critique of the medical model is its narrow scope, often neglecting to consider factors (positive or negative) related to the patient's whole being or the larger systems of influence when determining the patient's treatment plan (Barbour, 1995). Thus, Engel's (1977) biopsychosocial model of care emerged out of that critique. Borrell-Carrio, Suchman, and Epstein (2004, p. 581) highlighted that Engel's work was a "call to change our way of understanding the patient and to expand the domain of medical knowledge to address the needs of each patient." Essentially, this more holistic and systemic model helped to pave the way for addressing the complex relationship of "contributors to and influences on particular health outcomes" (Borrell-Carrio *et al.*, 2004, p. 578).

In addition to the movement toward utilizing a holistic view of the patient, there has also been a change in the level of collaboration that exists between various healthcare providers (Borrell-Carrio *et al.*, 2004). Over the past two decades, many medical settings have moved toward an integrated delivery of care, an emphasis on empowering clients around treatment decisions, as well as incorporating the role of family in service delivery (Hodgson & Lamson, 2016; Hodgson, Lamson, Mendenhall & Crane, 2014; McDaniel, Doherty, & Hepworth, 2014; McDaniel, Hepworth, & Doherty, 1992). These considerations will be addressed in this chapter for aiding families and other professionals in better understanding the medical perspective.

The primary provider for patients with IDD during childhood is the pediatrician, who typically serves as the gatekeeper for referrals to other medical professionals and specialty care providers. This is largely a by-product of our current health insurance structure, which will be addressed later in the chapter. Learning how the pediatrician's office handles the referral process and identifying the key support staff who facilitate the "behind the scenes" activities for this process is valuable in achieving the collaboration needed to meet healthcare needs and maximize insurance benefits for the patient, especially for those who suffer from chronic health conditions.

Foundations of Health Literacy

The United States is currently in a transformative time for healthcare. Issues related to affordability and access to healthcare are in the news on a daily basis. Americans spend more on healthcare than anyone in the world, and yet have poorer health outcomes (Squires & Anderson, 2015). To change this, we must move away from a system that rewards *volume* toward a system that rewards *value*. This process will involve many changes, which requires patient-families to possess a certain level of health literacy. What is health literacy? How does one gain health literacy? The U.S. Department of Health and Human Services, Office of Disease Prevention and Health Promotion (2010) defines *health literacy* as "the degree to which individuals have the capacity to obtain, process, and understand basic health information and services needed to make appropriate health decisions."

Families with children with IDD will need to develop their health literacy on several levels. Individuals with IDD will develop their health literacy at their own pace, but caregivers need to develop health literacy at a much brisker pace in order to provide knowledge and support to the individual with IDD as they navigate healthcare systems. There are many ways for patients to become informed, including books, scientific studies, and internet sites. However, in the age of social media, it is important to find as many resources as possible to verify information that is received. Other methods of learning are just as important, including discussions with other patients and families who have the same interests and medical issues. Regardless of the learning style, being available to discuss lessons learned is paramount to developing health literacy. It is wise to remember that everything on the internet is not factual and it is essential for families to understand the limitations of online information. Parents are encouraged to seek out information through credible websites, including national foundations for disability-specific populations. Ultimately, parents should work to develop a balance between being pro-active consumers of information related to best practices and standard treatments, combined with consultation and guidance from a trusted medical professional.

The Role and Perspective of the Physician

One important aspect of health literacy is understanding the healthcare visit. All doctors learn to approach a patient using the *SOAP* format, which stands for *S—subjective; O—objective; A—assessment; and P—plan* (Physician SOAP Notes, n.d.). It works like this: a nurse or assistant usually asks the patient the reason for that day's visit. The reason is called the "chief complaint." For example, a parent brings a child to the doctor with a chief complaint of sore throat. The nurse writes down "sore throat" as the chief complaint and measures the child's blood pressure, temperature, and weight. Then, the doctor comes in and asks more questions. By putting the timeline of the illness together, the doctor has created the "S" or *subjective* part of the visit. It is at this point, parents can help create an accurate story by asking questions, filling in timelines, and reminding the doctor of things s/he might not remember. In this example, a mom who reminds me that the child had strep throat six weeks ago is very helpful.

A critical part of the "S" is a series of questions called the *Review of Systems* (ROS). The ROS may be just a few questions. In the example of the sore throat, the ROS would include questions about fever, cough, and runny nose. When working up a more complex problem, doctors use a more complex ROS. When your child has a checkup, an ROS should be asked as well. The ROS starts at the top of the head and goes to the bottom of the feet. Sometimes these questions are answered as the patient sits in the waiting room. Parents may want to develop their own ROS before a checkup, hospitalization, or visit to a specialist. The Table 10.1 provides some examples of the types of concerns that a thorough ROS can raise that may be helpful in making a correct diagnosis.

Once the patient's history is taken, the doctor moves on to the physical exam, which makes up the "O" or *objective* part of the visit. The objective part of the visit can also include x-ray results or laboratory studies. In our example above,

Table 10.1 Sample Review of Systems (ROS) for a Medical Evaluation

SYMPTOM	*FREQUENCY/DURATION*	*SEVERITY*
headache	daily	cannot play due to headache
cough	three weeks	throws up after coughing
vomiting	daily	only after coughing
sleep	—	sleeping well, no concern
behavior	daily	tantrums at dinner table

the result of a throat culture would be included in the objective information. One of the most important elements of the "O" part of the visit is often skipped—a thorough physical exam. In an age where there are many different technologies available, some doctors skip ahead to lab and x-ray results without doing a complete physical exam. The following example will demonstrate why that can be a problem.

One time I saw a teenager diagnosed with an autism spectrum disorder who was unable to speak. Six months before I saw him, he had completely stopped walking. During the six months, he saw five other doctors and had to have blood drawn multiple times as well as numerous x-rays, including expensive medical scans and lab tests. What he did not have when I saw him was a health-related diagnosis. After taking the history, I was a little overwhelmed that I was being asked to evaluate this child after so many other doctors had been unable to come up with a diagnosis. So, I went back to the very basics taught in medical school. I had him undress to his underwear and I started a head to toe physical exam. His ears, nose, and throat were all normal, as were his heart, lungs, and abdomen. When I started pressing on his bones, I felt a crunch over his hip. He had stopped walking because he had a broken hip. He had a broken hip because he was taking a seizure medicine, which had thinned his bones. None of the previous x-rays, CTs, MRIs, or blood work had shown the fracture because his hip had not been identified as the problem by a thorough physical exam. I believe if another doctor had pressed on his hip six months earlier, they would have made the correct diagnosis. Again, I am not relaying this story to worry people, but to let parents and patients know what to expect from their doctor. Vague symptoms that occur in a patient with difficulty communicating need a thorough physical exam in order to obtain the most accurate and thorough information possible. This information is then used to guide what x-rays or medical tests need to be ordered.

The "A" or *assessment* is usually the most complex part of the evaluation. In the assessment, the doctor puts the puzzle pieces of the story together with her knowledge of medicine and develops a ***differential diagnosis***. A differential diagnosis is simply a list of conditions that could explain the symptoms the patient is having. In the sore throat example, a differential diagnosis might include strep throat, a viral illness, or allergies. With more complex symptoms, the differential diagnosis can become more complex as well.

The "P" or *plan* is the outline of steps needed to return the patient to the best baseline of health. In the earlier example, the plan might include an antibiotic for strep throat. The "P" should always be treated as a dialogue between the doctor and patient or their caregiver. For example, if a patient has strep throat and the doctor writes a prescription for an antibiotic to be taken three times a day for ten days, the parent might speak up and ask if there is an alternative that can be given fewer times a day or for a shorter period of time. This is a simple example. When I discuss the "P" with a person with a special healthcare need or their parent, I invite their thoughts. Often, I talk about standard care as well as any complementary and alternative therapies that are of interest to the family.

Finally, when the "A" and "P" are being created, doctors, patients and their caregivers should keep in mind another diagnostic pitfall, referred to as *diagnostic overshadowing* (Kanne, 2013; Reiss, Levitan, & McNally, 1982). Diagnostic overshadowing occurs when a healthcare provider allows bias to enter into his/her decision making. This can be conscious or subconscious. A couple of examples will clarify this concept. One time I was consulted and asked to see a young adult with Fragile X syndrome. He had become sullen and withdrawn. His doctor and family were at a loss to explain the change in his personality. Further history revealed that his brother had left for college three months earlier and this young man was the only sibling still at home. I referred him for counseling and some changes were made at home, and he ultimately improved. I do not mean to sound critical of the doctor, but to make the point that the doctor saw Fragile X syndrome and could not consider other sources of the patient's symptomology. This is an example of diagnostic overshadowing.

In another case, a young child with DS had a sudden onset of refusal to eat and presented with a fever. After a careful physical exam, I became concerned he had appendicitis. I referred him to a surgeon who was dismissive of the family's concerns. Referral to a second surgeon confirmed the diagnosis. The first surgeon experienced diagnostic overshadowing—he saw a child with DS and nothing more. The moral of the story is this: children with IDD have many unique healthcare needs, but they are susceptible to every other ailment that any child can have. Parents should request a second opinion if they believe something is wrong and they are not getting satisfactory answers. Another lesson from this anecdote is that families must nurture good working relationships with their primary care doctor, who can be an advocate for them with other healthcare providers and specialists, when necessary.

In addition to the *SOAP* notes that are kept for each medical visit, doctors have other notes or lists when children have ongoing health issues, often called *problem lists.* For example, a child with an autism spectrum disorder might also have a seizure disorder and a communication disorder. These would be listed in the problem list. Drug allergies and major procedures are also included in the problem list. These serve as quick reference lists so the doctor does not need to read each and every note, every time.

Finally, these notes and lists are part of the patient's medical record. Many doctors and most hospitals have electronic medical records, and while personal computers, cellular phone technology, and the internet have allowed for greater connectivity, the same is not always true with medical records. A great deal of difficulty remains with the electronic medical record system. One office may have one type of electronic medical record that may not 'speak' to the electronic medical record of another office. The reasons for the lack of interoperability are complex. This is an area where we expect to see great improvement in the next few years, but in the meantime, it is one of the reasons parents should keep complete shadow records at home, so that when their child goes to the hospital, parents can provide current information that may help ensure they receive quality healthcare services.

Importance of Shadow Medical Records

From the beginning, parents and caregivers of children with IDD should develop a shadow medical record for their child. This record can be digital, on a computer, thumb drive, or CD or can simply be a notebook that goes to each clinic visit. Important documents should be included in the record, such as vaccination records (including type, date, and lot number), current and previous medications, current and previous diagnoses, a list of all procedures (including surgeries, x-rays, medical scan reports, lab results), a list of doctors and therapists, and emergency contact information. Records of current and previous medications, including any that were not effective or that caused negative reactions, are often as helpful as a list of drug allergies of the child. The shadow record needs to be updated after every clinical visit so that a timeline emerges, which helps healthcare providers provide better care.

Families can prepare for medical appointments by writing down questions beforehand. If they have questions, families should ask for an additional appointment time if their questions were not fully addressed before the end of the original appointment. By being assertive in this situation, parents accomplish two things—most importantly, they get the attention of the healthcare provider, and secondly, if the provider fails to respond, they may need to seek a different healthcare professional.

Considerations for Parents and Caregivers

Care for the Caregiver

Years ago, I learned that in times of crisis, fundamentals must be taken care of first. The concept can be summed up as the caution given on airplanes to "apply your own oxygen mask first and then assist your children." Before parents and caregivers can help their child, they must help themselves. Many times when parents receive a diagnosis about their child, they are overwhelmed, frightened, alone, and often feel as though they have been thrown into the deep end of the pool and do not know how to swim. In those early moments, it is important to encourage parents to connect with family and friends for support and to directly ask for help. For example, everyday tasks, such as preparing meals and doing laundry, can be done by friends and family members, allowing parents to focus on their child. Additionally, friends and family members often appreciate finding ways to help. Caregivers may need to be reminded to eat, sleep, and spend time with their other children. Healthcare providers can offer help in discussing difficult topics with other family members and other children, as parents may not have the knowledge of how to begin these conversations.

It has been my observation that when a parent receives an IDD diagnosis, it is not uncommon for their questions to immediately go to long-term issues. I have had parents of newborn babies ask me what will happen to them when the baby is 50 or 60 years old. From my own personal experience, it is important to help the family focus on the immediate situation. These are common questions and worries parents of a child with IDD have and should be acknowledged by the professional, while also helping parents and family members attend to the present situation, which may involve medical issues beyond the IDD diagnosis. Helping connect families to their support network and working to offer concrete answers to their current needs is an important first step for healthcare providers.

Communication: A Shared Responsibility

Because of the many interactions with the healthcare system, there are multiple places where miscommunication can occur. While healthcare professionals know a great deal about symptoms and diseases, parents know their children *far* better than healthcare providers. Often, a family member is the one person who coordinates the healthcare—not the healthcare professional. It is crucial for parents to have a good understanding of their child's medical needs and to be able to speak up and ask questions. The following vignette serves as an example of a great parent intervention that will help illustrate this point:

> "Anne" is a 10-year-old girl who was born at 25 weeks gestation after a pregnancy complicated by hypertension and diabetes. Anne's intensive care nursery course was complicated by premature lungs which necessitated a ventilator; a stroke; and multiple episodes of infection. She began having seizures while hospitalized. Eventually Anne was discharged to go home. She was diagnosed with cerebral palsy and developmental delay when she was two years old. A psychological evaluation performed in elementary school revealed an intellectual disability.

The child mentioned in the vignette, Anne, was admitted to the hospital because of a severe case of pneumonia. Anne's epilepsy necessitated the use of a drug called *clonazepam* to stop her seizures. When I wrote her admission orders, I ordered *clonazepam*. However, because of poor handwriting, the pharmacist dispensed *clonidine*—a very different medicine that lowers blood pressure. Her mother noticed the pills had a different appearance from usual and questioned me. I recognized the mistake and corrected the order.

A landmark report by Kohn *et al.* (2000) raised the awareness of medical errors. Since that report, much has been learned about the prevention of medical errors. Informed and involved patients and caregivers help reduce these mistakes. I share this story not to scare people about medical errors, but to encourage caregivers and patients to speak up when they have questions. It is essential that parents see themselves as part of the team and contribute to their loved one's healthcare by speaking up. Patients with IDD and their families understand the negative consequences of inadequate health literacy, and many may have experiences where miscommunication between the patient and a provider have had a poor outcome. However, many parents celebrate the relationship between a patient and a gifted, beloved healthcare professional. Ultimately, communication is a key ingredient for developing a collaborative physician-patient relationship, but being informed about how medical systems function is also essential.

Understanding Hospitals and Medical Centers

Children with IDD often spend time as patients in hospitals and medical centers. Understanding how hospitals function is an important component of health literacy. This section will provide a description for patients and family members in order to understand hospitals and medical centers and to be informed prior to a time when their child may become a patient.

It is important to recognize that a children's hospital is very different from other hospitals or medical centers. Children are not simply small adults; there are disorders and diseases that are unique to children. For example, if a newborn baby becomes unresponsive and is taken to a non-children's hospital, there could be a delay in diagnosis, simply because the doctors are not familiar with inborn errors of metabolism, which present in the newborn period. In addition to different diseases, some diseases may present differently in children. It is not uncommon for a child with pneumonia to present with abdominal pain instead of the cough and fever usually seen in an adult with the same illness. In addition, medications are dosed differently for children and some medications are not approved for use in children. Children's hospitals have medical staff who have additional, specialized training related to pediatric medical issues. For children with IDD and special healthcare needs, obtaining healthcare services from a children's hospital should be a priority for their parents and caregivers.

Health literacy extends to an understanding of how hospitals work. The emergency room (ER) is one place a child with IDD may enter a hospital setting. One of the primary goals of an ER is to stabilize a critically ill patient. ERs often utilize very specific, standardized protocols. These protocols generally work very well in emergency situations; however, families who have children with IDD should be prepared to advocate in the ER as they do in other settings. For example, most ERs would know to check blood sugar levels on a patient with diabetes, but they may not know to check an ammonia level on a child with a seizure disorder or urea cycle disorder. Before an ER visit is necessary, parents should develop an ER game plan with their primary care physician, which includes a list of their child's diagnoses, medications, allergies, the primary care doctor's phone number, and a suggestion for tests that should be checked based on unique healthcare needs. As children get older, they can carry this card with them in case they have to go to the ER without a parent or caregiver. This is a simple but important step, because the child's well-being could depend on this critical information. The primary benefit from this exercise is that the parent will bring greater awareness to busy ER personnel, which may make them realize they have a unique situation that does not necessarily fit into their protocols. They may also recognize that they are in the presence of a very organized and knowledgeable parent or caregiver, which can be an asset to them as healthcare professionals.

Hospitalization can be a stressful time for families. Parents can advocate for their children in many ways, from checking on medications to providing consistency through the many shift changes that take place, as there may be numerous healthcare providers involved in their child's care. At discharge, parents should take notes about follow up appointments, medications, what signs to watch for, and what to do if problems arise.

Reimbursement of hospitals from insurance companies often depend upon the quality of care they provide. One part of these quality measures are through patient satisfaction surveys, which are usually sent to the patient or their family after discharge. Regardless of whether patients had an excellent experience or a problem, it is important for patients or a family member to complete these evaluations, as they are important to hospitals for continuous improvements to the quality of services they provide.

Unfortunately, there are times when things do not go smoothly and problems may result during a hospital stay. A parent may have a difference of opinion with a doctor, or a child may have problems with a specific medical provider. If patients are unable to work out these differences, it is important to know that hospitals always have an administrator on call, who serves as a patient ombudsperson. An ombudsperson is an official appointed to investigate complaints about an institution. The administrator on call can be paged to assist the patient and family to work out these differences and try to reduce any potential problems.

Maximizing Health Insurance Benefits

The insurance industry is the final system of care where improved understanding will benefit health literacy. Because of recent changes in federal laws, health insurance has changed significantly. In the United States, through the Affordable Care Act of 2010, insurance companies are no longer able to exclude people from insurance because of pre-existing conditions, and they are also prohibited from having life time limits on insurance (U.S. Department of Health and Human Services, 2015). Both of these provisions are vital to people with IDD and special healthcare needs (Feldman, Buysse, Hubner, Huffman, & Loe, 2015). Even though these protections now exist in the United States, health insurance remains an extremely complicated topic and currently is in a state of flux. It is possible the economics of healthcare will continue to change for some time.

In the United States, many people have insurance through their employer, which often covers their family members, including children. This insurance is provided by private insurance companies who contract with the employer to provide a set of services for a set cost. Most of these policies have some cost sharing provisions, including co-payments or co-insurance that is paid by the patient. Nowhere is health literacy more important than in understanding these cost sharing provisions. These provisions are the out of pocket costs *the patient* will pay for medications, medical appointments, and hospital stays. Co-payments are usually a fixed amount and apply to medications and medical appointments. Co-insurance is a percentage of the total cost of an item and is most often applied to expensive medications or other medical services. Contacting a human resource expert at their place of employment when selecting an insurance plan is crucial for families with a child with IDD. Failure to understand these cost sharing provisions can cost the family thousands of dollars.

Many children with IDD and special healthcare needs will have Medicaid as their insurance, either as a primary insurance or secondary to employer-based insurance. Medicaid is a public program where the federal government pays taxpayer dollars to each state, who then work with the insurance companies to provide health insurance to the Medicaid beneficiaries (Centers for Medicare and Medicaid Services [CMMS], n.d.). There are income-eligibility requirements for Medicaid that vary across populations as well as across states. The federal government places some requirements on states in terms of what services must be covered; however, individual states have the ability to determine which services will be covered, which is why a person may notice their Medicaid coverage changing when they move from one state to another.

The Children's Health Insurance Program (CHIP; CMMS, n.d.) is another program funded jointly by states and the federal government. Medicaid and CHIP have different enrollment criteria that vary from state to state. In addition, the programs can vary across different states in terms of what services are covered. This is a very complex area, but all hospitals have staff who can identify what is appropriate for each individual and family. In addition, many communities have non-profit agencies that help with enrollment in Medicaid or CHIP. Just as with employer-based health insurance, Medicaid and CHIP can have cost-sharing requirements, for which the individual can be held responsible, so it is important to understand the specific details of each individual insurance policy (For more information, see CMMS, n.d.).

Once the insurance company has paid their portion of the bill, they will send the patient and/or family an explanation of benefits (EOB) statement, which explains the insurance coverage. At around the time the EOB is received, a bill from the hospital has also been disseminated. At this point, parents may have many questions. First, it is important to understand that medical bills can have errors, which need to be brought to the attention of the clinic or hospital to be corrected. Sometimes, if financial stress is great, families can negotiate a payment plan with the clinic or hospital billing department. In addition, there can be a problem with the insurance company's payment, so it is important to contact the insurance company directly to discuss any problems or errors. There are insurance company employees who work specifically with patients to correct billing errors. If you find that an insurance company, Medicaid, or CHIP is not responsive, a claim appeal can be requested for review. In addition, every state has an insurance commissioner who works to ensure that insurance companies are following the law. And finally, elected officials are available to help families who have exhausted all of these steps and have not received adequate resolution.

Principles for Practice

How can a provider help individuals with IDD and their family members improve their health literacy in order to live a healthier life? The very decision to live a healthier lifestyle can put anyone on the path to better health. Providers can encourage patients to become as informed about health and illness as possible by providing developmentally appropriate and culturally competent materials and by being available to discuss health goals and options for improving health. By practicing motivational interviewing, providers can help their clients learn to take charge of their health (Rubak, Sandbæk, Lauritzen, & Christensen, 2005). Building positive and supportive physician-patient-family relationships helps to optimize health outcomes. A relationship built on trust and respect will serve as the foundation for working collaboratively and effectively. Trust and respect are rooted in seeing the patient as a person, first and foremost.

Utilizing People's First Language

A wise mentor once told me "Everyone wants to be loved." That sage remark is a key takeaway from this chapter. It can also be paraphrased to say that everyone wants to be treated with respect. Everyone wants their healthcare provider to recognize them as a person who *has* a disease or condition as opposed to *being* the disease or condition. Many times, parents of a child with IDD find themselves advocating for this position with the very people who are caring for their child. Some parents may feel intimidated by healthcare providers. A gifted healthcare professional will encourage parents to be assertive for their child and for all children.

Healthcare providers should be familiar with the concept of "people first language" (The Arc, 2016). For example, healthcare providers should not use terms such as "Down syndrome girl" or "Down syndrome boy;" instead, they should say "Mika, the girl with Down syndrome" or "Matt, the young man with Down syndrome." If a healthcare provider fails to use people first language, patients and their families can use this as an opportunity to educate. Often humor is a good way to get this point across. For example, a patient or family might explain that he certainly does not want to be called an "appendix," and he does not want to be called "Down syndrome," either. Once the ice is broken, the concept of people first language can be explained. Teaching others about people first language will have an additional benefit. Professionals who understand the importance of people first language are often better at listening in many different situations. In order to become comfortable using people first language, it may be helpful to practice ahead of time, possibly talking to family, friends, or colleagues about using people first language.

Fostering Self-Agency in Patients

Not having IDD or special healthcare needs myself, I can only report from the perspective as a parent with my own child, as well as my perspective as a healthcare provider. Patients with special healthcare needs related to IDD should be provided the opportunity to develop health literacy at a developmentally appropriate level. People with IDD often are not included in the discussion of their own healthcare. Healthy or typical individuals would not tolerate this treatment, and neither should people with IDD and special healthcare needs.

As soon as children are able to communicate, parents should encourage them to participate in their own medical care—keep in mind, not all communication is spoken. For very young children and those with severe IDD, this may be as simple as asking healthcare providers to speak to the individual directly, not only the parents or caregivers. By gently encouraging children to respond directly to the healthcare provider, rather than their parents, children learn to take responsibility for their own health and healthcare. This is a delicate balance, encouraging the child to speak up and trying to get the most out of a short medical visit. However, each time a parent allows the child and healthcare provider to speak directly to each other, the parent is contributing to the child's greater level of independence.

Some children, and those with IDD, can become very shy around healthcare professionals. In fact, some are fearful of healthcare professionals, often because of previous painful medical procedures. Situations such as these can be improved by speaking with the healthcare provider or their staff before the appointment. Likewise, talking to the child before the visit can allay some concerns. Role playing is a powerful tool to teach children and those with IDD how to get the most out of the healthcare visit, allowing the child to be the doctor and the parent to pretend to be the child. Because many people with IDD are visual learners, the use of visual supports may be helpful. A book or electronic document can be created by parents with their child about the healthcare visit, which may help the child review and practice prior to the visit, thus reducing the child's anxiety. The internet has several sites that can help a parent develop visual supports for a variety of situations that need additional help with communication (see Center on the Social and Emotional Foundations for Early Learning, 2010; Loring, & Hamilton, 2011).

Healthcare literacy and advocacy will improve as the child's development progresses. Healthcare providers should be encouraged to direct questions to the patient. Only when additional information is needed should the provider ask questions directly of the parent or caregiver. At times, in their rush to provide care, medical providers may speak only to a parent or caregiver. Parents need to ask the professional to slow down and speak directly to the child. Some parents have reservations about interrupting a medical professional. However, my advice to parents is be polite, but do it! There are very few medical emergencies when a provider cannot slow down to complete a thorough medical history, which includes speaking directly to the patient.

Each person with IDD has a unique set of healthcare needs. But they also need to receive the same care as everyone else. For example, most children with IDD will need to receive the same vaccines as other children. Some parents worry that their child might be more susceptible to a side effect from a vaccine. However, as a physician, I worry more about the converse of this—these children are more susceptible to the effects of the diseases the vaccines prevent (see Hassinck, 2015). Often children with special healthcare needs are behind on vaccinations because they were ill during the usual vaccination schedule, so all parents need to ensure their children are current on all vaccinations. There are certainly some health conditions that cannot be changed, but there are many preventative behaviors that can be implemented that support a healthy lifestyle.

As children grow and develop, their understanding of health and wellness also will grow. Learning about their medical condition will prepare children for independence. Some patients with IDD can learn to take medications with minimal supervision. A daily pill box, which can be purchased at any drug store, can help organize even the most complicated medical regimen. Many children can even learn to administer insulin to themselves. It may take a while to teach and master, but persistence will ultimately result in increased autonomy. While it is necessary for children with IDD to learn about caring for their specific medical condition, they also should learn about health and wellness. Proper nutrition, exercise, and adequate sleep are the keys to wellness and should not be overlooked in the IDD population. These health behaviors serve as keys to wellness but also as mechanisms for prevention of illness.

Conclusion

In closing this chapter, I want to tell all parents and professionals who work with them to remember that the child with IDD who possesses special healthcare needs is a child first. Healthcare professionals are to provide all individuals with quality healthcare, including individuals with IDD. Healthcare is a relational process that includes interactions between the physician-patient-family and the larger medical systems of care. Each party plays an important role and brings specific assets and skills to the relationship.

It is also important to remember that healthcare providers can and do make mistakes and parents should ask questions, explore resources for improving one's understanding of their loved one's condition, provide positive feedback when they appreciate the manner in which the healthcare provider addressed their needs, seek a second opinion when they do not feel heard or valued as a consumer, and elicit direct involvement between the child and their healthcare provider for building a trusting relationship. Being a well-informed healthcare consumer will help ensure that the care one receives is the care they deserve.

Key Messages from This Chapter

- **For individuals with IDD and their families**: It is important for individuals with IDD to become self-advocates—no one understands your needs better than you. Individuals with IDD and their family members should learn about their medical conditions and what healthcare services are necessary for those conditions. Finally, keep yourself healthy by eating healthy food, getting regular exercise, and getting enough sleep every night.

- **For professionals**: Professionals need to learn and practice people first language. Use your position not only to heal, but also to educate—including lessons in self-advocacy, maintaining health, and navigating complex healthcare systems. Listen to your patients and their family members—they are the true experts in their care.
- **For policy makers**: Policy makers should get to know a family with a child with IDD and special healthcare needs. It is important that they gain an understanding about how the family uses federal, state, and local resources to help their child. Investing in supports for a person with IDD will lead to better health outcomes and more independence, both of which will be good for the economy.

References

Barbour, A. (1995). *Caring for patients: A critique of the medical model.* Stanford, CA: Stanford University Press.

Borrell Carrio, F., Suchman, A., & Epstein, R. (2004). The biopsychosocial model 25 years later: Principles, practice, scientific inquiry. *Annals of Family Medicine*, *2*(6), 576–582. doi:10.1370/afm.245

Center on the Social and Emotional Foundations for Early Learning. (2010). *Tips and ideas for making visuals to support young children with challenging behavior.* Retrieved from csefel.vanderbilt.edu/modules/module3b/handout2.pdf

Centers for Medicare and Medicaid Services. (n.d.). *Medicaid.gov: Keeping America healthy.* Retrieved from https://www.medicaid.gov/

Engel, G. (1977). The need for a new medical model: A challenge for biomedicine. *Science*, *196* (4286), 129–136. doi:10:1126/science.847460

Feldman, H. M., Buysse, C. A., Hubner, L. M., Huffman, L. C., & Loe, I. M. (2015). Patient protection and Affordable Care Act of 2010 and children and youth with special health care needs. *Journal of Developmental and Behavioral Pediatrics*, *36*(3), 207–217. doi:10.1097/DBP.0000000000000151

Hassinck, S. G. (2015). *An important immunization message from the AAP.* Retrieved from https://www.healthychildren.org/English/safety-prevention/immunizations/Pages/An-Important-Immunization-Message-from-the-President-of-the-American-Academy-of-Pediatrics.aspx

Hodgson, J., & Lamson, A. (2016, September). *Medical family therapy in primary care: Research updates.* Presentation at the meeting of the American Association for Marriage and Family Therapy, Indianapolis, IN.

Hodgson, J., Lamson, A., Mendenhall, T., & Crane, D. R. (Eds.) (2014). *Medical family therapy: Advanced applications.* New York, NY: Springer.

Kanne, S. (2013). Diagnostic overshadowing. In F. R. Vokmar (Ed.), *Encyclopedia of autism spectrum disorders* (pp. 938–940). New York, NY: Springer.

Kohn, L. T., Corrigan, J. M., & Donaldson, M. S. (Eds.) (2000). *To err is human: Building a safer health system.* Washington, DC: National Academies Press. Retrieved from http://www.nationalacademies.org/hmd/Reports/1999/To-Err-is-Human-Building-A-Safer-Health-System.aspx

Laing, R. D. (1971). *The politics of the family and other essays.* New York, NY: Routledge.

Loring, W., & Hamilton, M. (2011). *Visual supports and autism spectrum disorders.* Retrieved from www.autismspeaks.org/docs/sciencedocs/atn/visual_supports.pdf

McDaniel, S. H., Doherty, W. J., & Hepworth, J. (2014). *Medical family therapy and integrated care* (2nd ed.). Washington, DC: American Psychological Association.

McDaniel, S. H., Hepworth, J., & Doherty, W. J. (1992). *Medical family therapy: A biopsychosocial approach to families with health problems.* New York, NY: Basic Books.

Physician SOAP Notes. (n.d.). *Physician SOAP notes.* Retrieved from http://www.physiciansoapnotes.com/

Reiss, S., Levitan, G. W., & McNally, R. J. (1982). Emotionally disturbed mentally retarded people: An underserved population. *American Psychologist, 37*(4), 361–367. doi:10.1037/0003-066X.37.4.361

Rubak, S., Sandbæk, A., Lauritzen, T., & Christensen, B. (2005). Motivational interviewing: A systematic review and meta-analysis. *The British Journal of General Practice, 55*(513), 305–312. Retrieved from https://www.ncbi.nlm.nih.gov/pmc/articles/PMC1463134/

Squires, D., & Anderson, C. (2015). *U.S. health care from a global perspective: Spending, use of services, prices, and health in 13 countries.* Retrieved from www.commonwealthfund.org/publications/issue-briefs/2015/oct/us-health-care-from-a-global-perspective

The Arc. (2016). *What is people first language?* Retrieved from https://www.thearc.org/who-we-are/media-center/people-first-language

U.S. Department of Health and Human Services. (2015). *Read the law: The Affordable Care Act section by section.* Retrieved from https://www.hhs.gov/healthcare/about-the-law/read-the-law/

U.S. Department of Health and Human Services, Office of Disease Prevention and Health Promotion. (2010). *National action plan to improve health literacy.* Washington, DC: Author. Retrieved from https://health.gov/communication/initiatives/health-literacy-action-plan.asp

11 Allied Health Professionals

Enhancing Potential through Early Childhood Intervention and Therapies

Jennifer J. Bekins, MS

Introduction

Child development is a complex process that intertwines physical, cognitive, communication, social/emotional, and self-help skills. The first years of life are marked by milestones in these areas which are celebrated by parents and monitored by healthcare providers. What happens if a child begins to miss these milestones or is born with a diagnosis frequently associated with developmental delays, such as Down syndrome, Fragile X syndrome, or fetal alcohol syndrome? A child may be eligible for early intervention supports, but determining how to balance these services in addition to other aspects of family life may become an overwhelming task; however, allied health professionals are in the position to help caregivers weigh intervention options that meet the child's needs in ways that are sensitive to the needs of the family as a whole.

Overview of Early Intervention Services

Early intervention (EI) is a general term for the services provided within the first three years of life that focus on the child's cognitive, motor, communication, social-emotional, and adaptive development (Rosenberg, Robinson, Shaw, & Ellison, 2013). EI services have been shown to facilitate improved developmental outcomes in children with an intellectual or developmental disability (IDD) and reduced cost to education systems as the child ages (Guralnick, 2011; Karoly, Kilburn, & Cannon, 2005; Lazara *et al.*, 2011). These services may include developmental intervention, speech-language pathology and audiology services, sign language services, occupational therapy, physical therapy, psychological supports, vision services, and assistive technology devices and services (Individuals with Disabilities Education Act, 2004). In the United States, there are several different ways families may access intervention for their child with an IDD diagnosis, including state-run early intervention programs, medically based services, and private practices. Each option has strengths and challenges including cost, time, and availability, which will be described later in the chapter.

It is understood that outcomes will differ among children based on the age they enter EI programming and their diagnosis (Early Childhood Technical

Assistance [ECTA] Center, 2016). Many children will achieve skills equal to their same-age peers by the time they begin preschool and will not require additional special education services. Children with more significant IDD diagnoses may progress more slowly. The purpose of EI is twofold: to help children reach their potential in communication, cognition, and social-emotional development and to help parents support their child's developmental needs. The role of allied health professionals during the early years of intervention includes but is not limited to: screening and evaluation; planning, implementing, and monitoring therapy services; transition planning from an early intervention framework; communication and consultation with other team members; and ongoing education related to EI best-practices in their related fields. Regardless of the type of service delivery model (state versus medically based), a child with a suspected IDD must go through an evaluation process to determine what services are appropriate to meet his/her own unique needs.

In the United States, the most commonly received therapy interventions include: speech-language pathology services, physical therapy, and occupational therapy (National Survey of Child and Adolescent Well-Being, 2007). While there are differences between the scope of practice for each of these professional areas, they share foundational knowledge in pediatric development and management of conditions affecting daily living. Each with their own area of focus, professionals from these three allied health groups work to educate and empower families to understand and meet the needs of their child through techniques that can be incorporated into everyday routines.

Speech-Language Pathology

A speech-language pathologist (SLP) is qualified to address delays or disorders in communication, language, speech, emergent literacy, and feeding/swallowing (American Speech-Language-Hearing Association [ASHA], 2008). Communication is the process of expressing information and understanding what is being conveyed by others. This includes understanding and using behaviors to relay and comprehend wants, needs, and preferences. In infants and toddlers, communication may be verbal, such as spoken words, or non-verbal including eye contact, body language, and gestures like waving or reaching toward a toy that interests them. Language is a shared code of communication that includes rules that govern the meaning of words and how words are created, combined, and used based upon the social situation (ASHA, n.d.). Speech is a verbal form of communication, which includes the production of words and their clarity. Speech-language pathologists work in conjunction with audiologists to ensure that the child is hearing all of the sounds necessary to understand and develop speech, especially for those children with diagnoses known to contribute to hearing loss or a history of frequent ear infections.

If feeding concerns are identified, an SLP with advanced training in swallowing disorders may be a key member of the child's feeding team (Lefton-Greif & Arvedson, 2016). The feeding team may also include a physician or advanced practice nurse, pediatric nutritionist, occupational therapist, and/or social worker. While feeding skills are part of childhood development, disorders related to feeding add a layer of complexity that requires increased communication and collaboration to ensure a successful outcome.

Physical Therapy

With an educational background in musculoskeletal and neuromuscular conditions, physical therapists (PT) provide intervention to improve or restore mobility and prevent or manage health conditions (American Physical Therapy Association, n.d.). During the first years of life, physical therapists help children develop the motor skills they need to engage in their daily routines for play and self-care. This includes helping children acquire the strength and coordination necessary for sitting and exploring the environment through crawling, walking, climbing, and playing with a variety of toys (Academy of Pediatric Physical Therapy, 2010). Physical therapists working with infants and young children with IDD are trained in conditions that affect muscles, nerves, heart, lungs, skin, and other tissues. This knowledge allows the PT to develop a treatment plan that addresses the child's individual needs. For instance, a child with Down syndrome with hypotonia (low muscle tone) and ligament laxity (loose ligaments) may use compensatory strategies during movement that, if persistent, may cause functional limitations later in life (Winders, 2013). The PT may show the parent how to use optimal patterns of movement during activities such as transitions from sitting to laying down. The PT may take a different approach when working with a child who has had a stroke in infancy. If the child has poor posture and fatigue as a result of paralysis, the PT may work to improve sitting endurance through a home exercise program focusing on trunk stability (Children's Hemiplegia and Stroke Association, n.d.).

Occupational Therapy

Occupational therapists (OT) working with infants and toddlers focus on teaching the family how to support their child's response to and participation in daily routines within the natural environment (American Occupational Therapy Association, 2011). For very young children, daily routines may include establishing a sleep/wake cycle, dressing, self-feeding, and play skills that require fine motor coordination, such as stacking blocks or putting together simple puzzles. Occupational therapists also address sensory aspects of development, specifically how a child's body responds and reacts to his or her environment through the senses of vision, hearing, smell, taste, and touch. This may include body awareness, movement, coordination, and balance. Finally, with knowledge in the oral motor, oral sensory, and positioning aspects of feeding/eating skills, OTs may be key members of a team supporting feeding concerns (Edwards *et al.*, 2015). For example, when working to transition to cup drinking with a toddler who has oral hypersensitivity, the OT may try a cup without a spout. An open or spoutless cup may prevent the feeling of an object in the mouth, which the child with hypersensitivity may reject.

Working Collaboratively

Allied health providers frequently work collaboratively to address the child's developmental needs and in some instances, they treat together. Co-treatment describes treatment sessions where the services are provided by two providers at the same time. This type of treatment session should not be for scheduling convenience of the provider or family. Instead, the rationale for co-treatment recommendation must be well documented to support the benefit to the patient and include the goals that will be addressed (ASHA, 2014).

Co-treatment allows providers to see the child simultaneously while addressing complimentary skills (Jordan & Lofland, 2016). Examples of co-treatment for children with IDD include:

- A toddler with poor endurance due to congenital heart disease is learning to climb stairs and is beginning to combine words together. The PT goals may focus on alternating feet when stepping up. When reaching the top of the stairs, the SLP may have an activity prepared to encourage the child to put two words together while resting from the physical activity.
- A child with autism, oral aversion, and history of aspiration is learning to self-feed. The OT may target sensory components of eating while the SLP follows a plan for decreasing thickener in liquids. They co-treat during a mealtime with the child to address all aspects of feeding.

Co-treatment is not available in all locations and may not be a covered service for all children. Caregivers who think this treatment approach may be beneficial for their child should discuss this with members of their EI team.

Early Intervention and Federal Law

In the United States, the Federal law known as the Individuals with Disabilities Education Act (IDEA) Part C mandates EI services for children from birth to two years, eleven months old who have a diagnosis associated with a high probability of developmental delay, or children with delay in at least one of five established areas: cognitive, motor, social-emotional, communication, or adaptive (IDEA, 2004). The goal of Part C is to help families understand how to meet the needs of their child, support development, and decrease costs later in life via early identification and intervention (Rosenberg *et al.*, 2013). This is completed through comprehensive, team-based services and supports that are coordinated for eligible children.

Children may be referred to early intervention by their parent or healthcare provider. The Early Childhood Technical Assistance Center (ECTA Center, 2015) provides a comprehensive list of State Part C coordinators overseeing the implementation of EI services. Eligibility criteria varies by state as do the availability of intervention services (ECTA Center, 2015). EI services provide family-centered education and support the child's participation in their natural environments, such as home, daycare, and within the community through an Individual Family Service Plan (IFSP). Containing measurable goals, the IFSP is written with permission of the child's caregiver. EI services are overseen by a service coordinator who helps establish a team of professionals, including speech, physical, and occupational therapists, to meet the child's specific developmental needs.

Through Part C, initial evaluations, assessments, and ongoing service coordination are provided free of charge. If a child is eligible to receive ongoing EI services, the cost for these services varies. With increases in the number of eligible children and decreases in funding streams, many states have looked at how they implement their EI services (Grant, 2005). While many states provide services free of charge, others bill for therapy services utilizing a sliding-scale fee, private insurance, or Medicaid. The frequency, location, and party responsible for service payment are included in the IFSP.

While allied health services are provided for under Part C, factors such as personnel shortage, dwindling budgets, and service difficulty delivering services in urban and rural areas has affected the way the states address the needs of children with IDD. To address this need, EI programs have responded in several ways (Grant, 2005). First, many states have elected not to cover those children seen as "at-risk" including those with low birth weight, foster care placement, or elevated lead levels and instead focus on those children with more significant developmental delays or those with an IDD diagnosis, such as Down syndrome. Second, some states have shifted the primary referral to state EI programs back to the primary medical provider or the child's guardian. This necessitates increased parent-physician partnership and for families to have a medical home, where coordinated healthcare is comprehensive, patient-centered, team-based, and focused on quality and safety (Adams, Tapia, & The Council on Children with Disabilities, 2013). Lastly, some states have shifted the costs of treatment, including speech, physical, and occupational therapy services, to families themselves. These cost-shifting measures may include billing the family's insurance directly or charging a fee-for-service using a sliding scale based on income level. Families are able to learn more about EI services in their state or jurisdiction by talking directly to their child's primary care physician or visiting the Center for Parent Information and Resources (2016).

Medically Based or Private Practice Services

Part C for EI services are funded in part through federal, state, and local dollars; however, many states have had to look for cost-cutting measures given budgetary constraints. This has led to an increase in families seeking therapy services at outpatient medical facilities or private practices. Despite many insurance companies covering allied health services, individual therapy appointments may involve a considerable out-of-pocket expense for families.

In the era of high deductible insurance plans and increased co-payments, weekly or bi-weekly outpatient or private services may be cost prohibitive, particularly if the child receives more than one type of intervention. Depending on state regulations some children may be eligible to receive therapy services covered by Medicaid or waivers (more information is available at Medicaid.gov); however, a limited number of allied health professionals are also Medicaid providers.

In contrast with state-run EI programs that provide services in the natural environment, outpatient medical offices and private practices are often the antithesis of a child-friendly setting. Areas for patient care are often designed to meet the needs of adult patients or are very medical in nature. Providers who work with infants and toddlers understand that early milestones are developed through relationships and play, which can take place in a variety of settings. Therefore, an effort is frequently made to stage the environment to encourage parent-child interaction in ways that mirror interactions at home. This may include open spaces and portable steps to work on walking, carpeted areas for play on the floor, and even kitchens to address learning during mealtime routines.

Regardless of where therapy services are provided, research has shown that outcomes in EI improve when families are included in treatment (Dempsey & Keen, 2008; Karoly *et al.*, 2005; McConnell, Parakkal, Savage, & Rempel, 2015). This allows caregivers to understand how to apply therapy techniques to their daily routines. Rather than have a dedicated "therapy time" for the child each day, families are encouraged to incorporate skills into their daily routines (Hwang, Chao, & Liu, 2013; Woods, Kashinath, & Goldstein, 2004). While intervention services are valuable, the bulk of practice and progress is made outside of the treatment sessions; therefore, parental understanding of goals and therapy methods is essential for skill acquisition.

Case Example

"Christopher" is a 10-month-old boy with Down syndrome who lives with his mother, "Shelia," and his three- and five-year-old brothers. Shelia is a single mother who works full-time to support her family. She has already missed a significant amount of work to support her family while Christopher underwent open heart surgery at six months old. He is just learning to sit on his own and does not crawl. Christopher loves holding onto his mother Shelia's hands while she claps and says the "Patty Cake" rhyme. He drinks well from a bottle and babbles with sounds like, "dada." Christopher recently started taking baby food from a spoon.

Christopher receives early intervention services through the county but due to budget cuts, he is seen by a physical therapist, acting as the primary service provider, at home every eight weeks. When Christopher was in the hospital recovering from surgery, members of the therapy inpatient team recommended that Christopher receive weekly occupational therapy, physical therapy, and speech-language pathology visits. They explained that consultative services through the county's early intervention program were not enough to support Christopher's multiple needs. Shelia's insurance covers outpatient therapy but each visit requires a $50 co-payment. Shelia will do anything for Christopher, but she does not know how she can manage the recommended level of care given her work schedule and financial constraints.

Despite her hesitation, Shelia is able to make appointments for Christopher in the outpatient therapy department of the regional medical center. She attempts to "do it all," adding three separate therapy visits to the calendar, but quickly burns out. Shelia starts to cancel and not show up to appointments. Christopher's therapists talk to her about the importance of treatment adherence and compliance with visits in order to ensure he progresses. Shelia feels overwhelmed but is not sure how to communicate her concerns or balance Christopher's therapy, work, and other life commitments.

Principles for Practice

For families of children with IDD, Christopher's story is a familiar one. With the intersection of evidence-based practice, healthcare changes, and cuts to state EI funding, families may experience frustration with knowing how to meet their child's needs in ways that are effective in terms of outcomes, time commitment, and cost (Adams *et al.*, 2013). As in Christopher's story, allied health professionals frequently work in silos, not considering the implications of their recommendations within the broader spectrum of the child's needs. When therapists make unilateral recommendations, the family is faced with the challenge of balancing multiple appointments in addition to work, family-time, and other life commitments.

Historically, allied health providers have fallen in line with their medical colleagues by providing directive treatment recommendations known as *informed consent*. The allied health provider indicates that the child should have weekly outpatient therapy; therefore, the family should make every effort to comply with this recommendation. This model is paternalistic and inadvertently reinforces the "good parent" vs. "bad parent" mentality of treatment compliance, rather than taking into account the many factors that influence parental participation including emotional readiness. Instead, providers should take a broad view, understanding that treatment for the child should be family-centered and take into account linguistic needs, cultural preferences, and personal values.

Frequently, providers set goals and estimate how much time it will take on a weekly or monthly basis to address the child's needs for their focused area. However, in the current healthcare climate, it is essential that the family be a part of what is known as "shared decision making" (Hubner, Feldman, & Huffman, 2016). Shared decision making is a concept borrowed from the healthcare field, which changes the process of receiving intervention from one of informed consent to one of dialogue with the family about treatment options and their personal values and priorities (Spatz, Krumholz, & Moulton, 2016). This is particularly important if there are two or more ways for a child to receive treatment or if multiple providers are making treatment plan recommendations. At the end of the evaluation or prior to starting a therapy program, providers should have a conversation with the family that includes:

- Social-emotional dynamics of the home.
- Socioeconomic aspects of treatment or financial burden of care.
- Time commitments for each type of therapy and the trade-offs involved.

- Readiness to implement treatment.
- Barriers to treatment options presented (transportation, limited time at home due to multiple medical appointments, and/or parental work schedule).

While these topics may look daunting, they can be answered naturally in conversation with the family. It is important for allied health professionals to communicate not only the recommendation for treatment, but the time, cost, and level of commitment outside the therapy session involved on the part of the family. Once enrolled in treatment, it is essential for providers to maintain a dialogue about self-management or the family's ability to understand and implement the child's goals outside of the treatment setting. This reinforces a collaborative relationship and allows for adjustments to meet the changing needs of the family.

In Christopher's case, his mother is trying to balance life as a single, working parent with the increased care needs of her son. While Christopher's mother expressed interest in receiving additional therapy, it is clear she is overwhelmed with all of the recommendations. It is important for providers to partner with parents and caregivers like Shelia to help them feel respected and supported in the decisions for their child's treatment.

Conclusion

This chapter outlined the roles and responsibilities of allied health professionals providing therapy services for individuals with IDD, including speech-language pathologists, physical therapists, and occupational therapists, as well as a description of EI services. Regardless of how a child receives therapy services, from state-mediated treatment to outpatient clinics, allied health professionals are responsible for delivering therapy in ways that are responsive to the family's needs. By partnering with families through shared decision making, allied health professionals are able to increase participation in treatment as the goals are built upon the caregiver's personal values and priorities and are mindful of barriers to successful implementation. This in turn empowers families as they carry over skills throughout the child's day. As early childhood education and healthcare changes, continued focus on supporting the individual with IDD and the family in treatment decisions is essential.

Key Messages from This Chapter

- **For individuals with IDD and their families**: It is important for families to know what supports are available to advance their child's development. Early intervention services are available in each state and many private options are available; however, eligibility criteria and availability of services varies regionally. The aim of EI is to address the child's development as soon as possible in order to improve lifelong outcomes.
- **For professionals**: Allied health professionals play an important role in supporting the development of children with IDD. Therapists should help families weigh the many treatment options available by partnering with caregivers, rather than providing directive recommendations.

- **For policy makers**: Policy makers have the advantage of nearly four decades of evidence supporting the role of early intervention in improving outcomes in young children with IDD. Continued funding is needed for early childhood development research and programs. The return on EI investment has already been shown to have societal benefits including increased academic achievement, decreased delinquency and crime, and increased labor market contribution.

References

Academy of Pediatric Physical Therapy. (2010). *Early intervention physical therapy: IDEA Part C.* Retrieved from https://pediatricapta.org/includes/fact-sheets/pdfs/IDEA%20EI.pdf

Adams, R. C., Tapia, C., & The Council on Children with Disabilities. (2013). Early intervention, IDEA Part C services, and the medical home: Collaboration for best practice and best outcomes. *Pediatrics, 132*(4), e1073–e1088. doi:10.1542/peds.2013-2305

American Occupational Therapy Association. (2011). Occupational therapy services in early childhood and school-based settings. *American Journal of Occupational Therapy, 65*(Suppl.), S46–S54. doi:10.5014/ajot.2011.656003

American Physical Therapy Association. (n.d.). *The role of physical therapy with infants, toddlers, and their families in early intervention.* Retrieved from https://pediatricapta.org/special-interest-groups/early-intervention/pdfs/Role%20of%20PT%20in%20EI.pdf

American Speech-Language-Hearing Association. (n.d.). *What is language? What is speech?* Retrieved from http://www.asha.org/public/speech/development/language_speech.htm

American Speech-Language-Hearing Association. (2008). *Roles and responsibilities of speech-language pathologists in early intervention: Position statement.* Retrieved from http://www.asha.org/policy/PS2008-00291/

American Speech-Language-Hearing Association. (2014). *Joint guidelines for therapy co-treatment under Medicare.* Retrieved from http://www.asha.org/Practice/reimbursement/medicare/Joint-Guidelines-for-Therapy-Co-Treatment-Under-Medicare/

Center for Parent Information and Resources. (2016). *Services in your state for infants and toddlers.* Retrieved from http://www.parentcenterhub.org/repository/services-ei/

Children's Hemiplegia and Stroke Association. (n.d.) *Physical therapy.* Retrieved from http://chasa.org/treatment/physical-therapy/

Dempsey, I., & Keen, D. (2008). A review of processes and outcomes in family-centered services for children with a disability. *Topics in Early Childhood Special Education, 28*(1), 42–52. doi:10.1177/0271121408316699

Early Childhood Technical Assistance Center. (2015). *States' and territories' definitions of/criteria for IDEA Part C eligibility.* Retrieved from http://www.nectac.org/~pdfs/topics/earlyid/partc_elig_table.pdf

Early Childhood Technical Assistance Center. (2016). *Outcomes for children served through IDEA's early childhood programs: 2014–2015.* Retrieved from http://ectacenter.org/eco/assets/pdfs/childoutcomeshighlights.pdf

Edwards, S., Davis, A., Ernst, L. Sitzmann, B., Bruce, A., Keeler, D., Almadhoun, O., Mousa, H., & Hyman, P. (2015). Interdisciplinary strategies for treating oral aversions in children. *Journal of Parenteral and Enteral Nutrition*, (*39*)8, 899–909. doi:10.1177/0148607115609311

Grant, R. (2005). State strategies to contain costs in the early intervention program: Policy and evidence. *Topics in Early Childhood Special Education*, *25*(4), 243–250. doi:10.1177/02711214050250040501

Guralnick, M. J. (2011). Why early intervention works: A systems perspective. *Infants and Young Children*, *24*(1), 6–28. doi:10.1097/IYC.0b013e3182002cfe

Hubner, L. M., Feldman, H. M., & Huffman, L. C. (2016). Parent-reported shared decision making: Autism spectrum disorder and other neurodevelopmental disorders. *The Journal of Developmental and Behavioral Pediatrics*, *37*(1), 20–32. doi:10.1097/DBP.0000000000000242

Hwang, A., Chao, M., & Liu, S. (2013). A randomized controlled trial of routines-based early intervention for children with or at risk for developmental delay. *Research in Developmental Disabilities*, *34*(10), 3112–3123. doi:10.1016/j.ridd.2013.06.037

Individuals with Disabilities Education Act, 20 U.S.C. § 1400 (2004).

Jordan, K., & Lofland, K. (2016). Collaborative teaming: OT and SLP Co-treatment of autism spectrum disorder. In T. A. Cardon (Ed.), *Technology and the **treatment** of children with* autism spectrum disorder (pp. 49–57). Cham, Switzerland: Springer International.

Karoly, L. A., Kilburn, M. R., & Cannon, J. S. (2005). P*roven benefits of early childhood education* (RAND Labor and Population Research Brief). Retrieved from http://www.rand.org/pubs/research_briefs/RB9145.html

Lazara, A., Danaher, J., Kraus, R., Goode, S., Hipps, C., & Festa, C. (Eds.) (2011). *Section 619 Profile* (18th ed.). Chapel Hill, NC: The University of North Carolina, FPG Child Development Institute, National Early Childhood Technical Assistance Center.

Lefton-Greif, M., & Arvedson, J. (2016). Pediatric feeding/swallowing: Yesterday, today, and tomorrow. *Seminars in Speech and Language*, *37*(4), 298–309. doi:10.1055/s-0036-1587702

McConnell, D., Parakkal, M., Savage, A., & Rempel, G. (2015). Parent-mediated intervention: Adherence and adverse effects. *Disability and Rehabilitation*, *37*(10), 864–872. doi:10.3109/09638288.2014.946157

National Survey of Child and Adolescent Well-Being. (2007). *Need for early intervention services among infants and toddlers in child welfare (Report No. 8).* Retrieved from http://www.acf.hhs.gov/opre/resource/national-survey-of-child-and-adolescent-well-being-nscaw-no-8-need-for-early

Rosenberg, S. A., Robinson, C. C., Shaw, E. F., & Ellison, M. C. (2013). Part C early intervention for infants and toddlers: Percentage eligible versus served. *Pediatrics*, *131*(1), 38–46. doi:10.1542/peds.2012-1662

Spatz, E. S., Krumholz, H. M., & Moulton, B. W. (2016). The new era of informed consent: Getting to a reasonable-patient standard through shared decision making. *Journal of the American Medical Association*, *315*(19), 2063–2064. doi:10.1001/jama.2016.3070.

Winders, P. (2013). *Gross motor skills for children with Down syndrome: A guide for parents and professionals* (2nd ed.). Bethesda: Woodbine House.

Woods, J., Kashinath, S., & Goldstein, H. (2004). Effects of embedding caregiver-implemented teaching strategies in daily routines on children's communication outcomes. *Journal of Early Intervention*, *26*(3), 175–193. doi:10.1177/105381510402600302

12 The Education System

Building Partnerships and Inclusive Communities

Grace Francis, PhD and Sarah Nagro, EdD

Introduction

The educational system is one of the most significant systems of care individuals with intellectual and developmental disabilities (IDD) and their families will encounter. As a result, federal special education law provisions extend beyond educational contexts to meet student needs. These services can include behavioral, social, and emotional information and support provided to students and their families. With the national climate focusing on student academic outcomes as the primary means of evaluation (Kidron & Lindsay, 2014), education professionals including administrators, teachers, and staff may come to view the educational system solely through the lens of student performance rather than student care. Consequently, the goals of professionals in the educational system may seem in opposition to those of students and families they serve. Yet because of the importance of these relationships, it is critical for families to develop positive communication and good working relationships with administrators, teachers, and staff.

The Education System: Two Perspectives

"Sandra Jackson" sits at her kitchen table, seemingly unaware of the ruckus her three boys are making as they wrestle in the living room. The written invitation to her middle son's school-aged annual education plan meeting lies in front of her. The meeting is scheduled for next Thursday, giving her a week to figure out her work schedule. She wonders if her presence will make a difference anyway. She was too bombarded with information and nervous to say anything last time she met for his disability evaluation and no one seemed to notice. She knows that her son's special education teacher wants the best for Adam, but dreads walking into a room by herself with five professionals (four of whom she has never met) telling her what Adam can and cannot do and how his behavior disrupts others. She can't help but feel defensive, even though she knows they are just doing their job. These meetings are so different from when Adam was in the early intervention program for children aged from zero to two years. Sandra remembers the professionals in her house working with Adam and teaching her and her husband how to encourage his spoken language and tolerance of routine changes and sensory input. Although it sometimes felt overwhelming having so many professionals in and out of the house, Sandra developed close relationships with some of Adam's therapists and believed that her entire family's needs, including their emotional needs, were addressed in Adam's early childhood education plan.

Just a few blocks away, "Miss Rembold" walks back to her classroom from leaving all but two of her students in the lunchroom. She knows the importance of building relationships with her students so she uses her 30-minute lunch, and only break for the day, to celebrate students who have earned enough stars to have lunch with a friend and the teacher—a coveted reward. When Miss Rembold gets back to the room, she quickly checks the "Notes from Home" cubby to see which parents have communicated about attending upcoming annual education plan meetings. She looks over the returned parent slips and only sees two families who agreed to join her for a meeting. Discouraged, she thinks about potential ways to increase parent participation. She considers calling the other ten families she invited to follow-up with each of them and personally invite them to attend the meetings, but then remembers the math tests that need grading, updating tomorrow's social studies learning objective given the confusion during class today, changing the reading centers for tomorrow morning, and writing in student behavior logs for three students who have goals to improve self-regulation—all tasks requiring attention before 3:45pm when she starts with her after school group. Miss Rembold decides she cannot feasibly call all the families, but she can send another copy of the meeting invitation letter home with the remaining ten students in the hope that these families will get the letters and respond. Miss Rembold sits down, opens her lunch, and asks the two students what they thought of the football game last night.

The educational system is one that almost all families with a child with IDD will experience. For some families, involvement with the educational system may begin as early as infancy. As a result, professionals partnering with these families must be aware of the inner workings of the educational system ranging from early childhood to the transition from high school to adult life. Developing positive family-professional collaboration throughout a student's academic career results in positive professional, family, and student outcomes (Burke & Hodapp, 2014; Tschannen-Moran, 2014), making it an essential, and as we will review, legally mandated component of the educational system.

Sandra and Miss Rembold's perspectives are likely familiar to many families and professionals. It is clear that both parties want to maximize student potential, but are unsure how to accomplish this shared goal as partners. Students with IDD bring unique needs that must be met by the school system, while the school system and all the individuals involved in the students' education can be a very complex system for families to understand and navigate. Further, research indicates that including students with IDD in general education settings among their peers without disabilities has numerous benefits, including academic gains (Kurth & Mastergeorge, 2012), increased social skills (Carter, 2011), and higher expectations for *all* students (Kurth & Mastergeorge, 2010). However, the degree to which students are included in general education settings or, as we will explain, the "least restive environment" can create tension between families and professionals due to several issues, including systemic barriers (Ryndak, Jackson, &

White, 2013), a lack of educator professional development, and misconceptions about inclusion (e.g., students will not receive appropriate services in general education settings; Cullen, 2010). This chapter provides an overview of the legal requirements of the Individuals with Disabilities Education Act (IDEA, 2004), as well as strategies that educators, families, and other professionals can use to effectively communicate and maximize student and family outcomes.

Special Education Law: Individuals with Disabilities Education Act

The Individuals with Disabilities Education Act (IDEA, 2004) is the most recent federal reauthorization of the Education for All Handicapped Children Act (1975), the first federal special education law. This law was designed to enhance equal opportunities for full participation, independent living, and economic self-sufficiency among individuals with disabilities (Turnbull, Stowe, & Huerta, 2007). IDEA is comprised of six foundational principles designed to bolster these student outcomes: (a) zero reject (*every* child is entitled to a free appropriate public education), (b) nondiscriminatory evaluation (students are entitled to fair, unbiased evaluation to determine if they have a disability), (c) appropriate education (students with diagnosed disabilities are entitled to an Individualized Education Plan designed to advance student progress), (d) least restrictive environment (educators must presume that students with disabilities will receive education in general education classrooms among students without disabilities), (e) parent participation (legal guardians of students can contribute to student educational plans), and (f) procedural due process (students and legal guardians can hold schools accountable for following IDEA provisions; Turnbull *et al.*, 2007). We expand on these principles by describing how they are outlined in Parts B and C of the statute (the parts that directly outline services provided to individuals with disabilities from birth to 21 years of age), and how they relate to the principle of "parent participation," which will be described in the following section.

IDEA: Part B

Part B of IDEA (20 U.S.C. Sec. 1411–1419) includes provisions of services for school-age children with disabilities aged three to 21. Part B authorizes schools to use federal funds to carry out the principles of IDEA (e.g., hire special education teachers, ensure that students who need adapted equipment, such as a specialized computer to receive an appropriate education). Part B also outlines provisions for educators, families (which may include the student with a disability), and other professionals (e.g., social workers, school psychologists, therapists) to collaborate and create an annual Individualized Education Program (IEP) for students with disabilities (Sec. 611:1411). The IEP is a crucial and legally binding written plan that documents a student's (a) present level of performance, (b) measurable annual goals, (c) the amount, location, and type of direct instruction from special education teachers, (d) related services (e.g., physical therapy, speech/language therapy), (e) supplementary aids and services (e.g., accommodations, assistive technology), (f) the degree to which the student will participate in the general education setting, (g) participation in assessments, and (h) secondary transition services (e.g., post-graduation goals, employment-related skill development; Turnbull *et al.*, 2007).

IDEA: Part C

Part C of IDEA (20 U.S.C. Sec. 1431:14444) includes provisions of services for infants and toddlers with disabilities from birth to two years of age. Similar to Part B, Part C authorizes state agencies and schools to use federal funds to carry out the principles of IDEA (e.g., provide in-home therapy, developmental assessments). Also like Part B, Part C outlines provisions for families and professionals (e.g., service coordinators, therapists) to create an annual Individualized Family Service Plan (IFSP) for infants and toddlers with a diagnosed disability (Sec. 631:1431). The IFSP is similar to the IEP developed in Part B, as both use a team-based approach and document the child's present level of performance and needed supports and services (e.g., nutrition, nursing, family training, occupational therapy). However, the IFSP differs from the IEP in several key ways. First, as the name of the document suggests, unlike the IEP, the IFSP focuses on goals and outcomes for the child and family. As a result, IFSP services reflect child and family needs (e.g., physical therapy, parent training) and occur in the family home, daycare, or other community setting instead of the school. Second, the IFSP delineates roles and responsibilities related to goal achievement to both families and professionals (Turnbull *et al.*, 2007). In short, the family unit is at the center of the IFSP and the IFSP is tasked with identifying and addressing family concerns and goals.

Parent Participation

As one of the six foundational principles of IDEA, *parent participation* is an essential component of the legislation found to maximize student outcomes (Tschannen-Moran, 2014) and is embedded in both Parts B and C of the statute. For example, parents are required members of the IEP team in Part B, and the IFSP in Part C focuses on the needs and goals of the entire family unit as an additional means of parent participation. Further, IDEA (2004) also outlines parental rights related to continuous information about their child's educational progress. Despite the requirements under IDEA and copious research demonstrating the benefits of family-professional partnerships, many families report a lack of involvement in their child's educational planning (Burke, 2013). This is due in some part to school professionals' limited knowledge of or support to engage in effective partnership practices (Epstein & Sanders, 2006).

Despite these barriers, families note that positive and frequent communication with professionals is the most effective way to build partnerships (Francis *et al.*, 2016). Therefore, it is imperative that professionals and families collaborate to maintain open, informative, and effective communication to maximize IDEA provisions and, ultimately, enhance student outcomes. The following section provides partnership strategies that professionals and families can use to increase communication and create positive and productive partnerships. But first, we revisit Sandra Jackson and Miss Rembold.

> Sandra takes out her son Adam's IEP from the previous year. Attached to the IEP is a thick document with the title "PROCEDURAL SAFEGUARDS" written in bold letters across the first page. Each year Adam's teacher gives her the same document, telling her that it contains information about her rights under IDEA. Sandra smirks as she flips through the first handful of pages. "This thing reads like stereo instructions," she thinks. Sandra sighs as she turns her attention back to Adam's IEP. She quickly reviews his present level of performance and annual goals from last year. "Wow," she thinks, "Adam has really come a long way since last year. Maybe I will respond to Miss Rembold's invitation to set an IEP meeting time so that I can make sure that Adam is challenged at school."
>
> Miss Rembold is initially excited by Sandra's response to the IEP invitation. However, it doesn't take long for a twinge of stress to set in once she realizes that she has two other IEP meetings scheduled the same day. She immediately sends an email to the school counselor, occupational therapist, speech and language pathologist, and principal to see if they can make Adam's meeting. She also drafts an email to Sandra thanking her for her response, encouraging her to invite anyone she wants to the meeting, and reminding Sandra to contact her any time with questions or concerns. Miss Rembold ends the email with a smiley face and genuinely hopes that it demonstrates her eagerness to build a positive relationship.

Communication Strategies to Create Partnerships

Effective communication is foundational for building positive relationships and working partnerships. School partners are tasked with developing communication systems that are both effective and efficient to balance the constant flow of information to share and the limited time available to do so. Creating class-wide communication systems is one strategy to inform families and obtain feedback in order to build partnerships. Specifically, class newsletters, notes home, blogs, and class websites are common and efficient ways that school partners can share information with families (Epstein, 2011). Written forms of communication may be most common but can include accessibility challenges, such as language used, document readability, clarity, complexity, and structure (Epstein, 2011; Epstein *et al.*, 2009).

Family members have varying literacy levels (Kutner *et al.*, 2007), and the excessive literacy demands placed on parents, particularly parents navigating the special education process, may impede meaningful family involvement (Mandic, Rudd, Hehir, & Acevedo-Garcia, 2012). Recognizing these potential accessibility barriers for families, IDEA (2004) mandates that information for parents is "written in language understandable to the general public" (34 CFR 300.503). School partners can improve written communication by writing at an eighth-grade reading level or below and using tools such as the PROSE Checklist (Nagro, 2015; Nagro & Stein, 2016) to enhance structure, readability, and clarity, as well as reduce complexity in order to reach a wider range of parents while maintaining the intended message of the original document.

Text messaging is emerging as a preferred way for families to communicate with professionals (Relch, 2015) and is a fast and easy way to transmit quick videos, photographs, or messages (e.g., "Ingrid is doing fine in art today"). However, professionals may be hesitant to provide personal phone numbers to families (Strauss, 2015). Fortunately, there are several programs that school partners can use to send texts from mobile phones without disclosing personal numbers (see RainedOut, n.d., and Remind, n.d. for examples). School professionals can use such programs to send photographs, reminders, invitations, class news, and other documents, and families can use the same programs to respond back to the instructor.

Although in-person or over the phone verbal communication is an excellent way for families and professionals to relay information and develop relationships (Francis *et al.*, 2016), some barriers may make this form of communication challenging. For example, some families may need transportation and/or childcare in order to attend meetings at school (Lawson & Alameda-Lawson, 2012) or may experience difficulty taking leave time from work (Reynolds, Crea, Medina, Degnan, & McRoy, 2014). Differing first languages, views of disability and education, or distrust may also create misunderstandings or otherwise disrupt parent-professional meetings (Haines, Summers, Turnbull, Palmer, & Turnbull, 2015). School partners can collaborate with each other, families, and community partners to provide free or reduced transportation or childcare at the school to make at-school meetings more accessible for families (Francis *et al.*, 2016). Partners can also consider conducting meetings in family homes or communities (e.g., the public library) to reduce the need for families to travel to the school for meetings (Stetson, 2012). Further, reaching out to families prior to meetings to review the purpose of the meeting, review specific information that will be discussed, and provide families with ideas for ways in which they can contribute (e.g., bringing artifacts from home, developing goals or additions to the student's present level of performance, or inviting advocates to meetings) can foster greater participation (Diliberto & Brewer, 2014) and mediate potential disagreements (e.g., the degree to which a student is included in general education, the necessary supports provided to the student; Nespor & Hicks, 2010).

Parent advocates, such as those available through Parent to Parent USA (2013), "act as bridging agents in generating networks, connecting parents with others, articulating their knowledge with other parents' knowledge, and bringing additional communicative resources to encounters," such as a three year re-evaluation meeting (Nespor & Hicks, 2010, p. 309). Professionals can encourage families to invite advocates or other people to the meeting who can provide relevant information about the student and ask important questions (Trainor, 2010). Similar to bringing someone to a medical appointment, this process may help families feel more comfortable sharing information and better comprehend information. Parent advocates can also share information about community resources that the family and school can access to support student outcomes, such as Centers for Independent Living (ILRU, 2016), which provide services including advocacy, peer counseling, and independence skills training.

Professionals must address differences in languages spoken by families, including American Sign Language, in order to keep them informed. For example, IDEA (2004) calls for school professionals to translate written information related to student educational planning in the "native language of the parent or other mode of communication used by the parent, unless it is clearly not feasible to do so" (34 CFR 300.503). The statute also mandates that school professionals arrange for interpreters, as needed, to ensure that parents understand and can contribute to their child's educational plan (34 CFR 300.322). If finding an interpreter proves challenging, professionals can connect with schools in nearby districts to determine if they have an interpreter available as well as other community resources (e.g., places of worship).

Treating families as the expert of the student with IDD by asking them to share their experiences and wisdom on what works (or does not work) for the student is an excellent way to gain valuable information and learn more about the family's perspectives (Collier, Keefe, & Hirrel, 2015). As with any communication between individuals, differing perspectives or even disagreements may occur between families and professionals. One strategy for addressing differing perspectives is to engage in person-centered planning. Person-centered planning is a team-based approach to engaging in a relaxed conversation about a student's future and is shown to enhance parent-professional partnerships (Shepherd, Giangreco, & Cook, 2013). Typically, all group contributions are written on large sheets of paper hanging on the walls. This process ensures that all perspectives are equally recognized and that the student remains at the center of the discussion. This process also provides an opportunity to invite community representatives (e.g., job coaches, advocates, social worker, physician, Social Security representatives) to attend the meeting in order to gain additional information and connect families to resources. It is important to recognize that some families may be hesitant to contribute to meetings for a variety of reasons, such as cultural beliefs and expectations or deference to the opinions of professionals (Marfull-Jensen & Flanagan, 2015). Therefore, professionals should afford families the opportunity to provide alternative viewpoints through statements such as, "I remember you expressing a concern about ..." or "Is this approach what you envisioned?" to ensure that all members of the team, including the student and family, are heard.

Professionals who maintain a relaxed, friendly, and enthusiastic disposition experience greater partnership among families and can increase family expectations for their children (Francis *et al.*, 2016). Addressing family members who seem anxious with statements such as, "I can see that you are pretty uneasy. How can I help you feel more comfortable?" or "Tell me about your favorite recent memory with your son," is an additional way to address family emotions and demonstrate care and concern (Francis *et al.*, 2016). School partners may also consider addressing family members who appear agitated or defensive with statements such as, "I know you feel that the school system has let you down in the past, but I will work with you to help your daughter succeed," or "I know that I will need to earn your trust and I am willing to do that."

With these strategies in mind, we return to Sandra Jackson and Miss Rembold one last time.

> Sandra takes a deep breath as she walks into the school, grateful that her husband was able to come to the meeting with her this time. Tucked under her arm is Adam's most recent IEP, his latest evaluation report, and the procedural safeguards document (now with key parental rights highlighted). Sandra has not yet met Miss Rembold and cannot afford to be caught off guard. She fully expects to have to defend her son's right to continue learning in the general education classroom. Sandra could not help but feel startled when Miss Rembold met her in the hallway, extending a hand and greeting her and her husband by name with a smile. Miss Rembold led the Jacksons into a private room off the library and introduced Amber Johnson (the school social worker), Randell Jacobson (occupational therapist), and Tonya Grant (principal). Sandra began to relax as she sat down at the small table with her husband on her right and Miss Rembold to her left. Miss Rembold began by telling a funny story about Adam and sharing examples of his work and a video of him square dancing in gym class. Miss Rembold clearly had read the notes that Sandra sent about strategies to use with Adam and the other professionals sought her opinion about every part of the IEP. "What a change from last year," Sandra reflects on the way home. "This meeting reminded me of the meetings we used to have in our home when Adam was in the 0–2 program."
>
> Miss Rembold felt proud during the meeting to share with everyone all the efforts she and Adam put in to help him make gains in reading fluency and math computation. She was particularly happy when Adam's mom shared that Adam has been talking about this new "copycat reading strategy" he is working on where he copies how the teacher reads each sentence to practice reading with feeling. Miss Rembold learned about embedding "echo reading" into her lessons during a recent professional development session and was thrilled Adam was responding to it. She left the meeting feeling relieved, motivated, and having a clear direction for Adam's education. Miss Rembold learned that Sandra prefers texting because she is unable to check emails or take phone calls at work. Miss Rembold wonders if other families might respond better to information sent through texts rather than letters sent home and added researching strategies for communicating with parents through text message to her to-do list for this weekend. As she walks back to check on her class before her next IEP meeting, Miss Rembold sees Adam walking back from the bathroom, smiles, high fives him, and says, "I just had a chance to meet your parents and we are all so proud of your efforts

in reading this year. I also noticed that your dad likes cars as much as you do since he was wearing a NASCAR hat." Adam laughs and explains that his dad is bringing him to a race this summer as they walk back into the classroom. "You know what?" asks Miss Rembold. "I think that you should be the one leading your next IEP meeting." Adam nods and beams with pride.

Principles for Practice

In order to ensure that family-professional partnerships are meaningful, successful, and sustainable, it is imperative that school personnel take a multi-tier approach by establishing strategies at the school, classroom, and individual level. We outline several best practice strategies that are helpful in developing partnerships between school professionals and the families of students with IDD.

Creating a Positive School and Community Culture

A positive school culture that welcomes and embraces *all* students and families is essential for partnerships to exist (Francis *et al.*, 2016; Mapp & Kuttner, 2014). In order to develop this culture, all school partners (e.g., educators, administrators, custodial staff, office staff) must maintain the belief that: (a) all families want their children to succeed; (b) all families can contribute to as well as benefit from partnerships; and (c) all students and families matter and are worth the investment of time and resources (Epstein *et al.*, 2009; Francis *et al.*, 2016). Further, the inclusion of students with disabilities in general education prevents students from feeling "like the odd man out" and, instead, helps them feel like "valued members of the school community because their needs were met alongside their peers in non-stigmatizing ways" (Francis *et al.*, 2016, p. 284). School professionals demonstrating an earnest dedication to educating students with and without disabilities side-by-side enhances trust and motivates families to become more involved in their children's education and to contribute to positive school culture and functioning (Tschannen-Moran, 2014).

In addition, it is important for professionals and families to recognize how their own cultures, values, experiences, and biases may influence how they perceive others in order to disrupt preconceived perceptions that may have a negative influence on a relationship. A school-wide mission statement that reflects a commitment to building partnerships (Bronhheim, Goode, & Jones, 2006) and professional development activities on partnering with families, including culturally responsive teaching and relationship development, benefits all stakeholders. Further, school partners can recruit cultural and religious leaders from the community to serve as cultural brokers to build relationships with diverse families, including immigrant or refugee families who have children with IDD (Kugler & Price, 2009).

Another strategy used to build a positive and inclusive school culture is to create school traditions that incorporate families and the community. For example, an annual "back-to-school event" is one way to increase student interest and motivation, as well as family partnership. School partners can keep these events interesting by inviting students and their families to contribute to the event(s) through simple activities, like selecting the theme or location through surveys, as well as more involved roles, such as serving on planning committees, securing community partners to attend or contribute to events, and publicizing events through various media. School traditions and events create a sense of pride and community within a school and also provide an opportunity for students with IDD, their families, and school professionals to meet in a relaxed setting and have discussions that allow them to get to know one another outside of the context of student progress (Epstein *et al.*, 2009).

Empowering Families as Team Members

True family-professional partnerships include strategies to empower families to share in decision-making as team members (Nagro, 2015). Family partnership may take many forms at a school and should contribute to the notion of reciprocity among partners. Particularly for families with a student with IDD, family members can identify or communicate known needs and interests of other families and the community and collaborate with school leaders to establish and serve on committees to address those needs (e.g., parent support committee, hiring committee, policy committee, curriculum development committee; Francis *et al.*, 2016).

Families also can orchestrate a family welcoming committee in which "veteran" or alumni families connect with families who are new to the school to invite them to school or community events (Francis *et al.*, 2016). Family members can collaborate with school administrators to provide relevant family training and workshop opportunities (e.g., stress management techniques, special education laws, transition to adulthood, advocacy), as well as personally contacting other families with invitations to contribute to or participate in school or community initiatives (Zionts, Zionts, Harrison, & Bellinger, 2003). However, serving on committees or in leadership positions is not appealing or possible for all families. Therefore, professionals and family members should communicate with other families and professionals (e.g., schools with strong partnerships with their families) to investigate varied and innovative strategies to develop and maintain partnerships, so every family has the opportunity to engage in the education system in ways that are meaningful to them.

Conclusion

The benefits of family-professional partnerships are well documented in the education literature and extend to students, educators, and families (Burke & Hodapp, 2014; Tschannen-Moran, 2014). As our vignette demonstrates, families and professionals are invested in student well-being and are willing (if not eager) to collaborate in order to maximize student outcomes. However, barriers such as distrust, cultural/linguistic differences, or differing opinions regarding educational services are sometimes unavoidable. Families and professionals can consider the strategies presented in this chapter to develop or repair relationships so that these stakeholders can collaborate to prevent or overcome barriers.

Key Messages from This Chapter

- **Individuals with IDD and their families**: Family-professional partnerships begin and are sustained by frequent, positive, reciprocal communication that occurs between the school personnel, the student with IDD, and their family members.
- **Professionals**: Professionals have a crucial role to ensure that all communication is accessible; however, communication extends beyond sending notes home and attending meetings, and includes addressing differing backgrounds, values, perceptions, and dynamic emotions among partners.
- **Policy makers**: Policy makers should consider changing the phrase "parent involvement" currently used in IDEA (2004) to "family involvement" in order to broaden the scope of partnership activities beyond parents or legal caregivers to a student's system of caregivers (e.g., uncles, grandparents) who play an active role in the development of the student.

References

Bronhheim, S., Goode, T., & Jones, W. (2006). *Policy brief: Cultural and linguistic competence in family supports.* Washington, DC: National Center for Cultural Competence, Georgetown University Center for Child and Human Development. Retrieved from https://nccc.georgetown.edu/information/families.html

Burke, M. M. (2013). Improving parental involvement: Training special education advocates. *Journal of Disability Policy Studies, 23*, 225–234. doi:10.1177/1044207311424910

Burke, M. M., & Hodapp, R. M. (2014). Relating stress of mothers of children with developmental disabilities to family-school partnerships. *Intellectual and Developmental Disabilities, 52*, 13–23. doi:10.1352/1934-9556-52.1.13

Carter, E. W. (2011). Supporting peer relationships. In M. E. Snell & F. Brown (Eds.), *Instruction of students with severe disabilities* (7th ed., pp. 431-460). Upper Saddle River, NJ: Pearson Education.

Collier, M., Keefe, E. B., & Hirrel, L. A. (2015). Preparing special education teachers to collaborate with families. *School Community Journal, 25*, 117–135. Retrieved from http://www.schoolcommunitynetwork.org/SCJ.aspx

Cullen, J. P., Gregory, J. L., & Noto, L. A. (2010). *The Teacher Attitudes Toward Inclusion Scale (TATIS) technical report.* Carrollton, GA: Eastern Educational Research Association. Retrieved from http://files.eric.ed.gov/fulltext/ED509930.pdf

Diliberto, J. A., & Brewer, D. (2014). Six tips for successful IEP meetings. *Teaching Exceptional Children, 47*(2), 128–135. doi:10.1177/0040059914553205

Education for All Handicapped Children Act, P.L. 94–142. (1975).

Epstein, J. (2011). *School, family, and community partnerships: Preparing educators and improving schools* (2nd ed.). Boulder, CO: Westview Press.

Epstein, J. L., & Sanders, M. G. (2006). Prospects for change: Preparing educators for school, family, and community partnerships. *Peabody Journal of Education, 81(2)*, 81–120. doi:10.1207/S15327930pje8102_5

Epstein, J. L., Sanders, M. G., Sheldon, S. B., Simon, B. S., Salinas, K. C., Jansorn, N. R., VanVoorhis, F. L., Martin, C. S., Thomas, B. G., Greenfield, M. D., Hutchins, D. J., & Williams, K. J. (Eds.) (2009). *School, family, and community partnerships: Your handbook for action* (3rd ed.). Thousand Oaks, CA: Corwin Press.

Francis, G. L., Blue-Banning, M., Turnbull, A. P., Hill, C., Haines, S. J., & Gross, J. M. S. (2016). Culture in inclusive schools: Parental perspectives on trusting family-school partnerships. *Education and Training in Autism and Developmental Disabilities*, *51*(3), 281–293. Retrieved from http://daddcec.org/

Haines, S. J., Summers, J. A., Turnbull, A. P., Palmer, S. B., & Turnbull, H. R. (2015). Fostering Habib's engagement and self-regulation: A case study of a child from a refugee family at home and preschool. *Topics in Early Childhood Special Education*, *35*(1), 28–39. doi:10.1177/0271121414552905

ILRU. (2016). *ILRU directory of centers for independent living (CILs) and associations, 2016* (vol. *38*). Retrieved from http://www.ilru.org/projects/cil-net/cil-center-and-association-directory

Individuals with Disabilities Education Act, 20 U.S.C. § 1400 *et seq*. (2004).

Kidron, Y., & Lindsay, J. (2014). *The effects of increased learning time on student academic and nonacademic outcomes: Findings from a meta-analytic review* (REL 2014–015). Washington, DC: U.S. Department of Education, Institute of Education Sciences, National Center for Education Evaluation and Regional Assistance, Regional Educational Laboratory Appalachia. Retrieved from http://ies.ed.gov/ncee/edlabs

Kugler, E. G., & Price, O. A. (2009). Go beyond the classroom to help immigrant and refugee students' success. *Phi Delta Kappan*, *91*(3), 48–52. doi:10.1177/003172170909100310

Kurth, J. A., & Mastergeorge, A. M. (2010). Individual education plan goals and services for adolescents with autism: Impact of age and educational setting. *The Journal of Special Education*, *44*, 146–160. doi:10.1177/0022466908329825

Kurth, J. A., & Mastergeorge, A. M. (2012). Impact of setting and instructional context for adolescents with autism. *The Journal of Special Education*, *46*, 36–48. doi:10.1177/0022466910366480

Kutner, M., Greenberg, E., Jin, Y., Boyle, B., Hsu, Y., & Dunleavy, E. (2007). *Literacy in everyday life: Results from the 2003 National Assessment of Adult Literacy* (NCES 2007–480). Washington, DC: U.S. Department of Education.

Lawson, M. A., & Alameda-Lawson, T. (2012). A case study of school-linked, collective parent engagement. *American Educational Research Association*, *49*(4), 651–684. doi:10.3102/0002831211427206

Mandic, C., Rudd, R., Hehir, T., & Acevedo-Garcia, D. (2012). Readability of special education procedural safeguards. *Journal of Special Education*, *45*(4), 195–203. doi:10.1177/0022466910362774

Mapp, K. L., & Kuttner, P. J. (2014). *Partners in education: A dual capacity building framework for school-family partnerships*. Austin, TX: Southwest Educational Development Lab. Retrieved from http://www.sedl.org/pubs/framework/

Marfull-Jensen, M., & Flanagan, T. (2015). The 2010 Chilean national disability law: Self-determination in a collectivistic society. *Journal of Disability Policy Studies*, *26*(3), 144–152. doi:10.1177/1044207314533384

Nagro, S. A. (2015). PROSE checklist: Strategies for improving school-to-home written communication. *Teaching Exceptional Children*, *47*(5), 256–263. doi:10.1177/0040059915580031

Nagro, S. A., & Stein, M. L. (2016). Measuring accessibility of written communication for parents of students with disabilities: Reviewing 30 years of readability research. *Journal of Disability Policy Studies*, *27*, 13–21. doi:10.1177/1044207314557489

Nespor, J., & Hicks, D. (2010). Wizards and witches: Parent advocates and contention in special education in the USA. *Journal of Education Policy*, *25*(3), 309–334. doi:10.1080/02680931003671954

Parent to Parent USA. (2013). *P2P USA: Parent to Parent USA*. Retrieved from http://www.p2pusa.org

RainedOut. (n.d.). *RainedOut: Know before you go*. Retrieved from http://www.rainedout.com/

Relch, J. (2015). *Thinking about texting parents? Best practices for school-to-parent texting*. Retrieved from http://blogs.edweek.org/edweek/edtechresearcher/2015/12/thinking_about_texting_parents_best_practices_for_school-to-parent_texting.html

Remind. (n.d.). *Remind: Safe classroom communication*. Retrieved from https://www.remind.com/

Reynolds, A. D., Crea, T. M., Medina, J., Degnan, E., & McRoy, R. (2014). A mixed methods case study of parent involvement in an urban high school serving minority students. *Urban Education*, *50*(6), 750–775. doi:10.1177/0042085914534272

Ryndak, D. L., Jackson, L. B., & White, J. M. (2013). Involvement and progress in the general curriculum for students with extensive support needs: K-12 inclusive-education research and implications for the future. *Inclusion*, *1*, 28–49. doi:10.1352/2326-6988-1.1.028

Shepherd, K. G., Giangreco, M. F., & Cook, B. G. (2013). Parent participation in assessment and in development of individualized education programs. In B. G. Cook & M. Tankersley (Eds.), *Research-based practices in special education* (pp. 260–271). Boston, MA: Pearson.

Stetson, R. (2012). Home visits: Teacher reflections about relationships, student behavior, and achievement. *Issues in Teacher Education*, *21*, 21–37. Retrieved from https://www.itejournal.org/back-issues/spring-2012/Spring_12_TOC.html

Strauss, V. (2015). *Teacher: Why I gave my cell phone number to my students' parents*. Retrieved from https://www.washingtonpost.com/news/answer-sheet/wp/2015/09/15/teacher-why-i-gave-my-cell-phone-number-to-my-students-parents/?utm_term=.323e02aa7e40

Trainor, A. (2010). Diverse approaches to parent advocacy during special education home-school interactions: Identification and use of cultural and social capital. *Remedial and Special Education*, *31*, 34–47. doi:10.1177/0741932508324401

Tschannen-Moran, M. (2014). *Trust matters: Leadership for successful schools* (2nd ed.). San Francisco, CA: Jossey-Bass.

Turnbull, H. R., Stowe, M., & Huerta, N. (2007). *Free appropriate public education: The law and children with disabilities* (7th ed.). Denver, CO: Love Publishing Company.

Zionts, L. T., Zionts, P., Harrison, S., & Bellinger, O. (2003). Urban African American families' perceptions of cultural sensitivity within the special education system. *Focus on Autism and Other Developmental Disabilities*, *18*, 41–50. doi:10.1177/10883576030180010

Part IV

Preparing for the Future

The Transition to Adulthood and Beyond

13 Special Needs Financial Planning

Optimizing Resources for the Future

Mitzi K. Lauderdale, JD, CFP®, Michael C. Walther II, CPA/PFS, CFP®, CFA®, and Nicole Piland Springer, PhD

Introduction

Individuals with intellectual and development disabilities (IDD) and their families need to plan for the future for a number of reasons. While no one can predict with certainty what the long-term costs are for an individual with special needs, in almost all circumstances the amounts can be daunting for a family to cover on their own. Therefore, it is critical for families with loved ones with IDD to plan as effectively as possible for their future financial needs. In many cases, the financial planning for a child with special needs is akin to planning for a "third retirement" in the family. In addition to the expenses that need to be covered for parent(s)' retirement, a third set of expenses, which usually arise when the school district supports end in the child's early 20s, must also be included in the family's planning. This is complicated further for those raising a child with IDD as a single parent and trying to plan with only one income.

The reality is, most families with children with IDD do not have a special needs plan in place. Special needs plans include financial, legal, housing and care plans. While helping professionals may not believe they play an important role in the financial planning process, they could actually be the catalyst for some families to take a step toward putting a plan in place. In fact, Lauderdale and Huston (2012a) found that families who were encouraged by a mental health professional to put a plan in place were approximately 16 times more likely to have a plan, which included a special needs trust, a legal foundation for a special needs financial plan. While there is no need to be an expert on all areas, it is imperative that professionals have a basic understanding of what resources and barriers exist for special needs planning and, at a minimum, encourage families to consider developing a plan.

In a series of focus groups conducted by Lauderdale, Durband, Scott, and Springer (2010), parents expressed many fears and identified emotional stressors related to future planning. Fears arose in relation to financial planning obstacles, such as where to start, where to go, what resources to access, volumes of paperwork, fear of losing benefits, fighting insurance claims, and out-of-pocket expenses. Emotional stressors were identified within immediate and extended families, as well as communities and within their schools. Parents expressed feelings of isolation and that others could not relate to their situation, as well as concerns related to the stigma of IDD (Lauderdale *et al.*, 2010). As if the daily functioning of a family with a child with IDD is not enough, planning for the future is crucial, both from a financial perspective but also for providing continuity of care for their loved one. The following quote by one parent captures the complex set of questions parents often face with regard to planning:

> What will happen to him when I'm gone? Where will he live? Who will he live with? Who will give him his allowance? Take him places he needs to go? All that, and there's just not a lot of people who will step up and take on a disabled child. So could he live on his own? I don't know. Who would pay his bills? Who would do that?
>
> (Lauderdale *et al.*, 2010)

Another parent expressed her concern about not yet establishing guardianship:

> I mean what if some freak thing happened, something happened to both of us at the same time, we'd be in trouble. I wouldn't want him to go to the state. So you know, he'd be a lot better off with family.
>
> (Lauderdale *et al.*, 2010)

Individuals are provided services and education in the public-school system through age 21 in most states. After aging out of the school district supports, families must have a plan in place for their young adult with IDD. The plan should include information about activities and jobs, living situation, and financial support for the individual. In most school districts, the years leading up to age 21 are termed "the transition years." During this time, it is essential for families to finalize the plans for their loved one with IDD, if the decisions have not previously been made. Timing and onset of the disability impacts the planning process. In cases where the disability arises after the start of adulthood, the urgency to develop and implement a plan increases and, in some cases, fewer financial planning tools are available.

With proper special needs financial planning, families can stretch their savings further and create opportunities for the best possible lives for their loved ones with IDD. Ensuring that loved ones with IDD receive the maximum benefits from government entitlement programs is a cornerstone of special needs financial planning. The government is required to provide housing, healthcare, and food; however, proper planning allows families to supplement what the government provides (Nadworny & Haddad, 2007). Ultimately, the goal of special needs planning is to ensure continuity of care is provided for the loved one with IDD.

While the lifetime expenses for an individual with special needs can be staggering, it is often the caregiving decisions that are the most stressful for the parents. Therefore, in addition to evaluating the lifetime expenses faced by families, special needs financial planning must also address how and by whom care will be provided in the future. Determining who will be designated as the future caregiver is the greatest barrier experienced by families during the steps towards planning. The reality is that even the best special needs financial planning cannot replace the care and love provided by the family members of individuals with IDD (Lauderdale *et al.*, 2010). Even when there are siblings of individuals with IDD, parents expressed not wanting their other children to foot the "burden" of care for the sibling. As one parent stated, "I don't want it to fall onto my other children because I want them to have a life. I want them to be there, you know, to see him, to love him, but not to take care of him." Some mothers described how hard it was to say out loud, but secretly hoped, that their child would die first or they all "die at the same time" so that such planning would not be needed (Lauderdale *et al.*, 2010).

With the word "financial" in the title of this chapter, it is fair to assume it is all about money and resources. However, the content here focuses more on the personal side of planning. While assets and income are necessary to meet future goals, the family goals are pointless without the people necessary to implement the plan and see it to fruition. First and foremost, communication is key with family members, healthcare professionals, schools, friends, professional partners, and communities. After discussing the most crucial role of communication, we will present legal and financial tools available for planning, followed by ways to fund the financial plan in order to care for a child with IDD over a lifetime. Lastly, we will conclude with keys to successful planning.

Communication

Communication is important in all relationships, and it is essential for families with children with IDD. From professional experience, a significant challenge to communicating effectively the needs and goals of the individual and the family to the extended family is the stigma many families feel about their loved one's disability. While it is unfortunate that some families are unable to share the details of their planning with relatives, knowledge that stigma is a barrier can help the family's advisors provide communication support (Mittan, 2010; Thompson, 2016). A common challenge experienced by families, in terms of communicating their wishes, was shared by one focus group participant (Lauderdale *et al.*, 2010).

> The hardest part was guardians and telling family [members] that they weren't on the list. That was the hard part for us. None of our guardians are family members because our families just don't understand all that goes into taking care of them medically.

From many years of experience, the stigma barrier seems to be strongest in families with loved ones with a mental illness, but it exists at some level in almost all families with a child with special needs (Greenstein, 2017; The Arc, 2016; University of Washington, 2016). Hopefully with time, the perceptions in society will change and stigma for families will diminish, but until then, recognizing and managing stigma are part of an effective communication strategy.

Key Elements of Quality Communication

There are three areas where quality communication can deliver positive results. The first is the ability to maintain government benefits. Letting family members know the preferred way for them to title gifts to the relative with IDD can be the difference between maintaining uninterrupted social services and losing government benefits for a month or longer (Social Security Administration [SSA], 2016). Unexpected gifts that are given outright to the individual with IDD can cause the individual's personal resources to exceed the limits, thereby suspending his/her benefits until the excess can be rectified. (See Chapter 15 for more information.)

Another positive outcome from effective communication is the alignment of estate planning documents. If the estate planning of the grandparents, parents, and other family members are all aligned, the flow of assets is not just enhanced from a tax planning perspective, but also from a special needs planning perspective. Knowing that siblings or other relatives are being named to play various support roles, when the parents of the individual with IDD pass away, can help the broader family plan for their future and avoid unnecessary surprises. In addition, the special needs trust(s) that are being established for the benefit of the loved one with IDD should be the named beneficiary rather than the individual him/herself in the family's estate documents (Nadworny & Haddad, 2007). The proper titling of beneficiaries in estate plans is only possible with proper communication.

A third reason for communicating broadly with one's family is the ability to identify future funding sources for the expenses of the individual with IDD. If a family member or grandparent is planning to leave an inheritance to the child with special needs, it can impact the amount of insurance and savings the parents set aside for the child's future care. While it could be careless to assume that all future needs will be covered by the gifts from the extended family, having knowledge about planned gifts is important. Based on our professional experience, even in cases in which there is an awareness that gifts are coming from relatives at death, it is rare when the amounts are known with certainty or specificity. As such, parents should still make firm plans for covering their child's future financial needs and document that additional resources are likely coming from other family sources.

Care Guides and Letters of Intent

One of the most valuable tools that a parent can develop and leave behind for their loved one is a *care guide*. The document is often referred to as a *letter of intent* (Hoyt & Pollock, 2003; O'Hara & Frishman, 2013). The primary focus of the document should be on the current and future care needs of the individual with IDD (Nadworny & Haddad, 2007; O'Hara & Frishman, 2013). Unlike a family's legal documents, which will detail how trusts are to be managed and distributed, or who the executor, guardian, and agents for the powers of attorney will be (See Chapter 15), the care guide is a non-legal, non-binding document. While an ideal plan would be to involve a special needs financial planner who focuses their practice on families with special needs, some families are simply not ready or cannot overcome their own barriers to take that first step. Lauderdale and Huston (2012b) suggested that professionals may help families through the process of creating a letter of intent. Oftentimes, the letter of intent is the ideal starting place for a family to use as a map or "to do" list to fill in the necessary information (Lauderdale & Huston, 2013a). A letter of intent can then be developed into a care guide, which outlines the essential details about the individual's needs, for the benefit of future caregivers. This information allows caregivers to help the individual live his or her life to the fullest extent possible.

The Arc Center for Future Planning (2016) provides a resource for the future planning process, which identifies seven broad areas to address in future planning: (a) daily routines, needs, and supports (e.g., assistance needed for activities of daily living); (b) living arrangements (e.g., with whom the person resides, is it rented/owned?); (c) finances (e.g., family and individual public benefits, assets, incomes, special needs trusts, and insurance policies); (d) medical details (e.g., contact information for healthcare professionals, medications, allergies, and medical history); (e) decision-making supports (e.g., does the person with IDD have a legal guardian appointed?); (f) education history (e.g., schools attended, courses/diplomas completed); and (g) vocational/leisure/social information (e.g., current and past employment, leisure activities, religious beliefs, behaviors, interests, friendships, and other important relationships). (See Mazzoni, 2013; Oak Wealth Advisors, 2017; O'Hara & Frishman, 2013, for additional information and sample care guides and letters of intent)

No two care guides are the same, as they are specific to each situation. The amount of detail that a family chooses to include is dependent upon their loved one's needs and their administrative diligence to document and update the information. Using an electronic document that prompts the family to address various topics is less daunting and more likely to be completed by families. The electronic format allows for ease of sharing and updating as the needs and circumstances of the individual change. Unlike estate documents, which families usually bury in a drawer or file in a safe deposit box at a bank, the care guide can and should be shared with family members and agencies who are expected to be future care providers. Providing this information in advance of when they are performing the role allows them to be prepared and ask questions when members of the family are still available to answer them.

Key Roles in Future Planning

One of the biggest challenges for families with a child with IDD is completing their estate planning and their care guide. The most significant barrier is often naming appropriate individuals or entities to serve in the key roles (Lauderdale *et al.*, 2010). Persons or entities being named must have the time, willingness, and ability to execute their roles. A proper special needs financial plan requires the following roles to be considered when the parents are no longer willing or able to perform them: (a) guardian, (b) attorney-in-fact (the agent named on a Power of Attorney (POA) document), (c) trustee, and (d) caregiver. We will briefly describe these roles here, but more information can be found in Chapter 15.

Legal Guardian

Guardianship carries the most legal responsibility. Guardianship is a court-approved appointment, which gives the rights of an individual to another individual (Hoyt & Pollock, 2003; Larson, 2016). Because the transfer of rights is significant, the choice of guardian should not be taken lightly. There are a variety of guardianship options from full guardianship (plenary guardianship), which entails the loss of all rights by the individual with special needs, to a variety of limited guardianships (Larson, 2016). A guardianship of the estate only gives the guardian the right to handle the financial affairs of the individual. A guardianship of the person transfers the rights including healthcare decisions, the right to vote, and the right to drive. For many families, the hope remains that their child can handle many of life's tasks with some supervision and perhaps the needs do not rise to the level of needing a guardian. While naming a parent as guardian is relatively common, if another family member is being named as guardian in the estate plan, it would be best if they were made aware of the family's intentions, as assuming this role involves a significant amount of responsibility. Professional guardians, who understand the role and have experience reporting to the courts, exist because most relatives find it to be too challenging (Larson, 2016).

Attorney-in-Fact

In lieu of establishing a guardianship, families may opt to utilize power of attorney documents, which name an agent as the attorney-in-fact with the right to assist the individual with IDD in a variety of areas (Larson, 2016). A power of attorney for property allows another person to make financial decisions and transactions on behalf of the individual. A healthcare power of attorney allows another person to access the health records, sign medical releases, and communicate with healthcare providers. If an individual has communication skills and an ability to indicate preferences, using power of attorney documents to support him or her is often easier and more flexible than going through a court proceeding to be appointed or removed as a guardian (Nadworny & Haddad, 2007).

Trustee

The trustee has the sole responsibility of managing the trust and the assets it holds (Hoyt & Pollock, 2003). The trustee must have strong administrative skills and investment management skills. While trustees can hire people to prepare the tax returns and invest the assets, they still bear the ultimate responsibility for the trust. In addition, the trustee of a Special Needs Trust (SNT) must document and report every distribution made from the trust as all distributions are scrutinized by the Social Security Administration (SSA) for compliance with the rules. A disqualifying distribution can cause the individual with special needs to lose his/her income benefits and Medicaid services until the distribution is rectified (SSA, 2016). The trustee also must be able to communicate with the individual with IDD to understand his/her wants and needs, although the trustee has the sole discretion for making or withholding a requested distribution. From professional experience, families sometimes opt for a professional trustee in conjunction with a family member co-trustee whose primary role is communication between the professional trustee and the family member with IDD.

Ironically, the caregiver has almost no legal authority despite having the most contact with the individual with IDD. Among the four roles, caregivers have the highest attrition rate (Easterseals, 2015; NAC & AARP Public Policy Institute, 2015). It takes a great deal of effort to provide care, and it is often a far more significant commitment than the person realizes when they initially accept the role. Studies of caregivers have revealed that caregivers experience higher levels of anxiety and stress, have less time for their own lives, and incur unreimbursed expenses in providing care (Easterseals, 2015; NAC & AARP Public Policy Institute, 2015).

It is important that whoever is chosen to serve in the various support roles is made aware of the responsibilities that come with it. Problems arise when a family member steps into a role such as trustee of a SNT and does not know which types of distributions will disqualify the person with IDD from government benefits. Similarly, if a family member serving as the agent on a power of attorney for property naively believes that the person with IDD cannot also transact on the accounts, she/he may get some unpleasant surprises, such as purchased vehicles, homes, or shopping sprees. A power of attorney provides someone else with the same permission to act on one's behalf but does not revoke the rights of the individual (Hoyt & Pollock, 2003).

Although there is often a cost, hiring a professional to serve in one or more of the key roles is often a family's best option. While the fees require additional planning and financial savings on the family's part, it also relieves the family of the concern that the relative they might have named is unable or unwilling to serve. Or, the designated relative might pre-decease the parents and they fail to update their estate planning documents with a new designated guardian. From professional experience, the best planning includes naming an entity to play the above roles at least in the capacity as a successor guardian, agent, or trustee should the family's preferred choice or choices not be available.

Funding Future Needs

One question you may be pondering is: How much does a family need to fund this so called "third retirement?" No one can truly define exactly how much is needed because it is very challenging to predict the combined costs associated with support-related expenses and for what period of time; however, there are many strategies employed by planners to make reasonable estimations. We focus less on how much is needed and leave that to the family's planner, and instead, address what resources may be available to utilize. Assets of parents and loved ones often serve as the primary resource but may be combined with other crucial resources, such as life insurance and government benefits.

Individuals with IDD are often eligible for a myriad of government benefits. Supplemental Security Income (SSI), Social Security Disability Insurance (SSDI), Medicaid, Medicare, and Medicaid waiver programs are most commonly utilized. These are complex benefits and one should consult an expert for planning for government benefits. More information can be found on the SSA (n.d.) website and in Chapter 15.

Special Needs Trusts

A trust is a legal entity created by one or more persons (settlor, grantor, or trustor) for the benefit of another (beneficiary) to hold, manage and distribute the settlor's assets by a third party that can be a person or financial institution (trustee). The trustee has a fiduciary duty to the beneficiary, whether one or more. A trust is a valuable estate planning tool for various reasons, including but not limited to the following: (a) to benefit from federal and state laws and regulations that can minimize estate tax obligations; (b) to manage assets for a minor child and for descendants in general; (c) to insure that the ultimate distribution of the settlor's assets is to the beneficiaries that he/she wants, especially in blended family situations; and (d) to provide for a beneficiary with disabilities that render him/her unable to appropriately manage his own assets. There are numerous types of trust agreements, many of which are governed by IRS regulations. Trusts must be drafted by attorneys that specialize in probate and trust law because of the complex fiduciary relationships, proper management and usage of trust assets, and special federal and state tax applications and reporting requirements that trust agreements create. If the trust is not administered according to its stated purpose and the terms of the trust, the intended protections may not apply, causing the imposition of serious IRS or other government agency penalties.

The purpose of a Special Needs Trust (SNT), also referred to as a Supplemental Needs Trust, is to supplement government benefits available to a person with IDD. SNT's were originally established by the Omnibus Budget Reconciliation Act (OBRA, 1993) and later modified by the Special Needs Trust Fairness Act of 2015 (Krooks & O'Hara, 2016). The key component is for the SNT to supplement and not supplant the benefits and serve as the legal cornerstone of a special needs plan. The trust assets should be for the sole benefit of the person with IDD. The trust provides government benefit protections, asset protection, and the often underestimated benefit of privacy. Families need to be encouraged to seek legal and financial counsel from professionals who specialize in serving families with disabilities. The complex nature of planning provides too many opportunities for error even when the best of intentions are present; thus, you are encouraged to seek additional guidance and information (see The Arc of Texas Master Pooled Trust, n.d., for examples of what needs can be provided from a SNT).

Third Party SNTs are ideal because a Medicaid payback provision is not required after the death of the beneficiary (Hoyt & Pollock, 2003). This allows remaining trust assets to pass to surviving heirs or successor beneficiaries. These trusts are funded with assets owned by someone other than the beneficiary. From professional experience, many plans include more than one trust because of unique situations, such as legal settlements, poorly planned inheritance, or income earned by the person with IDD.

While many attorneys believe that a SNT in a will as a part of a parent's estate plan is sufficient, this is often a point of disagreement between attorneys and financial planners. The trust should be a stand-alone document, whether it is fully funded or not, so family members can name it as a part of their own estate plan. Therefore, the Third Party SNT is the trust that can be shared with others wanting to leave a gift, inheritance, insurance policy, or other asset for the benefit of the loved one with IDD (Hoyt & Pollock, 2003; Nadworny & Haddad, 2007). While self-settled trust and pooled trust assets should also be considered as assets available to plan for the future, after the death of the beneficiary, the remainder is subject to state claims for reimbursement for benefits provided (Hoyt & Pollock, 2003). Gifts and inheritances should not be contributed to those trusts, which is another reason why family communication is essential for optimizing planning efforts. As stated previously, establishing a SNT is complex and requires families to work with well-qualified legal and financial professionals to develop these legal documents.

ABLE Accounts

One of the newest financial planning opportunities for the special needs community in the United States is the ABLE account. The Achieving a Better Life Experience (ABLE) Act legislation was passed by Congress and signed by President Obama in December of 2014 (more information can be found at www.ablenrc.org). After 18 months of public comments and the drafting of regulations by the Internal Revenue Service, the first account application was made available by the State of Ohio on June 1, 2016. As of August 17, 2017, 27 states had accounts available; it is expected that all 50 states will eventually have their own programs available (ABLE National Resource Center [ANRC], n.d.). The information presented here is from the ABLE National Resource Center website.

ABLE accounts provide a number of benefits for families who are trying to save for the short- and long-term needs of the individual with IDD. Much like a Roth IRA or College 529 Savings Plan, ABLE accounts are funded with after-tax dollars and the accounts grow tax-free. Assuming distributions are made for appropriate expenses, the distributions are also tax-free. In order for the distributions from the ABLE accounts to be tax-free, they must be made for the sole benefit of the individual with special needs and be what are deemed "qualified disability expenses" under the 26 U.S.C §529A(e)(5). The expenses can be for education, healthcare, housing, employment support, job training, assistive technologies, transportation, or other services or expenses directly related to improving the individual's health, independence, or quality of life.

In many cases, families have SNTs drafted that can receive contributions from family members, but not from the individual named as the beneficiary. Although self-settled SNTs can be created to hold the assets of the individual with IDD, they are far less common than the SNTs funded by others because they are crucial to proper planning (Hoyt & Pollock, 2003; Nadworny & Haddad, 2007). Prior to the ABLE legislation, when an unexpected gift was received by the individual with IDD or there were excess earnings in a given month, the family was faced with the dilemma of spending down the unexpected cash during the month or having the individual have their government benefits suspended until their holdings fell back below the $2,000 asset threshold. Now, the ABLE account is available to absorb the unexpected income and eliminate some of the stress involved with maintaining access to government benefits.

Each individual with IDD is allowed to have only one ABLE account. The account can be funded by a variety of different people, including the individual with IDD. The annual contribution limit is currently $14,000 per account. Therefore, families must be aware of how much has been contributed during the year to avoid the risk of overfunding the account and having to return contributions to those who made the excess gift(s).

The other financial limits to understand have to do with the maximum balances allowed in the ABLE accounts. The first $100,000 in an ABLE account is exempt from the Supplemental Security Income (SSI) resource limit of $2,000. When the ABLE account exceeds $100,000, the dollars in excess of the $100,000 threshold count against the $2,000 limit and will impact benefit eligibility, which is described in more detail later in this chapter. Therefore, as the balance in an ABLE account increases due to annual contributions (maximum $14,000 a year) and growth in the investments, families need to find appropriate expenses on which to spend down the ABLE account to avoid hitting the $100,000 limit.

Because the accounts are sponsored by the individual states, the investment options and account expenses will vary across states. An individual is able to open an account in any state that offers non-resident accounts, not just their state of residence. They also have the ability to transfer the account from one state to another once per year. It is important to compare the investment options, plan expenses, and quality of reporting and information available among the ABLE accounts before selecting one.

In order to be eligible for an ABLE account, an individual must have a disability diagnosis before turning 26 years of age. Individuals can be any age when opening an ABLE account, but their diagnosis must have preceded their 26th birthday. If they are already receiving SSI or SSDI benefits, they are automatically eligible to open an ABLE account. However, if they are not receiving government income benefits, they will need to be able to prove that they meet Social Security's definition of disability and have a letter of certification from a licensed physician.

Much like a self-settled SNT, the ABLE account has a Medicaid payback provision. Any monies remaining in the ABLE account at the death of the beneficiary must be paid to the government to reimburse the state for any Medicaid services provided. For ABLE accounts, the Medicaid payback provision relates to expenses incurred by the state for the individual following the date when the account was opened. With respect to a self-settled SNT, the payback provision is calculated based on the services received over the individual's lifetime regardless of when the trust was created or funded. If there is a balance in the ABLE account after the state is reimbursed, it can be distributed to other individuals.

As of August 2017, there are three pieces of pending legislation that would expand the usefulness of the ABLE accounts. The first enhancement would allow for the tax-free rollover of a College 529 Savings Plan to an ABLE account. Even if limited to transfers of $14,000 per year, the ability to move funds from a College 529 Savings Plan to an ABLE account would allow a large number of families to relocate assets to a more beneficial account. The second enhancement is the increase in the age by which the disability diagnosis must be made. Currently, the diagnosis must be in place by age 26. The legislation being considered would increase the age to 46, which would allow more individuals who have injuries, accidents, or later onset disabilities to benefit from an ABLE account. The final enhancement is a proposal to allow the individual with the disability to add up to $11,770 (the Federal Poverty Level) of earnings to the ABLE account in addition to the $14,000 of contributions that can be made from other sources. The ability to add the earnings in addition to the other contributions would only be allowed if the beneficiary is not participating in a company retirement plan.

Updates about additional states making ABLE accounts available and revisions to the rules for using ABLE accounts can be found by visiting the ABLE National Resource Center (n.d.) website. It is managed by the National Disability Institute (NDI, 2017) and is a valuable resource for families interested in learning more about the ABLE accounts and their availability in all states.

Life Insurance

Life insurance is almost always a necessary part of a plan to fund a SNT, but all circumstances need to be taken into account prior to purchasing life insurance. The need to fund the trust is a permanent need, which requires a *permanent* life insurance policy, often referred to as a *whole life policy.* While these types of policies can be more expensive to purchase than term life insurance policies, they provide coverage as long as the premium is paid and does not expire. Term insurance is either not available or prohibitively expensive when the insured is age 65 or older. One way to reduce the cost of the permanent insurance premiums is to purchase a second-to-die policy. This approach works if the funds are only needed after both parents are deceased. Second-to-die policies pay out benefits at the death of the second spouse, but are always less expensive than a policy on a single life.

While retirement plans may provide additional complexities, they can be used to fund a SNT. Retirement plans must be treated the same with regard to beneficiary designations naming the SNT as the beneficiary (Caudill, 2009). Savings accounts and brokerage accounts should be titled to transfer or pay on death through contract to the same Third Party SNT bypassing the individual with IDD. Residences also create potential complications, but they can be transferred to the individual with IDD without jeopardizing their benefits. Alternatively, residences can be sold with the proceeds transferring to a Third Party SNT. Careful attention must be paid to beneficiary designations. The Third Party SNT should be named the beneficiary rather than the individual with IDD to prevent assets from being counted for SSI means testing. By naming the trust as the beneficiary, the assets will not be counted.

In general, all assets can be used to fund a special needs plan, but proper care must be taken ahead of time to craft complimentary estate plans for all parties involved taking into consideration government entitlement protection, asset protections, client wishes, needs of the beneficiary and unique requirements of assets available and assets being utilized.

Principles for Practice: Keys to a Successful Special Needs Financial Plan

Successful special needs financial planning is a result of identifying challenges, seeking options, collaborating with experts, documenting your experiences, organizing your records, and regularly updating goals. It is not possible to achieve optimal results passively. The planning is ongoing and requires active participation from the decision makers in the life of the individual with IDD.

Sometimes the most difficult task is coming to grips with the challenges. While it may be upsetting to the family, acknowledging that a disability exists and pursuing professional diagnoses to identify the extent of the disability is a critical first step in the planning process. Proactive parents who ask questions as soon as issues arise give their children the benefit of more years in early intervention programs. Parents who assume the issues will resolve themselves as the child matures cost their children the opportunity for support that can be critical in their development. Similarly, spouses and children of loved ones who are showing signs of IDD can greatly benefit their loved one facing challenges by being proactive.

Families need to seek and evaluate all available resources as soon as a diagnosis is available. Helping professionals can play a key role in directing families to appropriate resources. Connecting with specialists and peers allows the family to educate themselves about planning options. While the internet can be a dangerous source for answers, it can also be a tremendous resource for identifying organizations and specialists in your community who can become part of the planning team and support network.

When choosing professionals to engage in the planning for the current and future needs of the family and individual with IDD, it is essential to seek fiduciaries. Fiduciary advisors have a legal responsibility to put their client's interest ahead of their own (Hoyt & Pollock, 2003). Attorneys are fiduciaries. A small percentage of financial advisors are fiduciaries. Traditionally, insurance agents are not fiduciaries. Ensuring that the advice given is objective and in the family's best interest is important. When the advice includes conflicts of interest, money is often wasted on products and recommendations that are either unnecessary or sub-optimal.

Implementing flexible strategies is another important element of successful planning. The individual with IDD is going to have different requirements, abilities, and interests in the future. The best planning will adapt to changes and allow for progress to be maintained across the life span of the individual with IDD. Remaining diligent in documenting the development of the individual is essential. Communicating the changes with the planning team will increase the likelihood that the best options will be pursued as new information becomes available.

Conclusion

Communication needs to extend beyond the professional advisors to the broad family network. Ideally, all family members with any contact or familiarity with the individual with IDD should be aware of the family's future planning for the individual. It can be devastating when a well-intentioned family member makes a gift or provides a service that causes the individual to lose eligibility for government benefits. Communicating about the future care and financial needs of the individual with IDD can make transitions easier. If family members are expected to provide care or supervisory services at some point in the future, it is appropriate to inform them of the requirements of the role(s). It is much better to learn of their lack of interest in performing the required tasks when there is time to investigate other individuals or service providers who can assume the role and responsibilities. If extended family members have a better understanding about the future expenses the individual with IDD may have and they understand that a SNT has been established, they will be better able to contribute appropriately to the individual's future support.

Key Messages from This Chapter

- **For individuals with IDD and their families**: Caregiving is not simply limited to daily tasks but also requires preparation for the future well-being of loved ones. It is essential that families seek professional guidance in order to properly establish letters of intent, care guides, special needs trusts, guardianship and wills, and develop a level of open communication necessary for preventing negative financial consequences for the family and loved one with IDD.
- **For professionals**: Helping professionals can serve as a catalyst for leading families to the appropriate services in order to achieve a comprehensive

special needs plan. Be persistent in your support by encouraging families to take the initial steps for planning by facilitating the difficult conversations needed when identifying appropriate guardians and trustees. Professionals can also highlight that planning is a process and is not completed within a single office visit, nor is it static; once a plan is developed, it should be reviewed and updated regularly based on changes in the individual's and family's needs.

- **For policy makers**: The time demands, emotional energy, and the complexity of decision-making associated with creating a special needs plan contributes to significant levels of stress for parents and guardians. Families benefit greatly from state and national clearinghouses, which offer 24-hour online support or hotlines for addressing questions or support for guiding families during the benefits application process and beyond.

Additional Resources:

- Special Needs Financial Planning: http://specialneedsplanning.com/
  - Provides information by life stage for families with special needs
- Oak Wealth Advisors have a number of documents and resources for special needs planning (http://oakwealth.com/special-needs-services-resources/):
  - Special Needs Resources: http://oakwealth.com/special-needs-resources/
  - Top 10 Recommendations for Special Needs Families: http://oakwealth.com/top-ten-recommendations-for-special-needs-families/

References

ABLE National Resource Center. (n.d.). *What we're about.* Retrieved from http://ablenrc.org/

Achieving a Better Life Experience Act of 2014 (ABLE). div. B of Pub. L. 113–295. 128 Stat. 4056.

Caudill, A. (2009). Funding special needs trust with retirement benefits. *Journal of Financial Service Professionals, 63(4)*, 15–17.

Easterseals. (2015). *Many faces of caregiving study.* Retrieved from http://www.easterseals.com/explore-resources/for-caregivers/caregiving-study-2015.html

Greenstein, L. (2017). *Beyond silence: Stopping stigma one story at a time.* Retrieved from http://www.nami.org/Blogs/NAMI-Blog/March-2017/Beyond-Silence-Stopping-Stigma-One-Story-at-a-Time

Hoyt, P., & Pollock, C. (2003). *Special people, special planning: Creating a safe legal haven for families with special needs.* Oviedo: Legacy Planning Partners.

Krooks, B. A., & O'Hara, A. C. (2016). *Special Needs Trust Fairness Act becomes law.* Retrieved from http://www.wealthmanagement.com/estate-planning/special-needs-trust-fairness-act-becomes-law

Larson, A. (2016,). *What is guardianship?* Retrieved from https://www.expertlaw.com/library/estate_planning/guardianship.html

Lauderdale, M., Durband, D., Scott, J., & Springer, N. (2010). *Special needs training: A focus group study.* Paper presented at the Academy of Financial Services Conference, Denver.

Lauderdale, M., & Huston, S. J. (2012a). Financial therapy and planning for families with special needs children. *Journal of Financial Therapy*, *3*(1), 62–81. doi:10.4148/jft.v3i1.1494

Lauderdale, M., & Huston, S. (2012b). *Special needs caregivers: An increased need for support and professional guidance.* Paper presented at the Academy of Financial Services Conference, San Antonio.

Lauderdale, M. K., & Huston, S. J. (2013). The team approach to financial planning for families with special needs dependents. *Journal of Financial Planning*, *26*(3), 46–52. Retrieved from https://www.onefpa.org/journal/Pages/The%20Team%20Approach%20to%20Financial%20Planning%20for%20Families%20with%20Special-Needs%20Dependents.aspx

Mazzoni, M. (2013). Letter of Intent & Life-Long Special Needs Planning. Retrieved from http://lifeafterieps.com/letter-of-intent-life-long-special-needs-planning/)

Mittan, R. J. (2010). Understanding and coping with stigma. *Exceptional Parent*, *40*(5), 37–41. Retrieved from http://www.eparent.com/

NAC & AARP Public Policy Institute. (2015). *Caregiving in the U.S.* Retrieved from http://www.aarp.org/content/dam/aarp/ppi/2015/caregiving-in-the-united-states-2015-report-revised.pdf

Nadworny, J. & Haddad, C. (2007). *The special needs planning guide: How to prepare for every stage of your child's life.* Baltimore: Paul H. Brookes.

National Disability Institute. (2017). *About us.* Retrieved from http://realeconomicimpact.org/about-us

Oak Wealth Advisors. (2017). *Special needs resources.* Retrieved from http://oakwealth.com/special-needs-resources/

O'Hara, A., & Frishman, S. (2013). *The voice newsletter: Special needs alliance.* Retrieved from http://www.specialneedsalliance.org/the-voice/letter-of-intent-3/

Social Security Administration. (n.d.). *Disability planner: Social Security protection if you become disabled.* Retrieved from www.ssa.gov/planners/disability

Social Security Administration. (2016). *Understanding Supplemental Security Income SSI resources — 2016 edition.* Retrieved from https://www.ssa.ov/ssi/text-resources-ussi.htm

The Arc. (2016). *The Arc's HealthMeet initiatives.* Retrieved from https://www.thearc.org/healthmeet

The Arc Center for Future Planning. (2016). *Future Planning 101: What is future planning?* Retreived from https://futureplanning.thearc.org/pages/learn/future-planning-101

The Arc of Texas Master Pooled Trust (n.d.). *Providing for supplemental needs.* Retrieved from thearcoftexas.org/trust/index.php

Thompson, B. (2016, March 4). *To move beyond stigma, we first need to understand it.* Retrieved from http://www.nami.org/Blogs/NAMI-Blog/March-2016/To-Move-Beyond-Stigma,-We-First-Need-to-Understand#sthash.cURCwQVg.dpuf

University of Washington. (2016). *Disability stigma and your patients.* Healthy Aging & Physical Disability RRTC. Retrieved from http://agerrtc.washington.edu/sites/agerrtc/files/files/Aging_Stigma_Final.pdf

14 Meaningful Employment

Fostering Opportunities for Adults with IDD to Thrive

Jennifer L. Jones, PhD and
Kami L. Gallus, PhD

Introduction

Employment is a central aspect of life for most adults (Bergqvist & Eriksson, 2015). Research suggests the benefits of work are similar for individuals with and without intellectual and developmental disabilities (IDD; Siperstein, Parker, & Drascher, 2013). Employment provides opportunities for socialization, financial independence, and fosters a sense of purpose (Schur, 2002). Yet, individuals with IDD are significantly underrepresented in the labor force (Butterworth *et al.*, 2011). Personal, systemic, social, and policy barriers create significant employment challenges for many people with IDD and their families (Nord, Luecking, Mank, Kiernan, & Wray, 2013).

Despite the many historical and current challenges, individuals with IDD and their families continue to forge innovative and creative employment paths. This chapter begins by introducing readers to several adults whose employment histories illustrate some of the most common employment opportunities for adults with IDD. These scenarios introduce key terminology and the services and supports individuals with IDD access in employment settings.[1] Similar to the experiences of adults without IDD, the employment narratives illustrate typical patterns of employment noting common transitions and changes as individuals' skills and interests develop. After introducing readers to common employment scenarios, the historical context that shaped the current employment landscape is explored. Specific attention is given to outlining potential benefits of and barriers to employment experienced by individuals with IDD. Finally, this chapter provides practical principles for helping professionals working with individuals with IDD and their family members as they navigate the process of obtaining and maintaining meaningful employment.

Employment Scenarios

The scenarios presented in this section provide four different employment situations that are common for individuals with IDD. Each scenario presents information about the adult as well as their specific work situation.

Bennett: Sheltered Workshop Employment

"Bennett" is 36 years old and has worked at the local sheltered workshop for 18 years. *Sheltered workshops* are center-based day programs for adults with IDD who are not working in the open labor market (Migliore, 2010). Workshops maintain contracts with private companies to complete relatively simple tasks (e.g., assembling, packing, woodworking) at rates below minimum wage. Sheltered workshops often provide additional educational or leisure activities for adults with IDD (Migliore, 2010). The sheltered workshop where Bennett works contracts with a large department store to assemble size labels onto plastic hangers. Bennett is paid a *piece rate* of $.01 per hanger; thus, if he completes 100 hangers per shift, he earns $1.00 for the day.

Ali: Supported Employment

"Ali" is 47 years old and works as a part of a janitorial team with a group of five other individuals with IDD. The team of co-workers meets every morning at the local sheltered workshop and rides together to the businesses they are contracted to clean that day. Each co-worker is responsible for individual tasks (e.g., emptying the trash, sweeping the floors) and earns $2.50 per hour. This team is often referred to as an *enclave,* where a group of individuals with IDD work together to complete a task with the guidance of a job coach. A *job coach* is an employment specialist who provides on-site training and supervision for adults with IDD in a variety of employment settings as part of *supported employment* (Mank & Grossi, 2013). Supported employment emerged in federal law through the Developmental Disabilities Act of 1984, in response to a growing desire for individuals with IDD to be able to work in the community.

Caroline: Supported Integrated Employment

"Caroline" is 21 years old and loves animals. She learned of a job opening at the local pet store and asked her vocational services caseworker for assistance in completing the application. Individuals with disabilities, including IDD, are eligible for services from their state department of rehabilitation services. Caroline's job at the pet store is considered *integrated employment* because she works primarily with individuals who do not have disabilities. Caroline needs some assistance learning new tasks, completing her bi-weekly time sheet, and developing her customer service skills; thus, supported employment services provide a job coach to work alongside Caroline for two hours every other week. Caroline typically works 15 hours a week and earns $5.75 an hour. Since beginning the job at the pet store, Caroline has learned to use public transportation and is learning to budget her bi-weekly paycheck of approximately $150.

Spencer: Competitive Integrated Employment

"Spencer" is 28 years old and has worked in a local café for two years. Spencer is paid minimum wage and is supervised solely by the manager of the café—just like his co-workers who do not have IDD. This is considered ***competitive integrated employment***, an employment setting in which individuals with IDD are part of the general labor market, work in the community, and receive competitive wages at, or above, minimum wage (Workforce Innovation and Opportunity Act, 2014). Spencer's path to competitive integrated employment included many transitions. Upon graduating high school, Spencer worked 30 hours a week at a sheltered workshop. After two years at the sheltered workshop, he began supported employment working as a dishwasher at a local restaurant with the intermittent assistance of a job coach. The skills Spencer learned in the restaurant helped give him the experience and confidence needed to apply for a position at the local café. Spencer no longer needs the support of a job coach. The increase from piece rate at the sheltered workshop to his current earnings of $8.25 per hour have been substantial for Spencer.

Employment for Individuals With IDD: A Historical Perspective

While current employment statistics show much room for improvement, progress has occurred in employment of individuals with IDD over the past century (Kiernan, 2015). Historically, where an individual worked was determined by caregivers, guardians, and professionals. This practice of assigning jobs to individuals without considering their unique skills and interests is a practice recurrent throughout history. Segregated employment (e.g., sheltered workshops) was initially thought to be best practice to assure safety and protection from the unpredictability of society (Dague, 2012). Since the 1980s, a significant shift has occurred within employment-related policy as research began to consistently find that securing jobs in the community (often referred to as ***integrated employment***) were preferable for individuals with IDD (Mank & Grossi, 2013). However, practice in the field often lags behind research and policy, as noted by the significant number of individuals who continue to work in segregated settings.

The history of segregated employment coincides with the practice of segregated living as institutionalization emerged as the primary residential setting for individuals with IDD in the 1800s (Smith, Noll, & Wehmeyer, 2013). The Fair Labor Standards Act of 1938 (U. S. Department of Labor, n.d.) was passed while the U.S. economy struggled in the midst of the Great Depression. On the brink of World War II, this act included section 14C, which stated individuals with disabilities could be paid below the national minimum wage. Allowing subminimum wages was originally considered beneficial to adults with IDD as it created jobs for individuals unable to meet productivity requirements of the general labor force and encouraged employers to hire adults with disabilities as opposed to children (Grossman, 1978). This near century-old federal policy continues to be cited as support for employers, including disability-focused agencies responsible for the provision of services (e.g., agencies operating sheltered workshops and enclaves), to legally pay individuals with disabilities significantly below minimum wage.

The Current Employment Landscape

While Bennett, Ali, Caroline, and Spencer illustrate the various employment services and supports utilized by individuals with IDD, these scenarios do not represent the experiences of most adults with IDD. Using a nationally representative random sample, Siperstein *et al.* (2013) found that only 34% of Americans with IDD aged 21 to 64 years were employed, compared to 76% of working-age adults without disabilities (Erickson, Lee, & von Schrader, 2012). Among the small percentage of individuals with IDD who are employed, most work part time and thus do not receive employee benefits, such as paid time off or health insurance (Siperstein *et al.*, 2013). The work setting also varies, with 18% working in an integrated setting similar to Ali, Caroline, and Spencer; 13% working in a sheltered workshop similar to Bennett; and 3% reporting either self-employed or their employment setting was not categorized (Siperstein *et al.*, 2013). With employment data of Americans with all disabilities, not just IDD, only being tracked by the Labor Department since 2008, the scope of national trends is shallow (U. S. Department of Labor, Bureau of Labor Statistics, 2010). However, what is clear is that the participation rate for individuals with IDD in the labor force is even lower than that of people with other disabilities (Kiernan, 2015).

Renewed National Interest in Employment Issues

Subminimum wage and sheltered workshops have become topics of national discussion in recent years as awareness to the pay rates of individuals with IDD has come to light among a national movement toward integrated employment (Hoffman, 2013). The National Disability Rights Network (NDRN, 2012) has voiced strong opposition to the continued funding of segregated work settings by the service systems that are charged with serving individuals with IDD. The NDRN (2012) acknowledges that programs such as sheltered workshops were started with good intentions and were originally designed to teach meaningful skills and protect individuals with IDD from public judgment and ridicule; however, public perception about disability and many laws have changed toward favoring workplace integration. Those in favor of sheltered workshops and laws allowing for subminimum wage are concerned about financially crippling small agencies and nonprofits that manage sheltered workshops, as they would not be able to pay their employees with IDD minimum wage without an increase to their agency funding (Hoffman, 2013). There also are fears that an increase in minimum wage will actually eliminate jobs and result in previously employed individuals being unemployed (Young, 2016). Many families rely on sheltered workshops to provide a safe and consistent place for their relatives with IDD to attend each day (National Core Indicators, 2015). Some families and adults with IDD report choosing sheltered workshop settings over integrated employment due to concerns regarding safety, transportation, long-term placement, work hours, disability benefits, social environment, and work skills (Migliore, Grossi, Mank, & Rogan, 2008). While research shows significant benefits among some individuals with IDD working in the community as compared to sheltered workshops (Rogan & Rinne, 2011), less is known about the impact policy changes will have on parents or other family caregivers.

Leaders and practitioners in the field of IDD continue to struggle with the complexities of employment (Chase *et al.*, 2016). Supported employment, such as Caroline's job at the pet store, provides desired inclusion in the community, but for most individuals, this type of employment does not pay minimum wage. Similarly, some disability-focused agencies operate businesses (e.g., thrift shops) that primarily employ individuals with IDD, thus limiting contact with co-workers who do not have disabilities, but provide respectable wages (Chase *et al.*, 2016). These practices have led to the ongoing examination of employment priorities and what constitutes meaningful employment for individuals with IDD (Chase *et al.*, 2016). Unfortunately, many individuals with IDD are employed in settings that offer neither a fair wage nor inclusion in the community, while others are forced to choose between a respectable income and being a part of their community (Nord *et al.*, 2016).

Benefits of and Barriers to Employment for Individuals with IDD

The many positive benefits of employment for individuals provides a supportive foundation for the value of work and employment for all adults. Researchers and scholars in the field of IDD have determined several unique benefits associated with employment among individuals with IDD, including enhanced quality of life (Mank & Grossi, 2013). Schalock (2004) explored quality of life for individuals with IDD and established the following domains as the building blocks of the construct: emotional well-being, interpersonal relations, material well-being, personal development, physical well-being, self-determination, social inclusion, and rights. Employment and employment-related income often are considered objective indicators of quality of life (Schalock, 2004). For example, employment is thought to improve one's quality of life by providing opportunities to develop new skills, build relationships, establish financial literacy, and increase overall health and physical well-being. Furthermore, research has demonstrated that employed individuals report significantly higher levels of quality of life than unemployed individuals (Eggleton, Robertson, Ryan, & Kober, 1999). However, research repeatedly demonstrates that the benefits may differ by the type of employment, with individuals in competitive and supported employment reporting significantly higher quality of life than individuals working in sheltered workshops (Eggleton *et al.*, 1999; Kober & Eggleton, 2005).

These findings highlight how the various types of jobs, work settings, and cultures of the workplace may result in more or less positive impact on the various domains of quality of life. For example, the nature of social relationships formed and the level of new skills developed on the job varies greatly based on the employment setting. For Bennett and Ali, working in a sheltered workshop and enclave offers them long-term placements that utilize basic skills and provides them the opportunity to develop long-standing relationships with their co-workers with IDD, whereas Caroline's and Spencer's employment in integrated settings provides them with opportunities to develop new, more complex skills, and an integrated, inclusive work environment that allows them to build relationships with co-workers without disabilities. Overall, the substantial benefits employment brings to individuals across all types of jobs and work settings makes the distinctive gap in employment rates between individuals with IDD and those without disabilities unsettling (Siperstein *et al.*, 2013). Low employment rates among individuals with IDD suggest significant barriers to employment remain for individuals with IDD.

In order to make gains in closing the employment gap for individuals with IDD, it is also important to recognize the potential barriers faced by individuals and their family members. Research has consistently shown adults with IDD desire economic self-sufficiency (Gray, McDermott, & Butkus, 2000) and the opportunity to work in the community (Migliore, Mank, Grossi, & Rogan, 2007). Yet, personal, systemic, social, and policy barriers are contributing factors to the troubling and wide employment gap that has been well documented for nearly 20 years (Nord *et al.*, 2013; Siperstein *et al.*, 2013). Individuals with IDD whose primary educational experience included segregated special education classrooms are often ill prepared for the social demands of an integrated work setting (The Arc, 2016). Segregated classrooms and workplaces (e.g., sheltered workshops) may inadvertently support the view that individuals with IDD do not belong in integrated settings, and thus, may reinforce families' fears regarding their loved ones working in the community (Dague, 2012).

While great strides have been made in policy making employment and a career among the principal intended outcomes of special education (Nord *et al.*, 2013), the practices needed to support and ensure desirable employment outcomes have not been widely implemented for students with IDD (Shogren & Plotner, 2012). Shogren and Plotner (2012) utilized data from a national study of students with disabilities in the United States and concluded that while schools are largely in compliance with legislation, there are numerous troubling practices that prevent students with IDD from transitioning successfully from high school to meaningful employment. Likewise, employers are often misinformed or unaware that individuals with IDD are potentially valuable employees (Luecking, 2011). Leading researchers in the IDD field with expertise in employment conclude that while numerous effective interventions exist to help people obtain and maintain employment, programs tend to be system-centric and inconsistently implemented (Nord *et al.*, 2016).

Principles for Practice

Obtaining and maintaining employment for adults with IDD is a personal and potentially emotional process for individuals and their families. The responsibility of locating meaningful employment opportunities and helping loved ones navigate challenges in the workplace often falls to family members. Helping professionals should understand the value of employment as well as the potential stressors for both individuals with IDD and their family members. We are keenly aware that employment is a deeply personal issue for individuals and families and a politically charged issue for individuals, families, and professionals in the field of IDD. We pose that the process of obtaining meaningful employment cannot be gained through a one-size fits all approach. The following principles reflect a person-centered approach to employment that acknowledges the significant role family members play in the lives of their loved ones with IDD.

Recognize the Unique Characteristics of Individuals With IDD

It is important to consider the individual's strengths, preferences, interests and needs. Individuals with IDD are as diverse and unique as their peers without disabilities. Historically, individuals with IDD have been placed in employment settings with little or no regard for their unique abilities or desires. Everyone has strengths. Helping professionals can work with individuals and families to identify the unique contribution an individual could bring to a job. Caroline's love for animals and vigilance in caring for them is an asset to her employers and co-workers at the pet store. Her responsibilities on the job capitalize on her strengths, preferences, and interests, while having the support of a job coach assist in meeting her needs for additional on-site training. By paying attention and inquiring about fixated interests, professionals can help individuals identify jobs that allow them to benefit from their fascinations. Specific attention to what the individual enjoys can be a path toward meaningful employment.

Think Outside the Box

Individuals, families, and professionals should be encouraged to think outside the box. There is no referral sheet or specific formula for families to follow regarding employment opportunities for their loved ones. Professional resources for employment, such as vocational rehabilitation, are available; however, families may need guidance in maneuvering the overwhelming and complex systems of support (Francis, Gross, Turnbull, & Turnbull, 2015). Helping professionals can serve as a guide to families, assisting them in accessing both formal and informal networks. Just as Caroline was made aware of a job opportunity through family friends, helping professionals can empower individuals and families to identify potential pathways to employment.

It is important for professionals to remember that a lifetime of limited choices may impede an individual's opportunities and even desires for integrated employment (Dague, 2012). Effective approaches to employment require an open mind and a respect for the individual. Accepting individuals with IDD as contributing members of the workforce is a crucial first step for both helping professionals and family members. While barriers to gaining and sustaining employment do exist, there are many examples that the times and expectations are changing. The American Association on Intellectual and Developmental Disabilities (AAIDD, 2015) published an excellent resource highlighting paths to employment for individuals with IDD. This book presents numerous examples of successful emerging practices that lead to meaningful employment.

Encourage Opportunities for Professional Growth

Individuals should plan for professional development and personal growth opportunities as it relates to their employment. New preferences and interests can evolve with exposure to new experiences. Individuals with IDD should be able to express changes in desires of where to work, just as people without disabilities do. This may result in job changes as it did for Spencer. Families and professionals should not fear these changes but rather allow space for an individual to outgrow a job and develop new goals and dreams. Helping professionals play a vital role in enhancing individuals' beliefs in their own abilities by empowering individuals to try new experiences and tasks. Professionals can engage individuals with IDD in similar career development conversations and interventions developed for individuals without disabilities (e.g., Burwell & Chen, 2006; Roeden, Bannink, Maaskant, & Curfs, 2009).

If at First You Don't Succeed—Try, Try Again!

Finally, attaining and sustaining successful employment may take multiple attempts. All individuals must develop good work skills, including learning responsibility and taking initiative. Professionals can assist individuals with IDD in cultivating a healthy self-image regarding their employability. This may be especially important after an employment attempt has failed. Individuals struggling to obtain and sustain employment may struggle with feelings of failure and need the support and validation of professionals and family members to try again. Professionals can normalize these challenges and assist individuals and family members with supporting and encouraging the individual with IDD. It is important to remember that a once successful employment setting may not be an environment that the individual flourishes in forever. This is especially difficult for individuals with IDD and their family members when the process to locate and secure employment is often taxing on the family's time and resources. It is vital for professionals to consider the impact of a perceived failure of a job placement on the individual as well as the family. Persistence, perseverance, and a belief that successful meaningful employment is possible is essential to gaining employment for individuals with IDD.

Conclusion

History has shown that society struggles with determining and defining best practices for employment for individuals with IDD. Yet, the known benefits of employment can have a positive effect on individuals, families, and society at large. Meaningful employment is a developmental journey that unfolds throughout the life span. There is no guidebook or one-size-fits-all model for individuals with IDD or their family members. The case scenarios involving Bennett, Ali, Caroline, and Spencer illustrate the diverse journeys individuals are on when searching for and securing employment. Individuals with IDD have unique skills and abundant potential. Time and again when given the opportunities for new experiences, individuals with IDD rise to and even surpass expectations. Professionals must grasp the complex nature of employment for individuals with IDD and their families. Empowering families to utilize the natural supports within their community and think outside the box will help individuals with IDD improve employment outcomes.

Key Messages from This Chapter

- **For individuals with IDD and their families**: Employment can be a mutually beneficial endeavor for both individuals with IDD and employers. Benefits for individuals vary based on the type of employment setting. While changes to and challenges with employment can evoke strong emotions, such as fear and worry, it is important for family members to remain supportive of individuals' desires regarding the workplace. Remain persistent and hopeful—meaningful employment is possible.
- **For professionals**: Changes to and challenges with employment are often a very emotional and overwhelming process for both individuals with IDD and their families. Individuals and their families may have a history of limited choices and opportunities and may be hesitant to seek new or diverse employment opportunities. It is important for professionals to assist individuals and family members with identifying personal strengths and goals for employment, while navigating the often-complex systems of services and supports using strength-based and career development interventions.
- **For policy makers**: While public perception regarding integrated employment for individuals with IDD has shifted in recent years, participation in the U.S. labor force remains significantly lower for individuals with IDD compared to adults without disabilities. Many families and individuals report a lack of consistency and increased ambiguity related to wages, benefits, and necessary skills for specific types of employment settings that increases their fears of integrated and supported employment. Policies guiding employment supports and services for individuals with IDD should be person-centered and acknowledge the significant role of family members.

Additional Resources

- **Federal and State Employment Supports and Services:**
  - Rehabilitation Services Administration—U.S. Department of Education
    Phone: 202-245-7488
    Website: https://www2.ed.gov/about/offices/list/osers/rsa/index.html
  - List of State Vocational Rehabilitation Agencies:

https://www.fda.gov/downloads/AboutFDA/WorkingatFDA/UCM277757.pdf
  - Administration on Intellectual and Developmental Disabilities (AIDD) State Councils on Developmental Disabilities - Program Contacts: https://acl.gov/programs/aidd/Programs/DDC/Contacts.aspx
  - List of State Intellectual/Developmental Disability Agencies: http://www.nasddds.org/state-agencies/
- **For more information about creative employment opportunities for individuals with IDD, consider the following books and websites:**
  - American Association on Intellectual and Developmental Disabilities (2015). *Way leads on to way: Paths to employment for people with intellectual disability.* Washington, DC: AAIDD.
  - Dlouhy, S., & Mitchell, P. (2015). *Upcycling sheltered workshops: A revolutionary approach to transforming workshops into creative spaces.* Athens, OH: Swallow Press.
  - *Real People, Real Jobs: Stories from the front line*
    - http://www.realworkstories.org/
  - *Think Work!*
    - http://www.thinkwork.org/about
  - *Innovative business models: Communities working together to create meaningful employment opportunities for adults with IDD*
    - Bitty and Beau's Coffee: https://www.bittyandbeauscoffee.com/
    - Finley's Barkery: https://finleysbarkery.com/
    - Puzzles Bakery: http://www.puzzlesbakerycafe.com/
    - Rising Tide Car Wash: http://risingtidecarwash.com/
    - Tim's Place: http://www.timsplace.com/the-restaurant/

Note

1 Our aim in the current chapter is to introduce professionals to the employment terminology used in the IDD field. Many of these terms may be state, federal, or program specific and may lack a formal operational definition. When possible, definitions of terms from U.S. federal law are cited.

References

American Association on Intellectual and Developmental Disabilities. (2015). *Way leads on to way: Paths to employment for people with intellectual disability.* Washington, DC: Author.

Bergqvist, T., & Eriksson, B. (2015). Passion and exploitation among young adults with different labor market status in Europe. *Nordic Journal of Working Life Studies, 5*, 17–31. doi:10.19154/njwls.v5i2.4791

Burwell, R., & Chen, C. P. (2006). Applying the principles and techniques of solution-focused therapy to career counseling. *Counselling Psychology Quarterly, 19*, 189–203. doi:10.1080/09515070600917761

Butterworth, J., Hall, A. C., Smith, F. A., Migliore, A., Winsor, J., Ciulla Timmons, J., & Domin, D. (2011). *StateData: The national report on employment services and outcomes*. Boston: Institute for Community Inclusion, University of Massachusetts Boston.

Chase, R., Bourne, M. L., Butterworth, J., Ryal, K., Bonardi, A., Hiersteiner, D., … Vierling, K. (2016, November). *Defining employment and community employment categories for individuals with intellectual and developmental disability*. Phone conference conducted with National Core Indicators, Stillwater, OK.

Dague, B. (2012). Sheltered employment, sheltered lives: Family perspectives of conversion to community-based employment. *Journal of Vocational Rehabilitation*, *37*, 1–11. doi:10.3233/VJR-2012-0595

Developmental Disabilities Act, 42 U.S.C. § 6000 *et seq.* (1984).

Dlouhy, S., & Mitchell, P. (2015). *Upcycling sheltered workshops: A revolutionary approach to transforming workshops into creative spaces*. Athens: Ohio University Press.

Eggleton, I., Robertson, S., Ryan, J., & Kober, R. (1999). The impact of employment on the quality of life of people with an intellectual disability. *Journal of Vocational Rehabilitation*, *13*, 95–107. Retrieved from http://content.iospress.com/articles/journal-of-vocational-rehabilitation/jvr00047

Erickson, W., Lee, C., & von Schrader, S. (2012). *Disability statistics from the 2010 American Community Survey (ACS)*. Ithaca, NY: Cornell University Employment and Disability Institute (EDI). Retrieved from www.disabilitystatistics.org

Francis, G. L., Gross, J. M. S., Turnbull, A. P., & Turnbull, H. R. (2015). An exploratory investigation into family perspectives after the family employment awareness training. *Career Development and Transition for Exceptional Individuals*, *38*, 68–77. doi:10.1177/2165143414528241

Gray, B., McDermott, S., & Butkus, S. (2000). Effect of job coaches on employment likelihood for individuals with mental retardation. *Journal of Vocational Rehabilitation*, *14*, 5–11. Retrieved from http://content.iospress.com/articles/journal-of-vocational-rehabilitation/jvr00061

Grossman, J. (1978). *Fair Labor Standards Act of 1938: Maximum struggle for a minimum wage*. Retrieved from http://www.dol.gov/dol/aboutdol/history/flsa1938.htm

Hoffman, L. C. (2013). An employment opportunity or a discrimination dilemma?: Sheltered workshops and the employment of the disabled. *University of Pennsylvania Journal of Law and Social Change*, *16*, 151–179. Retrieved from http://heinonline.org/HOL /LandingPage?handle=hein.journals/hybrid16&div=13&id=&page

Kiernan, W. E. (2015). Foreword. In American Association on Intellectual and Developmental Disabilities, *Way leads on to way: Paths to employment for people with intellectual disability* (pp. v–x). Washington, DC: American Association on Intellectual and Developmental Disabilities.

Kober, R., & Eggleton, I. R. C. (2005). The effect of different types of employment on quality of life. *Journal of Intellectual Disability Research*, *49*, 756–760. doi:10.1111/j.1365-2788.2005.00746.x

Luecking, R. G. (2011). Connecting employers with people who have intellectual disability. *Intellectual and Developmental Disabilities*, *49*, 261–273. doi:10.1352/1934-9556-49.4.261

Mank, D. M., & Grossi, T. A. (2013). Employment: Renewed investments. *Inclusion*, *1*(1), 7–16. doi:10.1352/2326-6988-1.1.007

Migliore, A. (2010). Sheltered workshops. In *International Encyclopedia of Rehabilitation*. Retrieved from http://cirrie.buffalo.edu/encyclopedia/en/article/136/

Migliore, A., Grossi, T., Mank, D., & Rogan, P. (2008). Why do adults with intellectual disabilities work in sheltered workshops? *Journal of Vocational Rehabilitation*, *28*, 29–40. Retrieved from http://content.iospress.com/articles/journal-of-vocational-rehabilitation/jvr00402

Migliore, A., Mank, D., Grossi, T., & Rogan, P. (2007). Integrated employment or sheltered workshops: Preferences of adults with intellectual disabilities, their families, and staff. *Journal of Vocational Rehabilitation*, *26*, 5–19. Retrieved from http://content.iospress.com/articles/journal-of-vocational-rehabilitation/jvr00358

National Core Indicators. (2015). *NCI adult consumer survey outcomes: Oklahoma report*. Retrieved from http://www.nationalcoreindicators.org/states/OK/

National Disability Rights Network. (2012). Segregated and exploited: The failure of the disability service system to provide quality work. *Journal of Vocational Rehabilitation*, *36*, 39–64. doi:10.3233/JVR-2012-0581

Nord, D., Butterworth, J., Carlson, D., Grossi, T., Hall, A. C., & Nye-Lengerman, K. (2016). Employment for people with IDD: What do we know and where are we going? In American Association on Intellectual and Developmental Disabilities, *Critical issues in intellectual and developmental disabilities: Contemporary research, practice, and policy* (pp. 71–88). Washington, DC: American Association on Intellectual and Developmental Disabilities.

Nord, D., Luecking, R., Mank, D., Kiernan, W., & Wray, C. (2013). The state of the science of employment and economic self-sufficiency for people with intellectual and developmental disabilities. *Intellectual and Developmental Disabilities*, *51*, 376–384. doi:10.1352/1934-9566-51.5.376

Roeden, J. M., Bannink, F. P., Maaskant, M. A., & Curfs, L. M. G. (2009). Solution-focused brief therapy with persons with intellectual disability. *Journal of Policy and Practice in Intellectual Disability*, *6*, 253–259. doi:10.1111/j.1741-1130.2009.00226.x

Rogan, P., & Rinne, S. (2011). National call for organizational change from sheltered to integrated employment. *Intellectual and Developmental Disabilities*, *49*, 248–260. doi:10.1352/1934-9556-49.4.248

Schalock, R. L. (2004). The concept of quality of life: What we know and do not know. *Journal of Intellectual Disability Research*, *48*, 203–216. doi:10.1111/j.1365-2788.2003.00558.x

Schur, L. (2002). The difference a job makes: The effects of employment among people with disabilities. *Journal of Economic Issues*, *36*, 339–347. doi:10.1080/00213624.2002.11506476

Shogren, K. A., & Plotner, A. J. (2012). Transition planning for students with intellectual disability, autism, or other disabilities: Data from the National Longitudinal Transition Study-2. *Intellectual and Developmental Disabilities*, *50*, 16–30. doi:10.1352/1934-9556-50.116

Siperstein, G. N., Parker, R. C., & Drascher, M. (2013). National snapshot of adults with intellectual disabilities in the labor force. *Journal of Vocational Rehabilitation*, *39*(3), 157–165. doi:10:3233/JVR-130-658

Smith, J. D., Noll, S., & Wehmeyer, M. L. (2013). Isolation, enlargement, and economization. In M. L. Wehmeyer (Ed.), *The story of intellectual disability* (pp. 1–15). Baltimore, MD: Paul H. Brookes.

The Arc. (2016). *Public policy and legal advocacy: Education issues for people with disabilities.* Retrieved from http://www.thearc.org/what-we-do/public-policy/policy-issues/education

U.S. Department of Labor. (n.d.). *Compliance assistance: Wages and the Fair Labor Standards Act (FLSA)*. Retrieved from https://www.dol.gov/whd/flsa/

U.S. Department of Labor, Bureau of Labor Statistics. (2010, August 25). *Data on the employment status of people with a disability.* Retrieved from https://www.bls.gov/cps/cpsdisability.htm

Workforce Innovation and Opportunity Act, 29 U.S.C. § 3101 *et seq.* (2014).

Young, E. (2016, May 17). *Disabled earn pennies as caregivers debate Clinton's raise plan.* Retrieved from http://www.bloomberg.com/politics/articles/2016-05-17/disabled-earn-pennies-as-caregivers-debate-clinton-s-raise-plan

15 Special Needs Legal Concerns
Guidelines for Families and Guardians

Michele K. Goldberg, JD

Introduction

Parents of children with disabilities will benefit from understanding legal issues pertaining to long-term planning for people with intellectual and developmental disabilities (IDD). There is sometimes tension between advocacy groups and attorneys specializing in areas of law related to the disability community, but this chapter will focus on the law, not on the discussion of what is right, correct, or best for any particular person or family. In my practice, I often hear parents exclaim that they cannot understand why they need legal counsel because "he's my child and I should be able to take care of him and make decisions that are best for him." This is an understandable reaction; however, some things are written into the law and must be acknowledged, but a lot depends on the age and needs of the child. If the child is a minor, the parents are considered the natural guardians and have full authority to make all decisions for the child. When the child turns 18 years old, s/he becomes an adult by law and is considered independent from the parents, becoming his/her own decision maker. If the adult child has an IDD diagnosis, s/he may need a surrogate decision maker. This chapter will explain different options for parents who need to assist their child with serious decisions about health needs (medical, dental, and psychiatric), financial concerns, residential placement, protection from predators who may prey on individuals with IDD, and advocating for the now adult child's best interest and welfare.

Another concern for families of a child with disabilities who, because of the disability will not be able to financially support him/herself, is how to apply for and obtain government benefits, including Medicaid and Medicare and how to maintain eligibility for these benefits. This chapter also will explain the need for long-term special needs planning, including the importance of guardianship and having a legal will.

Guardianship and Alternatives to Guardianship

In the United States, each state has its own laws concerning guardianship and alternatives to guardianship. This author lives in and is licensed to practice law in Texas, but the principles and considerations are similar in other states. Some of the terminology varies from state to state; it should be noted that the information provided here uses Texas terminology. I strongly suggest researching on the internet for your particular state's laws, being sure to take information from an official website, such as the state or city attorney's office or an agency that works with people with IDD. (For Texas residents, some reliable resources for information are: Texas Guardianship Association, 2015; Texas Department of Aging and Disability Services, 2016; The State of Texas Office of the Governor Greg Abbott, n.d.; these are just a few examples and other states will have similar resources).

In general, adult persons with cognitive disabilities, such as IDD, some severities of autism, brain injuries, a mental illness that seriously impairs the person's judgment and perception of reality, or a combination of these disabilities, may need someone with legal authority to make decisions and advocate on their behalf. This is referred to as a *legal guardian*; the *ward* is the person under guardianship. Individuals over the age of 18 with IDD or a mental illness that significantly impairs their judgment who are unable to manage their own affairs, care for, or protect themselves, may need a legal guardian.

Guardianship gives an adult the legal authority to care for a child after the age of emancipation (18 years old). In situations where consent is required, the guardian, by court order, is the surrogate decision maker for the person with IDD. Families with children with IDD are sometimes confused or uncertain as to what guardianship is and why they have to go through the (possible) stress and financial strain of a legal proceeding for their own child. By law, the parent is the natural guardian until the 18th birthday. Once the child turns 18, s/he becomes an emancipated adult. In the United States, citizens have the right to travel freely, move from place to place, and decide where to live. The direct relation of this fundamental right to the special needs community is evident if and when the family must consider residential placement for the adult child. Without legal guardianship in place, individuals with IDD have the right to leave a residential facility, and the home administrators cannot stop them; however, if there is a legal guardian, that person has the authority to make all arrangements with the home about if and when the adult child can leave the facility. Additionally, only the guardian can give instructions about who can visit, take the person off-site, which healthcare (medical, dental, and psychiatric) providers the person can see, which medications are allowable, and—most importantly—to advocate for the individual with IDD. When there is no legal guardian, the individual is legally an adult, and therefore, an independent person who can make all of his/her own decisions, even if s/he lacks the cognitive ability or knowledge needed. The individual must also advocate for him/herself, even if s/he is non-verbal, which can make the situation very complicated.

I have worked on numerous cases involving an adult living in a group home or facility that became the subject of a predator who had posed as a "friend" to take the person off-site. The police were not even able to stop the contact because the child was considered a "consenting adult" who had the right to leave. Other cases involved a person who was taken with the other home residents to the contracted dentist or doctor without the parents' knowledge and had dental work performed or medications changed. Parents were infuriated and terrified that the home administrator had not contacted them, but the home is not obligated to contact family of an adult, unless that adult is under legal guardianship. Guardianship is a legal process that takes several months to complete. If the adult child needs that level of legal protection, the parents or other family must consider the potential for exploitation or of not being included in plans for the child's care when deciding which legal protections to seek.

The constitutional right to enter into a contract is unlimited. Some examples in our daily lives illustrate the numerous contractual relationships that adults are often committed to, including banking, credit cards, home mortgages, apartment rental, car loans, cell phone plans, cable TV and internet plans, health insurance coverage, consent for healthcare treatment (medical, dental and psychiatric), consent to disclosure of healthcare records, employment, hotel stays, and more (United States Constitution, Article 1, section 10, clause 1). An adult who lacks the capacity to understand that getting a credit card involves incurring debt, that the necessary medical invasive procedure that s/he refuses may prevent serious medical problems or save his/her life, or that the predator presenting himself as a "friend" is taking advantage of him/her for his own benefit, may be best protected by the appointment of a legal guardian.

Once a person has entered into a contractual financial arrangement, it is legally binding and very difficult to break. I have received numerous panicked calls over the years from parents whose adult child found a "friend" who took them to the cell phone store, used their good credit to obtain a cell phone, disappeared with the phone and left the adult child responsible for the bills. Explaining to the cellular phone provider that the responsible person has an IDD diagnosis and did not understand the obligation will not suffice to terminate the contractual relationship. Someone is using that phone and someone has to pay for it.

If an adult refuses or consents to medical treatment because s/he lacks the cognitive capacity to understand the prescribed treatment and is not able to ask appropriate questions, the parent cannot override the adult child and make such consents. Many physicians work with the families when the individual with IDD has passed the age of 18, but the hospital risk management departments are increasingly reluctant to allow the parent to consent on behalf of the now adult child, unless there is some legal documentation allowing for a surrogate decision maker or legal guardian. It is essential that parents seek legal counsel to discuss and decide what is most appropriate for their child with IDD.

Basic Guidelines of Guardianship

Guardianship is a legal proceeding. In the United States, each state has its own guardianship laws. In the State of Texas, guardianship matters are governed by Title 3 of the Texas Estates Code (TEC, §1001–§1357) and are conducted in Probate Court. The person applying for guardianship must go to court and ask a judge to adjudicate incapacity and to appoint a legal guardian. The application for guardianship must be substantiated by a capacity assessment from a medical doctor licensed in the State of Texas or a Determination of IDD performed by a licensed psychologist certified to administer such evaluations. After a judicial determination of incapacity, the judge appoints a legal guardian and gives him/her full or partial authority over the ward's affairs, personal and/or financial. The guardian must file an annual report with the Court on the location, status, and well-being of the ward and report all receipts and disbursements of the ward's assets.

There are two primary types of guardianship: guardian of the person and guardian of the estate. The ***guardian of the person*** has the legal authority to decide where the ward lives, consent to healthcare services (medical, psychiatric, and dental treatments), be the representative payee of governmental benefits, and advocate on behalf of the ward (TEC, §1151.051). One may serve as guardian of the person only or as guardian of the person and estate, if the ward has property to manage. The ***guardian of the estate*** who manages the ward's assets under supervision of the court must also obtain the court's permission for expenditures and then provide the court with receipts for the expenses. The guardian of the estate also has authority to bring a lawsuit on behalf of the ward (TEC, §1151.101). The guardian of the estate must be bonded, usually by an insurance policy, to protect the ward's assets (TEC, §1105.101–§1105.257).

Guardianship may be transferable from one state to another. The specific state requirements must be met upon transfer. Within the State of Texas, guardianships are transferrable from county to county. Texas law allows for interstate guardianships (TEC, Chapter 1253), which can transfer to or receive and accept a guardianship from another state. In some situations, there can be co-guardians. For example, both parents can serve as co-guardians; in some states (but not Texas), a parent and the ward's adult sibling can serve as co-guardians (TEC, §1104.001). In most states, once appointed guardian, the parent can designate the preferred person to serve as successor guardian when the parent is unable to continue serving as legal guardian. The succession is not automatic because a judge must appoint the guardian and grant guardian powers, but the courts try to honor the serving guardian's request. A guardian has full legal authority, which is binding on the third parties who interact with the adult child, while a power of attorney (POA) may not be binding (powers of attorney will be described later in this chapter). Costs of establishing a guardianship vary depending on the filing fees of the ward's county of residence, because the guardianship must be established in the county where the ward resides (TEC, §1023.001[a]) and the fees an attorney might charge.

Once the guardianship has been granted, it continues for the ward's lifetime. It can be terminated in a *restoration proceeding*, so named because the ward's rights are restored (TEC, §1202.051. *et seq*). A judge can grant a full or partial restoration if a medical doctor makes the recommendation. An illustrative example of a partial restoration allows the ward driving privileges and/or the right to manage finances, but maintains the guardian's right to make all healthcare (medical, dental, and psychiatric) decisions and to advocate for the ward.

In Texas, the guardian is not liable for the acts of the ward. If the ward commits a criminal act, destroys property, or does anything that creates liability, the guardian will not be personally liable, unless the guardian's negligence directly influenced the ward's behavior. For example, if the ward suffers from mental illness and refuses to take his/her medications, but the guardian allows him/her access to the family car and an accident occurs, the guardian could be held responsible. However, the guardian is liable for not adequately caring for the ward, such as not obtaining government benefits or appropriate medical treatment, or not advocating for the ward who cannot protect him/herself.

In my practice, I have listened to parental concerns about taking the child's rights away. The rights are actually given, by court order, to the guardian. The ward is not left without rights, but remains in the legal status of a minor child, so that the guardian can care for him/her just as when s/he was under the age of 18. Guardianships can be limited in some cases, allowing the ward to maintain the right to vote, ability to drive, or make financial decisions. One must realistically assess the adult child's abilities and limitations to determine the actual need for protection, supervision, ability to intervene, and communicate on behalf of the adult child. The family dynamics can and should continue to foster as much growth and independence as possible for the adult child, and guardianship should not hinder that independence.

Disability advocacy groups may discourage guardianship, asserting the significance of taking someone's individual rights (TEC, Subtitle E). But if an emergency arises, such as medical, financial, social, or a predator taking advantage of the person with IDD, the courts may be the only means to protect the person. On occasion, I have asked parent-clients which specific rights they are concerned about, and I have yet to hear a specific example, other than the right to vote, which can be maintained. I sympathize with these discussions but still ask the parents to see guardianship as a practical tool in long-term planning for their child, if guardianship is appropriate. There is no one-size fits all answer.

It is essential for parents and families of individuals with IDD to obtain legal advice from an attorney who specializes in guardianship law and long-term planning for persons with special needs. Many attorneys can help obtain guardianship, but only some have sufficient training and experience to adequately counsel on the many considerations in caring for a person who may be fully or partially dependent for life. When determining how best to protect an adult child with IDD, the adult child's abilities to make appropriate decisions, to provide for him/herself, to protect him/herself, and to tend to the daily functions of independent living must be considered. The legal documents that families need to assist the person who cannot function with total independence can be tailored, to some extent.

Due to the concern about limiting a person's constitutional rights, Texas guardianship laws were revised in September 1, 2015 (Texas Estates Code, 84th Legislature). Before a guardian can be appointed, clear and convincing evidence must be proven to the court that less restrictive alternatives were considered and determined not feasible to protect the best interests and rights of the proposed ward, and that supports and services available to the proposed ward that would avoid the need for the appointment of a guardian have been considered and determined not to be feasible (TEC, §1101.101). These alternatives to guardianship will be described next.

Alternatives to Guardianship

There are two primary alternatives to guardianship: (a) powers of attorney (POA), and (b) the Supported Decision Making Agreement (SDMA). Each of these procedures have a different purpose and legal limitations.

Powers of attorney (POA). A power of attorney (POA) is a directive whereby a person over the age of 18, who has the mental capacity to understand the document (called the *principal*), grants someone (called the *agent* or *attorney in fact*) the authority to make decisions on his/her behalf. There are several different POAs or directives; a list of those that are especially useful for an adult with a cognitive impairment, but who is high functioning, follows. There are specific POAs, including the Medical POA, HIPAA Release, and Statutory Durable Power of Attorney, as well as some other specific directives. In a Medical POA, the principal grants the agent the authority to make healthcare decisions for the principal with the healthcare provider. The healthcare provider must determine if the principal is competent to make decisions for himself/herself and if the principal was or could have been competent when the POA was executed. The principal always retains the right to refuse or consent to medical treatment even with the Medical POA (Texas Health & Safety Code, §§166.151–166.166).

A HIPAA Release—Authorization to Disclose Protected Health Information—is given by the principal to the authorized person allowing the medical care provider to disclose and release medical records, which would otherwise be confidential. This document is needed when billing health insurance or transferring a patient from a hospital to another facility because it authorizes the healthcare provider to send the medical records (Texas Health & Safety Code, §181.154). In a Statutory Durable POA, the principal grants the agent or attorney in fact the authority to make decisions concerning his/her property and financial matters, including, but not limited to, transactions concerning real estate, banking, insurance, taxes, and personal business (TEC, Chapter 752).

Finally, there are other directives that may be provided with a POA. These may include: (a) Advance Directive to Physicians, Family, or Surrogates, which states the person's preference about end of life decisions for artificial intervention; (b) Do Not Resuscitate (DNR), which states the person's preference for emergency care in the event of cardiac or other organ failure; (c) Designation of Guardian in the Event of Later Incapacity or Need of Guardian, which states the person's preference for a guardian of the person and guardian of the estate; the disqualification of a person can also be stated; and (d) Appointment of Agent to Control Disposition of Remains, which allows the person to designate someone to make funeral arrangements, including cremation.

Powers of attorney have limitations that are important to understand: they can be revoked in writing or orally, and they can be declined by the third party to whom they are presented. For example, if an adult child with IDD executes a Medical POA appointing his/her mother as agent, but tells the medical doctor that s/he will not allow the recommended and necessary procedure, the adult child's word overrides the mother's authority in the Medical POA. In contrast, a Letter of Guardianship is binding because it is a court order; only a state judge has the authority to appoint a guardian and grant the guardian powers.

Supported Decision Making Agreement (SDMA). Texas was the first state to enact SDMA. The purpose of the SDMA is to recognize a less restrictive alternative to guardianship for adults with IDD, who need assistance with decisions regarding daily living but are not considered incapacitated persons for purposes of establishing a guardianship (TEC, §1357.003). The adult with IDD must voluntarily, without coercion or undue influence, enter into a SDMA with a *supporter* that allows the supporter access to information, including medical, financial, educational, psychological, or treatment records from any source, to assist the adult with IDD in understanding the information and consequences of a decision. The supporter may assist the adult in communicating with appropriate persons. The supporter is not authorized to make the decision, only to assist in the decision making process. (TEC, §§§1357.051, 1357.052, 1357.054). The SDMA extends until terminated by either party to the agreement. The SDMA can be terminated if the Department of Family and Protective Services finds that the adult with a disability has been abused, neglected, or exploited by the supporter, or the supporter is found criminally liable of such conduct (TEC, §1357.053). The supporter must obtain a HIPAA Release for medical records and FERPA Release for educational records. A person who receives the original or a copy of the SDMA shall rely on the agreement (TEC, §1357.101). If the person receiving the SDMA has any reason to believe that the adult with IDD is being abused, neglected, or exploited by the supporter, that person must report the alleged abuse, neglect, or exploitation to the Department of Family and Protective Services immediately (TEC, §1357.102).

The SDMA can be used together with POAs and limited guardianships. SDMA is a useful alternative to guardianship for a person who is not totally incapacitated. It can help promote independence and teach the person skills to promote independent living. It allows the person the right to advocate for himself and make his own decisions, which fosters dignity and right of self-determination. (All provision for the Texas SDMA and the actual agreement are found in Texas Estates Code, Chapter 1357.) An experienced special needs attorney should be consulted on all aspects of legal guardianship and alternatives to guardianship.

Government Benefits

An essential component of long-term planning for persons with IDD is understanding what government benefits are available, how to obtain them, and prepare for maintaining the person's eligibility for the benefits. In the United States, the federal government and many individual states offer various benefits that can provide actual money, funding for housing, attendant care, transportation, other support services, and medical insurance coverage to the individual with IDD. The most basic and available benefits are described next.

Supplemental Income Sources

Supplemental Security Income (SSI) is a cash benefit from the general funds of the United States Treasury, not from taxes paid by workers, and is based on financial need. The federal maximum monthly payment is $735. Some, but not all, states add additional supplemental funding. SSI beneficiaries are automatically eligible for Medicaid coverage, which is described in the next section (Social Security Act, §1611 *et seq.*; 42 U.S.C. §1382 *et seq.*).

Supplemental Security Disability Income (SSDI or SSD) is a government-sponsored disability insurance based on the claimant's work history, earnings record, and amount of taxes paid over the course of the person's work history. SSDI recipients are eligible for Medicare after a 24-month (up to 29 month) waiting period. Some life-threatening illnesses have shorter waiting periods (Social Security Administration [SSA], 2015).

Medical Insurance Sources

Medicaid is a comprehensive medical insurance and prescription medication coverage program that also pays for programs and housing (with some limitations) for people with disabilities. Medicaid is available in limited circumstances for pregnant women and children, which is a separate topic, not included in this chapter. Individuals who are eligible for Medicaid can also have Medicaid and private insurance coverage; private insurance can remain primary, with Medicaid covering co-payments. (All benefits available through Medicaid are found in Title XIX to the Social Security Act, codified at 42 U.S.C. §1396 et seq.)

The Health Insurance Premium Payment Program (HIPP is a Medicaid program that helps pay for private medical insurance and is available for a parent or spouse with private medical insurance and a child or spouse with Medicaid. HIPP will reimburse the monthly premium even for the entire family with certain conditions, such as having employer sponsored medical insurance coverage. (For Texas, see Get HIPP, n.d.; for other states, search for the state and "HIPP.")

Similarly, Medicare is a government issued medical insurance, which includes hospital and limited nursing home care, for people over or under 65 years with disabilities; some prescription medication coverage also is available. Recipients of Medicare pay a premium and co-payment. An individual with IDD can be eligible for both Medicare and Medicaid if determined to be a "Disabled Adult Child," which is described in the following paragraph (Centers for Medicare & Medicaid Services, 2017).

Disabled Adult Child (or "DAC") is an additional benefit for an adult child with a disability that onset prior to the age of 22 (see SSA Program Operations Manual System [POMS], 2013a). When a parent of the adult child is eligible for Social Security Disability (SSD) or retirement benefits, the DAC can benefit from the parent's earning record with an increased monthly dollar award and the right to receive Medicare after a 24-month waiting period. A DAC also is entitled to a death benefit when the parent dies, also based on the parent's earning record. The additional monthly cash award is not taken from the parent's Social Security benefit, but given in addition to what the parent receives. The DAC can only receive this additional benefit from one parent (1 T.A.C. §358.107(b)(3); MEDP A-2310; Texas Health and Human Services, 2013). [CAVEAT: The DAC's Medicaid may be automatically canceled upon eligibility for the additional monthly cash award because the DAC's monthly income is too high to qualify for Medicaid. One must immediately appeal the loss of Medicaid under the provisions of the Pickle Amendment (see Mayo & Poland, 2017), named for Texas Senator Pickle who helped initiate this protective legislation, which allows for a person once eligible for Medicaid to be reinstated (42 U.S.C., §1396a).] Many programs and housing are Medicaid sponsored and losing Medicaid benefits can negatively impact a DAC who lives in a group home or other facility that is paid for by Medicaid. It is therefore imperative to look for Medicaid notifications and timely appeal, asking for reinstatement of Medicaid and a retroactive award. Once the Medicaid is reinstated, the DAC can keep Medicare and have Medicaid to cover medical insurance premiums and co-payments. Establishing an individual with disabilities, including IDD, as a DAC is a valuable long-term planning tool because having both Medicaid and Medicare coverage allows for 100% medical insurance coverage, and housing and day-program allocations. (see Farrell & Lesher, 2014).

Other Programs

Medicaid Waiver Programs are community-based alternative programs that offer assistance to keep a child or adult child with disabilities at home, rather than in an institution. Medicaid Waiver Programs are not based on assets or income; there is a long waiting period called the *interest list*. Medicaid Waiver Programs include Community Living Assistance and Support Services (CLASS), Deaf-Blind Multiple Disabilities (DBMD), Home and Community-based Services (HCS), and Medically Dependent Children Program (MDCP). Medicaid Waiver Programs are made on a first-come, first-served basis from a state-wide interest list. In addition to Medicaid, which is provided for medical expenses with no required premiums or co-payments, these programs provide the following, depending on the exact program: attendant care, therapy services, medical equipment, accommodations for the home, and transportation, in addition to Medicaid which is provided for medical expenses, with no required premium or co-pays. I always advise families to enroll their child for the Medicaid Waiver Programs, which are administered by state agencies. Although there is a long waiting period to qualify, the benefits can significantly improve the quality of life for the person with IDD.

Program Eligibility Requirements

In the United States, adults who have not accumulated a federal tax earnings record, because their disability has rendered them unable to self-support, should apply for SSI, which is linked with Medicaid. The federal monthly dollar award is capped as stated above, but Medicaid can add significant funding for medical, housing, and program support. The federal rules for qualifying for these benefits include citizen/immigration/residency status, age, medical eligibility, and financial eligibility. Not everyone living in the United States can qualify for government benefits. Certain requirements must be met, such as citizenship or immigration status. American citizens are always eligible, and permanent residents are eligible under certain requirements; immigrants who are in the United States illegally are not eligible for these benefits. Under the age of 18, the Social Security Administration (SSA) considers parents' combined income; thus, only families living below the poverty level are eligible. Over the age of 18, SSA considers the child an adult by law and parents' income cannot be considered (SSA, 2017).

In addition to these demographic eligibility requirements, individuals must meet medical eligibility. The claimant cannot engage in any substantial gainful activity because of a physical or mental impairment that will result in death or lasts more than 12 months. Claiming a disability alone will not qualify a person for SSI and Medicaid. The applicant (or the parent) must present the manifestations of the disability to prove why the claimant cannot become employed or maintain employment.

Finally, in order to obtain government benefits, the individual must meet financial eligibility requirements. The SSI claimant cannot have more than $735 combined income from all sources per month. Income is defined as earned, unearned, or deemed. *Earned income* is income earned by work. *Unearned* or *deemed income* includes all income that is not earned, including annuities, pensions, alimony, child support, dividends, life insurance proceeds, gifts, inheritances, and prizes. The SSA also considers *in-kind support and maintenance*, which is food and shelter provided for the SSI applicant by someone else. There are various rules and exceptions for calculating such provided support. Additionally, the SSI claimant cannot have more than $2,000 in combined assets. SSA counts U.S. Savings Bonds, custodial accounts, investment accounts, real property, as well as other assets (SSA, 2017). There are some exemptions, such as state-sponsored educational accounts and a homestead. Strict regulations apply to the disposal of the child's assets and income to qualify for SSI and Medicaid. Families should consult with an expert before disposing of assets belonging to the child. Improper transfer and usage of a child's assets to qualify for government assistance is considered fraud on the federal government, with criminal consequences.

Another serious consideration that requires expert advice is how to handle the payment of indefinite child support for an adult child. Because the SSA considers child support as the child's unearned income, the monthly SSI payment may be reduced or the adult child may be disqualified from benefits entirely. Many family law attorneys are not informed about government benefits and may unwittingly put provisions in divorce decrees that disqualify the child from eligibility for the benefits. However, both federal and individual state laws allow the creation of an irrevocable Medicaid Reimbursement Child Support SNT that provides both indefinite child support and eligibility for government benefits. Once again, the parent must consult with an attorney who is an expert in this very specialized type of planning. Federal and state laws allow child support to be payable to the trustee of a properly drafted child support SNT, which is not considered income to the child. The adult child can then receive SSI and Medicaid and have funds in a trust that supplements any government benefits. There are different types of SNTs. It is critical for parents to consult with an expert for proper drafting and instructions on how to set up and manage a SNT. A brief description of estate planning will be provided next; however, more information on financial planning, including SNTs, is provided in Chapter 13 of this text.

Estate Planning and Other Sources of Financial Support for Individuals with IDD

Among the concerns I hear in my practice is how to ensure quality of life for the child when the parents or family are deceased. Any estate plan must include a legal will, and for families with a child with IDD, a trust. Both are described in this section.

Legal Will

A legal will is the best vehicle to transfer ownership of property, both real and personal, after death, and to designate whom the person writing the will (called a *testator*) wants to serve in the various fiduciary roles, such as the executor, trustee, and/or guardian for the children. It is essential to have a will because without one, the testator's property will be divided according to the provisions of his/her particular state's laws. Additionally, if one dies *intestate* (without a will), his/her heirs will have additional legal work and expenses before they can dispose of the homestead, accounts in financial institutions, and/or other assets. A will is especially important for blended families, when the testator wants to provide for his current spouse, his children with the spouse, and/or his children from a previous relationship. In contrast, a *trust* is a legal document that specifically designates who will manage assets left for the benefit of another person. A more thorough explanation is provided in the next section. Most important to our discussion is how to provide for a child with IDD after the death of the parent or grandparent. I watch parents struggle over who to designate to care for the child with IDD and who to appoint as trustee of a trust set up for the benefit of that child. A brief overview of the specific fiduciary roles that should be enumerated in a will is provided next.

The will should name a person to serve as *executor* of the deceased's estate. The executor, or personal representative, is responsible for petitioning the court to admit a will to probate, to gather estate assets, pay last bills and expenses, address creditor claims, file the final income tax return, pay outstanding taxes, sell real estate and personal property, and distribute the assets to the beneficiaries according to the terms of the will. The executor must work with an attorney to accomplish his/her duties.

If a will does not exist or the person named in a will to serve as executor has died or is not willing to serve, a qualified person can petition the court to serve as *estate administrator*, because there is a need to take care of all or some of the above-mentioned duties. This estate administrator is also referred to as a "personal representative." The court can order a dependent or independent administrator, depending on the needs of the estate; often, when there are minor children, the judge will only allow a dependent administrator which maintains court supervision on all transactions.

A judge can appoint more than one person to serve as a personal representative. Appointing more than one personal representative can sometimes be a burden or create problems because both individuals are required to be present to sign closing documents at the sale of real estate, paperwork pertaining to accounts in financial institutions, employee benefits, and other documents. How to appoint these individuals as fiduciaries should be discussed in detail with a qualified attorney.

A *trustee* is the person or financial institution who manages the funds on behalf of another person (the *beneficiary*) and distributes the funds to the beneficiary according to the terms enumerated in the trust documents. Children under the age of 18 years cannot receive an outright inheritance and the surviving parent does not automatically have access to the minor child's inheritance; any assets designated for a minor child must be placed in either a court-supervised guardianship account or trust, which is managed by a trustee. A well drafted will allows the testator to indicate at what age his/her child may directly receive his inheritance and until what age the assets should be managed by the trustee. In cases involving minor children or a child with disabilities, including IDD, the testator names the person(s) s/he wants to be appointed guardian in the will. The appointment of a guardian or successor guardian is not automatic. Although the courts try to honor the testator's wishes, the named person must apply for appointment as guardian (guardianship was described more thoroughly in the beginning of this chapter).

Trusts must have a purpose. For a person without a disability and in need of government needs-based benefits, a common usage is for "health, education, maintenance, and support." These terms are broad enough to allow the trustee flexibility in using trust funds for the child's needs until s/he has reached the age to personally manage the assets. If the beneficiary is a person with a disability, including IDD, the portion of the assets designated for him/her must be assigned to a trust for which the purpose is to "supplement and not supplant" government benefits, called a Supplemental Needs Trust (SNT).

Supplemental Needs Trusts

SNTs are used to protect eligibility for benefits. For example, if the person with IDD would be eligible for SSI and Medicaid, except he/she does not meet the financial eligibility requirement because of existing assets, transferring the assets into a self-settled SNT can allow him/her to qualify for and receive the needs-based assistance. Additionally, if the individual with IDD has family members or friends that want to make financial contributions to that individual, they can direct an asset into a Third Party SNT while alive (called an *intervivos trust*), or upon death with a testamentary SNT (see SSA POMS, 2013b).

For clients who have no appropriate family members or friends to appoint for the various fiduciary roles, I often suggest meeting with an officer of a financial institution who has a special needs trust department to inquire into the fiduciary services that the bank can offer. However, corporate trustees often have high minimum initial funding requirements. In Texas, The Arc of Texas Master Pooled Trust (n.d.; 42 U.S.C. §1396(d)(4)(c)) is an option for management of a SNT. In many situations, the court can appoint a professional personal representative, usually an attorney who practices in the area of probate law. Fees for such professional services are paid from the estate or SNT. Again, a thorough description of financial planning is provided in Chapter 13 of this text and should be referred to for its valuable information.

Fundraising

Fundraising websites, such as GoFundMe.com, YouCaring.com, Indiegogo.com, FundAnything.com, and others have become increasingly popular. Considering the enormous financial expenses facing a family with a child who will never be independent or fully independent, it can be tempting to fund raise. Sometimes, well-meaning people other than the immediate family set up fund raising sites without informing the parents, such as another family member, friend, or co-worker. Families should be aware that such fund raising can result in the loss of the government needs-based benefits, including Medicaid, with more difficult financial consequences and possible claims for reimbursement to the SSA.

Conclusion

This chapter provided an overview of specific legal matters that directly pertain to the special needs community. It serves as an introduction to these areas of special needs planning, and is not a comprehensive description. Each topic requires its own full book to fully explore and explain, but I hope our readers have gained a general understanding of the legal aspects involved in long-term planning. I emphasize the need to work with an attorney who specializes in this area of law because mistakes in drafting can result in serious consequences, such as losing benefits because an improperly drafted SNT is counted as a personal resource or Medicaid could place a claim on a Third Party SNT that included unnecessary payback provisions. I often suggest that families seek legal counsel when considering their will and trusts. I also recommend employing or (at least) consulting with an experienced care manager because the SNT should be managed prudently to last for the life of the beneficiary. Some well-meaning trustees initially spend significant amounts from the SNT because the parent makes compelling requests for distributions, leaving little money for future needs. Because the long-term needs of the beneficiary must be weighed with immediate requests for distributions, seeking professional counsel is a wise investment and an allowable expenditure from a SNT. While these topics can be overwhelming, addressing them in segments and with qualified, experienced professional guidance can provide essential long-term benefits for individuals with IDD and their families.

Key Messages from This Chapter

- **For individuals with IDD and their families**: Common concerns of all families with a child with IDD, such as naming the person to care for the child when the parent is no longer able, how to provide for the child's needs, how to access government benefits, and how to balance the needs of the other children, must be addressed. There are many misconceptions about these legal matters that can cloud the family's ability to make appropriate long-term planning decisions.
- **For professionals**: It is essential for all professionals working with persons with IDD and other disabilities and their families to understand the various germane legal issues and how they can interact. Legal documents, such as powers of attorney, an Order Appointing Guardian, wills, SNTs and other trusts, are the essential tools for long-term planning for this community. The documents must be carefully and correctly drafted to accomplish the family's goals. In court and in practice, we often see improperly drafted documents that can jeopardize the person's eligibility for government benefits, and which fail to protect the individual, inadvertently waive legal rights, or interfere with family relationships.
- **For policy makers**: Recent legislation, specifically the ABLE Act, is just the beginning of the types of federal policies that can support individuals with IDD and their families. Collaborations between policy makers, IDD advocates, families of individuals with IDD, and other professionals are necessary to ensure that continued state and federal legislation and regulations continue to be developed that will have a positive impact for individuals with IDD.

References

Centers for Medicare & Medicaid Services. (2017). *Medicare & You 2017.* Retrieved from https://www.medicare.gov/pubs/pdf/10050-Medicare-and-You.pdf

Farrell, H. C., & Lesher, C. (2014, February). *Protecting and maximizing public benefits.* Paper presented at the meeting of the 2014 Changes and Trends Affecting Special Needs Trusts, The University of Texas School of Law, Austin, TX. Retrieved from https://utcle.org/ecourses/OC4791/get-asset-file/asset_id/31864

Get HIPP. (n.d.). *GET HIPP: Employer sponsored coverage through Medicaid.* Retrieved from www.gethipptexas.org

Mayo, P.-Y., & Poland, B. (2017). *Pickle people: Using the Pickle Amendment to obtain Medicaid eligibility.* Paper presented at the meeting of the 13th Annual Changes and Trends Affecting Special Needs Trusts, The University of Texas School of Law, Austin, TX. Retrieved from https://utcle.org/elibrary/download/a/40445/p/1

Social Security Administration. (2015). *Social Security disability benefits.* Retrieved from https://www.ssa.gov/pubs/EN-05-10029.pdf

Social Security Administration. (2017). *Understanding Supplemental Security Income SSI eligibility requirements—2017 edition.* Retrieved from http://www.socialsecurity.gov/ssi/text-eligibility-ussi.htm

Social Security Administration, Program Operations Manual System. (2013a). *SI 01715.015 special groups of former SSI recipients.* Retrieved from https://secure.ssa.gov/apps10/poms.nsf/lnx/0501715015

Social Security Administration, Program Operations Manual System. (2013b). *SI 01120.200 trusts.* Retrieved from https://secure.ssa.gov/poms.nsf/lnx/0501120200

Texas Guardianship Association. (2015). *Guardianship information.* Retrieved from texasguardianship.org

Texas Department of Aging and Disability Services. (2016). *A Texas guide to adult guardianship.* Retrieved from https://www.dads.state.tx.us/news_info/publications/brochures/pub395-guardianship.pdf

Texas Health and Human Services. (2013). *MEPD, A-2000, mandatory coverage groups.* Retrieved from https://hhs.texas.gov/node/4456

The Arc of Texas Master Pooled Trust. (n.d.). *About the master pooled trust.* Retrieved from thearcoftexas.org/trust/index.php

The State of Texas Office of the Governor Greg Abbott. (n.d.). *Guardianship.* Retrieved from gov.texas.gov/disabilities/resources/guardianship

16 When the Journey Ends

Parental Caregiving and Later Life Planning

Elizabeth A. Perkins, PhD and Lieke van Heumen, PhD

Introduction

This chapter will address issues at later stages of the life span for aging parents of adult children with intellectual and developmental disabilities (IDD). Families and professionals will be provided with an understanding of how to successfully prepare for this point in the life span as they encounter the physical, social, and psychological challenges that may arise. The importance of sibling caregivers in this caregiving scenario will also be discussed. The concept of future planning is described along with resources that can be utilized to implement this critically important process. The chapter concludes with summarizing important principles of practice.

Aging and IDD: A Rapidly Changing Landscape

A positive consequence of better healthcare, better treatment of chronic health issues, and better understanding of the impact of diet, exercise, and lifestyle choices, is vastly increasing all of our chances of living longer and aging well. Globally, in 2017, the number of adults who are aged 65 and older will, for the first time in human history, outnumber children up to age five (World Health Organization [WHO], 2012). In the United States, people aged 65+ currently comprise 13% of the population, a figure that will increase to 18% by 2030 (Cohn & Taylor, 2010). Every day, an estimated 10,000 baby boomers (the generation born between 1946 and 1964) reach age 65, and the current overall life expectancy (LE) in the United States is 79 years (Cohn & Taylor, 2010). Life expectancy at birth is the statistic that describes the age by which 50% of the population will have died, and 50% still survive. Thus, of all babies born in the United States today, half will live to age 79 and beyond.

Compared with the general population, overall LE of people with an intellectual and developmental disability (IDD) is lower. However, it can be misleading to state one specific LE figure, as there is considerable variation based upon IDD type(s), the severity of the disability, and other related medical issues. As a general rule though, milder disability, and less complexity of associated medical issues, generally results in higher LE. For example, the population with mild intellectual disabilities (about 85% of the population with ID) can expect to live into their mid-70s (Bittles *et al.*, 2002). Life expectancy for people with moderate ID reduces to 67 years and to 59 years for people with severe/profound ID (Bittles *et al.*, 2002). Individuals with autism spectrum disorder (ASD) also have a slightly reduced life expectancy, even after excluding those with ASD who have additional intellectual or developmental disability and/or mobility difficulties (Shavelle & Strauss, 1998). Life expectancy for people with cerebral palsy (CP) can vary significantly—for example, more functional independence (e.g., ability to eat, control their head, sit, or walk unaided) can impact life expectancy by as much as 30 years (Strauss, Brooks, Rosenbloom, & Shavelle, 2008). People with Down syndrome are also noted to have a much-reduced life expectancy, between 49–60 years (Bittles *et al.*, 2002; Yang, Rasmussen, & Friedman, 2002).

Overall, though disparities remain in LE between the general population and the IDD population, the aging population with IDD is growing and the gap between their LE and that of the general population has been quickly diminishing, especially in recent decades. Thus, people with IDD are a small but rapidly emerging segment of the aging population. This population is particularly noteworthy because they already have support needs ranging anywhere between intermittent (occasional) to highly intensive (continuous) levels of care. Furthermore, over 71% currently live with a family caregiver, and almost 25% of these family caregivers are already aged 60+ (Braddock *et al.*, 2013). In 2000, there were an estimated 650,000 Americans with IDD aged 60 years, which is projected to double to 1.2 million by 2030 (Heller, Stafford, Davis, Sedlezky, & Gaylord, 2010). Thus, because of their increasing longevity, more people with IDD than ever before will now face the prospect of life after the death of their caregiving parents. For caregiving parents of people with IDD and professionals who support them, there are unique challenges that aging in this context brings. The following section will highlight the physical, psychological, and social issues that can arise and includes strategies for how they may be addressed.

Aging Caregivers: Physical, Psychological, and Social Concerns

Caregiving is commonplace—almost ubiquitous—with over 40 million Americans providing 37 billion hours of care to a family member (AARP, 2015). However, when people think of caregivers, the image so often conjured is someone taking care of an elderly parent. Less imagined are caregivers who support children with significant disabilities, and even less would think of aging parent caregivers of adult children with IDD. And yet aging caregivers of people with IDD have unique issues—very different from what we may consider "general" caregiving.

Physical Issues in Caregiving

Haley and Perkins (2004) highlighted that the aging process can create difficulties for both the caregiver and their aging care recipient with IDD. Caregivers have had decades of providing care to their child with IDD and certainly have the advantage of a lifetime of experience to be adaptable to changing circumstances (Haley & Perkins, 2004). However, the development of new aging-related health issues in addition to lifelong disabilities, can exacerbate the aging-process in people with IDD, and unfortunately, there are few professionals appropriately educated to provide much guidance to caregivers (Haley & Perkins, 2004; Perkins & Moran, 2010). Though beyond the scope of this chapter, readers interested in more information on the aging process, aging-related health issues, and specific IDD concerns are recommended to refer to Saxon, Etten, and Perkins's (2014) book, *Physical Changes and Aging: A Guide for the Helping Professions.*

Individuals with IDD may require intensive support for basic needs (e.g., bathing, dressing, and toileting), eating/drinking, assistance with mobility/transfers, and other activities of daily living. Such support needs may require considerable physical exertion and stamina from a caregiver. Conversely, individuals with IDD who are receiving care may also develop a new health condition (e.g., diabetes, heart disease) that results in entirely new and significant care needs in addition to their pre-existing needs. The development of new chronic health conditions in both caregiver and care recipient is very likely; at least 50% of all adults in the United States have at least one chronic condition (Ward, Schiller, & Goodman, 2014), rising to 92% in those aged 65+ (Hung, Ross, Boockvar, & Siu, 2011). Some common aging-related health issues, such as osteoarthritis, vision/hearing loss, frailty, and heart disease, can adversely impact a caregiver's physical strength and stamina. Caregivers need to recognize these pitfalls for themselves and be comfortable admitting they need help, which may be difficult after decades of independence.

Given that caregiving for one person can be physically exhausting, imagine becoming a caregiver to another family member! A lifelong caregiver of an adult child with IDD who has become a caregiver to another family member has been described as "***compound caregiving***," because of the extra caregiving responsibilities it brings (Perkins, 2010). Previous research has reported that one third of older caregivers (aged 50+) of adult children with IDD were in fact compound caregivers, and perhaps even more telling, 68% had been caregivers sometime previously, and 34% anticipated the need to do so within the next few years (Perkins & Haley, 2010). The vast majority of compound caregivers provide care to other older family members (e.g., their parents, parents-in-law) or loved ones of similar ages (e.g., spouses and siblings), and the most common major issue in that new compound care recipient is often Alzheimer's disease (Perkins & Haley, 2010). The additional care recipient may have previously assisted in caregiving duties, thus magnifying the impact upon the compound caregiver (Perkins, 2010). A common example would be a grandparent who develops dementia who used to be actively involved with his/her grandchild with IDD, providing respite breaks to the caregiving parents.

With increasing age, the distinction between who is the caregiver and who is the care recipient may blur especially in those who have mild intellectual disabilities. In some cases, the caregiver and care recipient become more mutually dependent, or potentially have role reversals (Perkins & Haley, 2013). One study found that 22% of older caregivers of adult children with IDD actually reported receiving more physical help from their child than they actually gave (Perkins & Haley, 2013). Although it can be positive for a caregiver to receive help from his/her child with IDD, there is a need to be vigilant in order to recognize when both caregiver and care recipient capacities are extended beyond their mutual capabilities to safely assist each other. Professionals may need to advocate for increased assistance against potential reluctance from a caregiver to relinquish some of these responsibilities. An intriguing finding from one study indicated that aging caregivers of people with IDD rated their health to be better than same aged non-caregivers despite reporting more health challenges (Yamaki, Hsieh, & Heller, 2009). For some caregivers, after decades of providing care, the thought of not being a caregiver anymore may be simply unthinkable. For others, finally admitting the need for help may be a liberating relief.

Psychological Issues in Caregiving

Preparing for our own death is something we universally acknowledge as something we should do, but in reality, the chances that we attend to such a task usually only increases with advancing age. One survey of the general population in the United States aged 50+ found that approximately 60% have completed a will (AARP, 2000). Regarding more specific end-of-life instructions, 60% of all adults would like them to be respected, yet only one third actually complete advance directives (Pollack, Morhaim, & Williams, 2010). When one considers the reluctance for end-of-life planning for the general population with no intellectual/cognitive difficulties, such a task might seem more difficult for people with IDD and their family caregivers, yet paradoxically, it is even more critical that their wishes are correctly identified, respected, and implemented. Identifying family members' wishes may be some of the most poignant and compelling decisions they will make and the process of clarifying them provides invaluable insight for all individuals (Friedman & Helm, 2010).

Traditionally, many adults with IDD have had all major decisions in their life made by their caregiving parents who have also been their legal guardians. There is an emerging movement towards *supported decision-making,* which avoids the need for more restrictive guardianships (Blanck & Martinis, 2015). This model promotes better collaboration and discussion of the issue so the individual with IDD is assisted in making an informed decision with others, rather than decisions being made by others. Professionals and caregivers alike may find the book, "*People Planning Ahead: Communicating Healthcare and End-of-Life Wishes*" (Kingsbury, 2009), provides a useful framework to use with their care recipient with IDD, as well as initiating their own process in tandem.

Aging parent caregivers are often very fearful regarding the future life of their surviving children with IDD (Haley & Perkins, 2004). Though some caregivers will make meticulous arrangements, many others may never even formalize a plan. In a study of mothers (aged 58–87 years) of adult children with intellectual disabilities, less than half had made future residential plans for their adult child (Freedman, Krauss, & Seltzer, 1997). The concern is that these figures have not improved over the years. It is easy to unfairly judge such caregivers who have avoided making plans, but many become effectively paralyzed with indecision because they may perceive few available options or solutions (Grant, 1990). Indeed, unremitting apprehension and frustration with obstacles encountered in the planning process continue to be recurrent themes reported by aging caregivers (Taggart, Truesdale-Kennedy, Ryan, & McConkey, 2012).

Social Needs of Caregivers

As one ages, thoughts begin to revolve around the major transition from work-life to retirement. For some, retirement is a process that is accomplished in a series of small transitions (e.g., from full to part-time work or voluntary work). For others, it can be very abrupt. Consider the implications for caregivers of adult children with IDD. Retirement may be indefinitely postponed for some, due to the need for additional income—recognizing that across the life span, some caregivers are unable to work or save enough for retirement due to their caregiving responsibilities (Parish, Seltzer, Greenberg & Floyd, 2004). They may never experience an "empty nest" (Seltzer & Krauss, 1994) and some of the benefits that brings, including more personal freedom, time, ability to focus on one's own hobbies and interests, and more opportunity to socialize with others, yet they see friends and other family members embracing this change (Seltzer, Floyd, Song, Greenberg, & Hong, 2011). Some caregivers who retire from their employment may have competing demands and obligations. For example, their own desire for a more relaxed pace may be at odds with their continuing caregiving demands (e.g., helping their child have a fulfilled life with many activities). Other activities that they may have neglected include time with other children and grandchildren or other family members and friends.

Overall, although there are undoubted physical, psychological, and social concerns that can be distressing to caregivers, the majority of issues are amenable to being addressed or modified. Furthermore, the support of other family members, and especially the siblings of the adult with IDD, can be indispensable. Thus, further exploration to the unique role and support siblings can provide is warranted.

Recognizing the Importance of Sibling Caregivers

Adults with IDD generally have long-lasting close relationships with their siblings—indeed, across their respective life spans, a sibling relationship may be the most stable and enduring given the closeness of age and shared life experiences (see Chapter 8 in this text). Although mothers usually provide the most hands-on-care, siblings often provide considerable support and companionship to both parents and the adult with IDD (Bigby, 2000). When there are multiple siblings, it is often the case that one sibling in particular will have more prominent involvement in the life of the adult with IDD (Bigby, 1997). Unsurprisingly, individuals with IDD name their siblings among their most important family members (Arnold, Heller, & Kramer, 2012). Likewise, siblings also value the relationship with their brother or sister with IDD (Bigby, Webber, & Bowers, 2015).

As individuals with IDD live longer and their parents reach advanced age, the role of siblings becomes increasingly important. Between 40–60% of siblings of adults with IDD expect to assume the primary caregiving responsibility in the future (Amado, 2013; Heller & Kramer, 2009). Siblings tend to be among the key people informally nominated by a parent to assume future responsibility for safeguarding the well-being of their sibling with IDD, and thus are likely to become the new primary caregiver of the adult with IDD after the death of their parents (Heller & Arnold, 2010). In some cases, the sibling and the adult with IDD may live together, either temporarily or permanently (Bigby, 1997). As women tend to be most involved in the lives of adults with IDD, it is most often a sister rather than a brother who becomes the new primary caregiver (Prosser & Moss, 1996). Adults with IDD who have a brother as their only sibling may be at risk to receive only limited family support after the death of their parents (Bigby, 2002).

Many prominent IDD advocacy groups were initially formed by parents (e.g., in the United States The Arc, 2016; in the United Kingdom, Mencap, n.d.), along with the latest rise of self-advocacy organizations (e.g., Self-Advocates Becoming Empowered, n.d.). More recently, there has been much-needed recognition of providing sibling support and advocacy. A notable example, the Sibling Leadership Network (SLN, 2016), was formed in 2007 and has rapidly grown to provide siblings of individuals with disabilities the information, supports, and tools to advocate with their brothers and sisters and promote attention to the issues important to them and their families (SLN, 2016).

Planning for the Future

Given the reluctance of many parents to do otherwise, promoting the importance of future planning in this caregiving context cannot be over-emphasized. Fundamentally, any form of future planning is desirable, as the alternative can result in crisis situations and inappropriate nursing/group home placements, while families and professionals scramble to coordinate new supports. It is important to consider how traumatizing it may be to the individual with IDD to lose a parent, and simultaneously, have a multitude of other transitions to make during this difficult time. Any prior preparation and planning for the time after a caregiver dies, becomes incapacitated, or for some other reason needs to relinquish the caregiving role, is time well spent in aiding a smoother transition to new life circumstances for adults with IDD.

Some parents and caregivers may have never accessed formal support services for their children beyond their childhood/school years, so there may be a steep learning curve with identifying the range of services available, the application/eligibility requirements, out-of-pocket expenses, and other information about establishing an alternative residential placement. If the person with IDD has no siblings and no other potential family support, it is even more critical to ensure this person has been identified by the appropriate formal long-term services and support systems that provide residential/in-home and community-based care. This may include disability specific agencies or may require communication/liaison between aging and disability service networks, depending on the age of the individual. Being identified by the relevant support system can help ease caregiver burden if the person with IDD is eligible for services immediately. And regardless of whether immediate help is provided, being connected to and securing a position on a waitlist for services through these caregiving support systems is important.

Components of Future Planning

Future planning is very comprehensive and includes details about aspects of a person's life, reflecting the wishes of the person with IDD, as well as his/her parents, siblings, and other important people who are involved in his/her life (The Arc Center for Future Planning, 2016a). Recognizing the need to address this critical situation, The Arc Center for Future Planning (2016a) developed a web-based resource to guide families and professionals who are interested in implementing a future planning process. Developing each of these areas into a written document or plan will be beneficial to families of individuals with IDD. (See Chapter 13 for more information on future planning, including care guides and letters of intent.)

Professionals may also want to utilize and implement "*The Future is Now,*" a future planning training curriculum specifically developed for family caregivers and their adult relatives with IDD (Factor *et al.*, 2010). Designed to be conducted in person over five 2.5-hour sessions, this curriculum includes class exercises and homework assignments that result in a comprehensive letter of intent that describes how individuals with IDD want their future life to be, and more importantly, identifies the actions needed to meet their expectations. Caregivers who have undergone this future planning process often benefit from a significant reduction in caregiving burden (Heller & Caldwell, 2006). Therefore, although there might be reluctance on the part of the caregiver to tackle the subject of future planning and actually initiate the process, professionals who advocate for future planning should be encouraged that caregivers ultimately feel relief by addressing their fears and formulating an actual plan of action.

Sibling Involvement in Future Planning

As previously stated, many parents do not make future plans. Unfortunately, even when they do, surprisingly, many do not directly discuss the future plans with their children without disabilities, even though these siblings often take on caregiving roles (Bigby, 1997; Freedman *et al.*, 1997; Heller & Caldwell, 2006).

One study found that 64% of children without disabilities did not know their parents' future plans for their sibling with IDD (Griffiths & Unger, 1994). Even if included in the planning process, many siblings report having low involvement in future planning activities (Heller & Kramer, 2009). Of the different future planning tasks, siblings are most likely to be involved in identifying a future caregiver and in making residential plans (Heller & Kramer, 2009). They are less likely to be involved in tasks such as establishing a special needs trust or establishing power of attorney for their sibling with a disability (Heller & Kramer, 2009). However, the reason for lack of sibling involvement is often a benevolent one, as some parents may not want to burden the siblings with additional responsibilities (Griffiths & Unger, 1994).

Future planning is an ideal process for getting all family members convened to address specific questions and potential issues and to get everyone on the same page and in agreement with the specific plan. Siblings of individuals with IDD are necessary to include in all future planning activities and can greatly assist in the effort to identify important aspects in the planning process. Siblings can bring unique perspectives of the wishes and desires of their sibling with IDD that may not be apparent or have never been discussed with their parents and other professionals. As siblings are closer to each other in age and shared life experiences, they often share similar cultural/generational perspectives. Some subjects (e.g., intimate relationships) may be easier to discuss between siblings rather than between parents and adult children with IDD. Thus, future planning that specifically includes siblings in addition to parents and individuals with IDD can better inform the whole process (Arnold *et al.*, 2012; Bigby *et al.*, 2015; Heller & Caldwell, 2006; Heller & Kramer, 2009).

An advantage of the involvement of siblings, who participate in a robust future planning process when their parents are alive, is that they will also be better prepared for the same process when they are the primary caregiver. Siblings will need to consider their own family network to plan for their own replacement and to ensure that someone else (such as a niece or nephew) will have a similar commitment to the well-being of the person with IDD in the future, if such a scenario becomes necessary (Bigby, 1997, 2000; Bigby *et al.*, 2015).

Depending on their respective ages, siblings may not be as connected with their sibling with IDD than in previous years, due to the demands of their own family/work life. Thus, when siblings are not included in future planning tasks as a stakeholder, they may be less effective in their future caregiving roles (Heller & Kramer, 2009). Siblings need to be involved in discussions and they can often be a catalyst to encourage the future planning process within the family (Heller & Kramer, 2009). The SLN (2016) and the Arc Center for Future Planning (2016a) provide information to siblings related to future planning. The Arc Center for Future Planning (2016b) created a sibling tip sheet to serve as a resource for siblings to initiate conversations around future planning. The tip sheet describes the importance of siblings understanding the history of services received by their sibling with a disability, their support needs, and their future wishes.

Principles for Practice

We recommend the following guiding principles for professionals who support individuals with IDD and their aging caregivers with respect to implementing future planning. It is important to support the autonomy and self-determination of individuals with IDD in conveying their needs and desires, and always promoting their right to full inclusion in all aspects of community living. Professionals need to recognize the physical, psychological, and social impacts of aging on the capacity of older parents of adult children with IDD to continue their caregiving role and yet broach the topic with caregivers about the value in future planning. It is never too early to approach the subject and it may actually prompt immediate changes that are also beneficial. Recognizing that several attempts at encouraging future planning may be needed, individuals with IDD and their caregivers need to be allowed time to become comfortable with the idea of planning for what happens when parents are no longer able to care for their children.

It will be necessary for families to determine whether future planning is best implemented by the family members independently or as part of a group process. Discussions with peers, other caregivers, and other professionals can result in more possibilities and innovative solutions being generated, but some caregivers may prefer a more private process. Every effort should be made to accurately identify and involve all members of the family (especially siblings) and friends who should be included in future planning, while recognizing the family dynamics that may be at play and being prepared to advocate or negotiate between opposing ideas. While some planning is better than no planning at all, professionals should encourage completion of the major decisions (e.g., who will be the new primary caregiver), even if other plans are not fully completed. Individuals and families should be provided information about formal supports and services in their area, as well as other informal organizations (e.g., recreational and social clubs) that can be utilized to enhance the quality of life of the person with IDD.

We strongly advocate for the importance of future planning—and the earlier the better—because we believe it can enhance a caregiver's current life by removing perennial and unresolved concerns (see Chapter 13 in this text). Family discussions that include siblings (and others close to the person with IDD) will ultimately optimize the future planning and make the transition to post-parent life more seamless and less disruptive. Professionals who support these families are advised to broach the subject, and to be persistent, if necessary, in their encouragement of families to complete a future plan. Aging can be a time of harsh pragmatism, but it can also engender renewed vigor to complete those "bucket list" items. Aging caregivers who have future plans in place may be better positioned to pursue some of their own personal lifetime wishes too—content in knowing their adult child's future life and well-being is secured.

Conclusion

Aging is often viewed very negatively, as a time of loss of physical and cognitive ability, financial challenges, separation from family and friends, and the likelihood of the development of new health issues. We named this chapter "*When the Journey Ends: Parental Caregiving and Later Life Planning*" to address the reality that the majority of aging parent caregivers of adult children with IDD will die before their child does. This should be a welcomed reality, as in the general scheme of things, it is expected that individuals with IDD can and should survive their parents. For parents with considerable and lifelong caregiving responsibilities, it may seem that facing one's mortality and the consequences that it brings is almost too much to even contemplate. However, it is a shared reality experienced by the vast majority of us—and yet life teaches us that we are all quite adaptable and resilient beings, that we can honor and then embrace that reality through planning, and then continue on with the life that remains, more peacefully.

Key Messages from This Chapter

- **For individuals with IDD and their families**: People with IDD and their caregivers benefit from careful future planning for the transition to life beyond parent-provided care. Involvement of all family members in formulating robust plans will prepare everyone for their new support roles and responsibilities, which can be implemented without delay and confusion.
- **For professionals**: Professionals can have a crucial role to advocate and help facilitate future planning for people with IDD and their family caregivers. Professionals can help initiate the planning process and offer impartial guidance on overcoming potential issues as they are identified.
- **For policy makers**: Policy makers should consider the provision of service supports and funding structures that can help identify future needs and promote seamless transitions of appropriate and responsive supports across the life span. Furthermore, they need to recognize aging caregivers of adult children with IDD as a priority population, who are deserving of the peace of mind that guaranteed continuity of quality care can provide.

References

AARP. (2000). *Where there is a will ... Legal documents among the 50+ population: Findings from an AARP survey.* Retrieved from http://assets.aarp.org/rgcenter/econ/will.pdf

AARP. (2015). *Valuing the invaluable: 2015 update.* Retrieved from http://www.aarp.org/content/dam/aarp/ppi/2015/valuing-the-invaluable-2015-update-new.pdf

Amado, A. N. (2013). *Friends: Connecting people with disabilities and community members.* Minneapolis, MN: University of Minnesota, Institute on Community Integration, Research and Training Center on Community Living. Retrieved from http://rtc.umn.edu/docs/Friends_Connecting_people_with_disabilities_and_community_members.pdf

Arnold, C. K., Heller, T., & Kramer, J. (2012). Support needs of siblings of people with developmental disabilities. *Intellectual and Developmental Disabilities, 50,* 373–382. doi:10.1352/1934-9556-50.5.373

Bigby, C. (1997). In place of parents? The sibling relationships of older people with intellectual disability. *Journal of Gerontological Social Work*, *29*, 3–22. doi:10.1300/J083v29n01_02

Bigby, C. (2000). Informal support networks of older adults. In M. P. Janicki & E. F. Ansello (Eds.), *Community supports for aging adults with lifelong disabilities* (pp. 81–95). Baltimore, MD: Paul H. Brookes Publishing Company.

Bigby, C. (2002). Social roles and informal support networks in mid life and beyond. In P. Noonan Walsh & T. Heller (Eds.), *Health of women with intellectual disabilities* (pp. 121–136). Oxford, UK: Blackwell.

Bigby, C., Webber, R., & Bowers, B. (2015). Sibling roles in the lives of older group home residents with intellectual disability: Working with staff to safeguard wellbeing. *Australian Social Work*, *68*(4), 453–468. doi:10.1080/0312407X.2014.950678

Bittles, A. H., Petterson, B. A., Sullivan, S. G., Hussain, R., Glasson, E. J. & Montgomery, P. D. (2002). The influence of intellectual disability on life expectancy. *Journal of Gerontology Series A: Biological Sciences and Medical Sciences*, *57*, M470-2. doi:10.1093/gerona/ 57.7.M470

Blanck, P., & Martinis, J. G. (2015). "The right to make choices": The National Resource Center for Supported Decision-Making. *Inclusion*, *3*, 24–33. doi:10.1352/2326-6988-3.1.24

Braddock, D., Hemp, R., Rizzolo, M.C., Tanis, E.S., Haffer, L., Lulinski-Norris, A., & Wu, J. (2013). *The state of the states in developmental disabilities 2013: The great recession and its aftermath.* Washington, DC: American Association on Intellectual and Developmental Disabilities.

Cohn, D., & Taylor, P. (2010). *Baby boomers approach 65—glumly.* Retrieved from http://www.pewsocialtrends.org/files/2010/12/Boomer-Summary-Report-FINAL.pdf

Factor, A., Debrine, E. J., Caldwell, J., Keiling, K., Kramer, J., & Heller, T. (2010). *The future is now: A future planning training curriculum for families and their adult relatives with developmental disabilities* (3rd ed.). Chicago, IL: The Rehabilitation Research and Training Center on Aging with Developmental Disabilities, Department of Disability and Human Development, University of Illinois at Chicago.

Friedman, S. L., & Helm, D. T. (Eds.) (2010). *End-of-life care for children and adults with intellectual and developmental disabilities.* Washington, DC: American Association on Intellectual and Developmental Disabilities.

Freedman, R. I., Krauss, M. W., & Seltzer, M. M. (1997). Aging parents' residential plans for adult children with mental retardation. *Mental Retardation*, *35*, 114–123. doi:10.1352/0047-6765(1997)035 0114:APRPFA 2.0.CO;2

Grant, G. (1990). Elderly parents with handicapped children: Anticipating the future. *Journal of Aging Studies*, *4*, 359–374. doi:10.1016/0890-4065(90)90005-S

Griffiths, D. L., & Unger, D. G. (1994). Views about planning for the future among parents and siblings of adults with mental retardation. *Family Relations*, *43*, 221–227. doi:10.2307/585326

Haley, W. E., & Perkins, E. A. (2004). Current status and future directions in family caregiving and aging people with intellectual disabilities. *Journal of Policy and Practice in Intellectual Disabilities*, *1*(1), 24–30. doi:10.1111/ j.1741-1130.2004.04004.x

Heller, T. (2010). People with intellectual and developmental disabilities growing old: An overview. In T. Heller, P. Stafford, L. A. Davis, L. Sedlezky, & V.

Gaylord (Eds.), *Impact: Feature issue on aging and people with intellectual and developmental disabilities* , *23* (1). Minneapolis, MN: University of Minnesota, Institute on Community Integration. Retrieved from https://ici.umn.edu/products/impact/231/2.html

Heller, T., & Arnold, C. K. (2010). Siblings of adults with developmental disabilities: Psychosocial outcomes, relationships, and future planning. *Journal of Policy and Practice in Intellectual Disabilities*, *7*, 16–25. doi:10.1111/j.1741-1130.2010.00243.x

Heller, T., & Caldwell, J. (2006). Supporting aging caregivers and adults with developmental disabilities in future planning. *Mental Retardation*, *44*, 189–202. doi:10.1352/0047-6765(2006)44[189: SACAAW]2.0.CO;2

Heller, T., & Kramer, J. (2009). Involvement of adult siblings of persons with developmental disabilities in future planning. *Intellectual and Developmental Disabilities*, *47*, 208–219.

Hung, W. W., Ross, J. S., Boockvar, K. S., & Siu, A. L. (2011). Recent trends in chronic disease, impairment and disability among older adults in the United States. *BMC Geriatrics*, *11*(1), 47. doi:10.1186/1471-2318-11-47

Kingsbury, L. C. (2009). *People planning ahead: A guide to communicating healthcare and end-of-life wishes*. Washington, DC: American Association on Intellectual and Developmental Disabilities.

Mencap. (n.d.). *Mencap: The voice of learning disability*. Retrieved from www.mencap.org.uk

Parish, S. L., Seltzer, M. M., Greenberg, J. S., & Floyd, F. J. (2004). Economic implications of caregiving at midlife: Comparing parents with and without children who have developmental disabilities. *Mental Retardation, 42*, 413–426. doi:10.1352/0047-6765(2004)42 413:EIOCAM 2.0.CO;2

Perkins, E. A. (2010). The compound caregiver: A case study in multiple caregiving roles. *Clinical Gerontologist*, *33(3)*, 248–254. doi:10.1080/07317111003773619

Perkins, E. A., & Haley, W. E. (2010). Compound caregiving: When lifelong caregivers undertake additional caregiving roles. *Rehabilitation Psychology*, *55(4)*, 409–417. doi:10.1037/a0021521

Perkins, E. A., & Haley, W. E. (2013). Emotional and tangible reciprocity in middle and older-aged caregivers of adults with intellectual disabilities. *Journal of Policy and Practice in Intellectual Disabilities*, *10*, 334–344. doi:10.1111/jppi.12061

Perkins, E. A., & Moran, J. A. (2010). Aging adults with intellectual disabilities. *Journal of the American Medical Association*, *304(1)*, 91–92. doi:10.1001/jama.2010.906

Pollack, K. M., Morhaim, D., & Williams, M. (2010). The public's perspectives on advance directives in Maryland: Implications for state legislative and regulatory policy. *Health Policy*, *96*(1), 57–63. doi:10.1016/j.healthpol.2010.01.004

Prosser, H., & Moss, S. (1996). Informal care networks of older adults with an intellectual disability. *Journal of Applied Research in Intellectual Disabilities*, *9*(1), 17–30. doi:10.1111/j.1468-3148.1996.tb00095.x

Saxon, S. V., Etten, M. J., & Perkins, E. A. (2014). *Physical change and aging: A guide for the helping professions* (6th ed.). New York, NY: Springer.

Self-Advocates Becoming Empowered (n.d.). *Learn about SABE*. Retrieved from www.sabeusa.org

Seltzer, M. M., Floyd, F. J., Song, J., Greenberg, J. S., & Hong, J. (2011). Midlife and aging parents of adults with intellectual and developmental disabilities:

Impacts of lifelong parenting. *American Journal on Intellectual and Developmental Disabilities*, *116*(6), 479–499. doi:10.1352/1944-7558-116.6.479

Seltzer, M. M., & Krauss, M. W. (1994). Aging parents with co-resident adult children: The impact of lifelong caregiving. In M. M. Seltzer, M. W. Krauss, & M. P. Janicki (Eds.), *Life-course perspectives on adulthood and old age* (pp. 3–18). Washington, DC: American Association on Mental Retardation.

Shavelle, R. M., & Strauss, D. J. (1998). Comparative mortality of persons with autism in California, 1980–1996. *Journal of Insurance Medicine*, *30*, 220–225. Retrieved from https://www.aaimedicine.org/journal-of-insurance-medicine/jim/1998/030-04-0220.pdf

Sibling Leadership Network. (2016). *Sibling leadership network*. Retrieved from http://siblingleadership.org/

Strauss, D. J., Brooks, J., Rosenbloom, L., & Shavelle, R. (2008). Life expectancy in cerebral palsy: An update. *Developmental Medicine & Child Neurology*, *50*, 487–493. doi:10.1111/j.1469-8749.2008.03000.x

Taggart, L., Truesdale-Kennedy, M., Ryan, A., & McConkey, R. (2012). Examining the support needs of ageing family carers in developing future plans for a relative with an intellectual disability. *Journal of Intellectual Disability Research*, *16*, 217–234. doi:10.1177/1744 629512456465

The Arc. (2016). *Who we are*. Retrieved from http://www.thearc.org/who-we-are

The Arc Center for Future Planning. (2016a). *Future Planning 101: What is future planning?* Retreived from https://futureplanning.thearc.org/pages/learn/future-planning-101

The Arc Center for Future Planning. (2016b). *Tips for siblings: Getting the future planning conversation started*. Retreived from https://futureplanning.thearc.org/assets/CFP_TipsForSibs-510e2c3f92ed05e3152130222f3deacf3cbf95bae6855e1a854422db548d630d.pdf

Ward, B. W., Schiller, J. S., & Goodman, R. A. (2014). Multiple chronic conditions among US adults: A 2012 update. *Preventing Chronic Disease*, *11*, 130389–130393. doi:10.5888/pcd11.130389

World Health Organization. (2012). *Are you ready? What you need to know about ageing*. Retrieved from http://www.who.int/world-health-day/2012/toolkit/background/en/

Yamaki, K., Hsieh, K., & Heller, T. (2009). Health profile of aging family caregivers supporting adults with intellectual and developmental disabilities at home. *Intellectual and Developmental Disabilities*, *47*, 425–435. doi:10.1352/1934-9556-47.6.425

Yang, Q., Rasmussen, S. A., & Friedman, J. M. (2002). Mortality associated with Down syndrome in the USA from 1983 to 1997: A population-based study. *Lancet*, *359*, 1019–1025. doi:10.1016/S0140-6736(02)08092-3

Index

A&E TV, *Born This Way* series 26
ABLE accounts 181–3
ABLE National Resource Center 181, 183
Achieving a Better Life Experience (ABLE) Act (U.S., 2014) 181, 214
activity, as criterion of disability 4
Actor–Partner Interaction Model 19
adaptive behavior 63
advice to new parents from parents 46–56; principles for practice 54–8
advocacy, by siblings 221; groups 26, 28, 201, 206, 221; parent and family 49, 53–6, 64, 82, 133, 163–4, 221; professional 144, 164, 167; self-advocacy 64–5, 146, 202, 221
Affordable Care Act (U.S., 2010) 141
aging, of caregivers 216–25; of population 216–17
allied health professionals, and EI (early intervention) 149–56; working collaboratively 151, 154–5
alternative therapies 136
Alzheimer's disease 218
ambiguous loss theory 22–3, 79–80, 91–6; mastering, connecting and thriving 92–3, 95
American Association on Intellectual and Developmental Disabilities 63, 68–9, 194–5
American Psychological Association 85
American Sign Language 164
Applied Behavior Analysis (ABA) 6
The Arc 64, 69, 221; Centre for Future Planning 177, 222, 223
The Arc of Texas Master Pooled Trust 181, 213
assessment, capacity 204; medical 20–1, 85, 121, 133, 135, 136, 161
attorneys-in-fact 178
Australian Department of Social Services 98
autism spectrum disorders (ASD) 3, 5–6, 38; behavior and communication 6; diagnosis 23; and guardianship 202; life expectancy 217; and loss theory 17; medications 7; parents and 10, 92, 95; and physical examination 136; and relationship satisfaction 94; siblings and 104, 108, 111; and stigma 80; support groups 3, 111; treatment 6

Bader, S. H. 109
Barry, T. D. 109
Baxter, D. 35
Beart, S. 67
Behavior Analyst Certification Board 6
behavior-changing model 40
belief systems 34–5
benefits, government 176, 179, 180, 201, 207–8, 208–11, 213
Benson, P. R. 109
Bentley, G. 22

Bentley, G. E. 94
bipolar disorder 37
birth defects *see* congenital disabilities
Board-Certified Behavior Analysts 6
body function and structure, as criterion of disability 4
Bogden, R. 36
books, by parents 27; educational 51–2
Borrell-Carrio, F. 133
Boss, Pauline 17, 22, 95
Bronfenbrenner, U. 36
Brown, M. 91, 95
Buchan, L. 67

caregivers, aging 216–25; care for 138–9; "compound caregiving" 218; and future planning 222; lack of legal authority 179; mothers as primary 76–9; physical issues 217–19; psychological issues 219–20; retirement 220; siblings as 69, 105, 110, 220–1, 222–3; social needs of 220; stress affecting 46, 78, 83, 84–5, 179; as term 133; *see also* guardianship
care guides 176–7, 222
Center for Parent Information and Resources 152
Centers for Independent Living 164
cerebral palsy 5, 7–8; and chronic sorrow 24; life expectancy 8, 217; and loss theory 17; parents and 10; treatment 8
chief complaint 135
"Child First" theme 49–50, 54, 56, 145
Children's Health Insurance Program (CHIP) (U.S.) 142
China, children with IDD in 80–1
chronic illness health models 17, 19–21
chronic sorrow 23–4; and grief 24
Cless, J. 19
closure 25
coherence 35
College 529 Savings Plan 181, 183
communication 34, 35, 110; barriers to 163, 175; and financial planning 175–6, 185; in infants and toddlers (verbal and non-verbal) 149; as shared responsibility 139–40; skills 133; strategies to create partnerships 162–7
community inclusion 70
community support groups 24
complementary therapies 136
Condon, J. 118
congenital disabilities 21, 23–4
Congenital Malformations Surveillance Report 21
coping strategies 19, 35, 42, 94–5, 98, 109, 111
Costigan, C. L. 107
couple relationship 97–8
criterion reference 34, 36–8, 39, 41

Dads Appreciating Down Syndrome (DADS) 98
Darling, R. B. 79
data analysis procedures 48–9
decision making, shared 154, 155; supported 219
deinstitutionalization 64–5
dementia 218
Department of Family and Protective Services (U.S.) 207
Department of Health and Human Services (U.S.), Office of Disease Prevention and Health Promotion 134
Determination of IDD 204
developmental disability 5; as term 63
diagnosis, and ABLE accounts 182, 183; of ASD 23; at birth 121–2; conflicting emotions over 121–2; differential 136; of Down syndrome 23, 52; and effects of stigma on mothers 80–1, 84–5; families and 24–5, 138–9; and fathers 96, 98;

and grandparents 117, 118, 121, 122–3; initial 25, 65; in later life 122–3; stages of reaction to 96
diagnostic overshadowing 137
DiClemente, C. C. 40
disability, classification criteria 4; social-ecological model of 63; as term 4, 61–2
disability-specific organizations 24, 28, 64
Disabled Adult Child (DAC) 208–9
discrimination, race- or ethnicity-related 80–1
Double ABC-X model 18; and IDD research 18–19
Down syndrome (DS) ix, 5, 9–10, 38–9; advice from other parents 48–54, 50 (Table 4.2); case example 153–4; causes 63; "Child First" theme 49–50, 54, 56; and chronic sorrow 24; demographic information 48, 49 (Table 4.1); and developmental delays 148; diagnosis 23, 52; and diagnostic overshadowing 137; and early intervention 152; families and 20, 46, 47; fathers of children with 91, 92, 95, 98; life expectancy 9, 217; and motor skills 150; prenatal screening 9; and relationship satisfaction 94; and siblings 108; and stigma 80; and stress 19; support groups 51, 111; treatment 9–10
Down Syndrome Guild 52
Durtschi, J. A. 19
drug allergies 137, 138

Early Childhood Technical Assistance Center 151
early intervention 148–56, 158; eligibility for 151–2, 155; evaluation process for 149; and Federal law (U.S.) 151–2; medically based or private practice services 152–3
ecological systems 36, 41, 43
Education for All Handicapped Children Act (1975) (U.S.) 160
education system 158–68; perspectives 158–9
employment of adults with IDD 188–96; benefits of and barriers to 192–3, 194–5; competitive integrated employment 189–90; current landscape 191; employment supports 70, 189, 192; historical perspective 190–2; integrated employment 189, 190, 193; meaningful 188, 192–6; person-centered approach 194–6; programs for 193; resources 196–7; scenarios 188–90; segregated 190, 191, 193; wages legislation 190
empowerment, of families 40–1, 55, 56, 68, 134, 149, 155, 167, 194, 196; of individuals 67, 68, 194, 195; of mothers 77; of professionals 68
enclaves (in supported employment) 189, 190
end-of-life planning 219–20
Engel, G. 133
errors, medical 139–40, 145
estate administrators (personal representatives) 212
estate planning 211–13
executors of wills 211–12

Fair Labor Standards Act (U.S., 1938) 190
families of children with IDD 10–11; communication 65–6, 161–7; dealing with conflict 124; empowerment of 40–1, 55, 56, 68, 134, 149, 155, 167, 194, 196; and financial planning 185; inheritance plans 176, 181; regenerative 35, 38, 40, 42; rhythmic 34–5, 40, 42; and terminology 61, 62–4; *see also* professionals, and parents/families

family dynamics and disability 21, 125–6
family empowerment 41
family functioning 46
family–professional partnerships 167–8
family stress 17–19, 24, 68, 84–5; and crisis 18
family systems 17–19
Family Systems Illness model 20–4
Fatherhood Institute (UK) 98
fathers, bonding activities 96–7; of children with DS 91, 92, 95, 98; and couple relationship 97–8; father-focused programs 99; and IDD 91; involvement of 90–1, 120; mastering, connecting and thriving groups 95; perspectives from 90–9; and professionals 96–7; support programs for 98
Federal law (U.S.) 151–2, 160
Federal Poverty Level (U.S.) 183
feeding skills 149–50
FERPA Release 207
fetal alcohol syndrome 5, 63; and developmental delays 148
fiduciaries 185
financial planning 173–86; key roles in 177–9; keys to success 184–5; specific areas 177
Fisman, S. 108
Floyd, F. J. 107
Fragile X syndrome 137; and developmental delays 148
fundraising 213
The Future Is Now 222
future planning 201, 221–3; components of 222; person-centered 164; principles for practice 224; *see also* financial planning

Gau, S. 108
gender roles 76, 78, 120
GiGi's Playhouse—Down Syndrome Foundation 26
Goff, Dalton ix
Goldstein, T. 107
grandparents 117–27; activities with grandchildren 119–20, 123, 126, 218; becoming a grandparent 118; experiences of 117; and family relationships following IDD diagnosis 124; gender roles 120; grandparent drive 123; identity, latent and functional 123; multiple generations of 118; reactions to IDD diagnosis 118, 121, 122; relevant skills 125; as resources 125; roles of 119–20, 123, 126; sense of pride 124
Great Depression 190
grief and loss 21–5, 80, 85, 91–2, 121; *see also* chronic sorrow
guardianship 174, 178, 179, 201–6; and aging caregivers 219; alternatives to 206–7; basic guidelines 203–6; and individual rights 205; legal guardians 202; as legal process 203; restoration proceedings 204; roles of legal guardians 202; siblings and 204; terminology 201–2; transferable 204; types of 178, 204

Haley, W. E. 217–18
Hardy, G. 67
Harrison, J. 93
Hastings, R. P. 35, 108
health, aging-related issues 218; literacy 133, 134–5, 139, 140, 144; physical 46
healthcare, coordinated 152; expenditure on 134; visits 135–7
health insurance 133, 134, 141–2, 152, 208; employer-based 141–2; EOB (explanation of benefits) statement 142
Health Insurance Premium Payment Program (HIPP) 208

Hey, Dad! For Fathers Who Have a Child with a Disability (program) 98
HIPAA Release (Authorization to Disclose Protected Health Information) 206, 207
holistic approach 19, 85, 133–4
Hornby, G. 93
hospitalization 141
hospitals and medical facilities 133, 140–1; administrators as ombudspersons 141; emergency room (ER) 140
Huston, S. 173, 177

identity 62; ambiguity 23; bicultural 70–1; formation 67, 69, 70–1
Idiodycentric 15 (genetic disorder) 36–7
Individual Family Service Plan (IFSP) 152, 161
Individualized Education Plan or Program 160–2
Individuals with Disabilities Education Act (IDEA) 160–4; Part B 160–1; Part C (U.S.) 151–2, 161
informed consent 154
institutionalization 25
insurance *see* health insurance; life insurance
integrated care 20, 133, 134
intellectual and developmental disabilities (IDD) ix–x; definition of terms 4–5, 26; families of children with 10–12
intellectual disability 5; language of 63, 70–1; as term 63, 66–7
intellectual functioning 63
Internal Revenue Service (IRS, U.S.) 180, 181
internet 47, 135, 137, 184
interoperability, lack of 137
interventions 40
interviewing, motivational 143

job coaches 189

Karlof, K. L. 109
King, G. 35
Kingsbury, L. C., People Planning Ahead: Communicating Healthcare and End-of-Life Wishes 219
Kingsley, Emily Pearl, "Welcome to Holland" 42, 43, 93
Knestrict, T. 34, 36, 37–9
Kohn, L.T. 139
Kuchey, D. 34, 36, 37–9

labels 4, 61, 62–4
language, differences in 164; double bind of 66–7; grandparents and 122; and identity 62–3; and initial diagnosis 65; "people first" 143, 146; professionals and 68–9; sign language 164; *see also* terminology
Lauderdale, M. 173
Lauderdale, M. 173, 177
legal concerns 201–14
Leopold, T. 118
Letter of Guardianship 207
letters of intent 176–7, 222
Levine, K. A. 77
Levine, S. P. 107, 111
life expectancy 8, 9, 217
life insurance 183–4
loss theory 17

McCubbin, H. 34, 38
McCubbin, H. I. 18
McCubbin, M. 34, 38
McDaniel, S. H. 20, 21
marital satisfaction 46
Marriage and Family Therapy (MFT) 20
Masterson, M. 24
mastery 92, 94–5, 99
meaning making process 25, 27–8, 34, 67, 69, 70–1, 82–3, 95
Medicaid 142, 152, 153, 179, 180, 201, 208–11, 213; and fundraising 213; Payback provision 181, 183
Medicaid Reimbursement Child Support SNT 211

Medicaid Waiver Programs 209
Medical Family Therapy (MedFT) 20
medical model, traditional 133
medical perspective 133–46
medical records, electronic 137; shadow 137–8, 140
Medicare 180–1, 208–9
Mencap 221
mental health 20
mental retardation (as term) 4, 61, 63
milestones, developmental 7, 24, 47, 52, 53, 82, 148, 153
mothers, bonding activities 96; employment among, and financial problems 78–9; empowerment of 77; joy, happiness and personal growth in 81–2, 85; and meaning making 82–3; perspectives from 76–86; as primary caregivers 76–8, 83, 96–7, 97, 120; psychological well-being and coping 79–83; relational benefits 82; single 76, 77–8
motor skills 150
MRDD (Mental Retardation and Development Disabilities) 51

National Disability Institute (NDI) 183
National Down Syndrome Congress (NDSC) 23, 68–9, 111; Brothers & Sisters Conference 111
National Down Syndrome Society (NDSS) 68–9
National Institutes of Health 4
Nelson Goff, B. S. 19
norm referenced view 37

Obama, Barack 181
O'Brien, M. 22–3
occupational therapy (OT) 150–1, 153
Olshansky, S. 23–4
Omnibus Budget Reconciliation Act (OBRA, U.S., 1993) 180
organizational processes 34, 35
Orsmond, G. I. 109

Parent to Parent USA 163
parents, aging 216–25; literacy levels 162–3; parent advocacy 49, 53–6, 64, 163–4; parent attitude, "tough skin" response 52–3; parent education 50–2, 54–5; parent-provider relationship 40, 138; parent-to-parent support 47; participation or activation 40, 41–2, 160; as term 133; *see also* caregivers; families of children with IDD; professionals, and parents
Parker, T. 18–19
participation levels, as component of disability 4
Patterson, J. M. 18
patients, activation 41; fostering self-agency in 143–5; history 135
pediatricians 134
Perkins, E. A. 217–18
person-centered approach 63, 164, 194, 196
person-first language 26
personal growth opportunities 195
personal representatives 212
pervasive developmental disorder 108
physical examination 135–6
physical health 46
physical therapy 150, 153
physician, role and perspective of 135–8
Pickle Amendment 209
Pickle, Senator J. J. 209
Pisani, R. 21
plan, medical 136
Plotner, A. J. 193
poems, educational 51–2
policy makers 43, 56, 72, 86, 99, 112–13, 127, 146, 156, 168, 186, 196, 214, 225
positive attitude 34, 35, 42, 52–3, 55

positive illusions (as concept) 35
positive school culture 166–7
poster children 64
powers of attorney (POAs) 178, 179, 206; directives 206; limitations 207
pregnancy ix, 27
problem lists 137
Prochaska, J. O. 40
professional development opportunities 195
professionals, and aging caregivers 224–5; avoiding bias about family dynamics 125–7; communication about IDD 65; communication with children 144; empowerment of 68; and fathers 96–7; and financial planning 184–6; and grandparents 125–6; and identity process 67–8, 72; and legal issues 214; and mothers 83–5; and parents/families 11, 17–22, 28, 36, 39–41, 42–3, 55, 56, 69, 79, 136–7, 161–6; and siblings 111, 112; support and validation by 195–6; and terminology 62, 68; viewed as ultimate experts 64
PROSE checklist 163
psychological well-being and coping of mothers, negative effects 79–81; positive effects 81–3

quality of life 192, 209, 211

Ramisch, J. 19
reconfiguration 34, 41
reflection and reconfiguration 39–40, 41
reframing strategy 95
residential care facilities 77, 80
resilience 18, 32–43; of fathers 95; individual 33; parental and family 33–4, 91; principles for practice 39–40; research 26–7, 33–5, 40–2; of single mothers 77–8
retard, retarded (as terms) 4, 26
retirement plans 184
Review of Systems (ROS) 135 (Table 10.1)
Richardson, S. S. 107
rituals 34, 43
Rolland, John 20
Rossiter, L. 105–6
Roth IRA 181
routines 34, 43

satisfaction, relationship 19, 34, 35, 46, 91, 93–4, 141
Saxon, S. V., Physical Changes and Aging: A Guide for the Helping Professions 218
Schalock, R. L. 62, 192
schizophrenia, and chronic sorrow 24
Scorgie, K. 82
Selective Serotonin Re-uptake Inhibitors (SSRIs) 7
self-advocacy 64–5, 146, 202, 221
Self-Advocates Becoming Empowered 221
self-agency 143–5
self-determination 64–5
Seligman, M. 79
Sharpe, D. 105–6
Shearn, J. 66
Shogren, K. A. 193
Sibling Leadership Network (SLN) 221, 223
siblings, adult 107–8, 110–11; advocacy by 221; and ASD 104, 108, 111; behavior problems among 108–9, 110, 112; as caregivers 69, 105, 110, 220–1, 222–3; demographic characteristics and other variables 106–7; experience of 104–13; family and personal factors 82, 109–10, 110; gender and birth order 106–7, 110; groups, comparing 108; with IDD 107–9; as legal guardians 204; and planning for future 175, 176; positive and negative effects on 105,

110; and professionals 111, 112; research into outcomes for 105–6, 112; support programs for 111–12
single-parent households 77–8
Skinner, B. F. 6
Skopek, J. 118
Skotko, G. B. 107, 111
Smith, L. O. 109
SOAP format (of healthcare visit) 135–7, 135 (Table 10.1)
Sobsey, D. 82
Social Security Administration (U.S., SSA) 179, 210
Social Security Disability Insurance (SSDI) 180
Social Security Disability (SSD) benefit 209
special needs plans 173–86
Special Needs Trust Fairness Act (2015, U.S.) 180
Special Needs Trusts (SNTs) 179, 180–4; Medicaid Reimbursement Child Support 211; self-settled 182, 183; Third Party 181, 184
Special Olympics 61, 64
speech-language pathology (SLP) 149–51, 153
spirituality 21, 34
statistics, people with IDD 216–17
stereotypes 26
sterilization 64
stigma, effects of 80–1, 84–5; managing 176
stress, affecting caregivers 46, 78, 83, 84–5, 94, 94–5
students with IDD 158–68
Supplemental Needs Trusts (SNTs) 180, 211, 212–13; Third Party 213
Supplemental Security Disability Income (SSDI or SSD) 208
Supplemental Security Income (SSI) 180, 182, 208–10; eligibility requirements 210, 212
support groups 24, 47, 55, 70, 83; autism 3, 111; Down syndrome 51, 111
Supported Decision Making Agreement (SDMA) 207
supported employment 70, 189
systems theory 79

Taunt, H. M. 35
Taylor, S. 36
technology 47
tenacity 38
terminology, changes in 4, 61, 62–4; *see also* language
Texas, guardianship in 201–2, 203–4, 205, 207
Texas Tech University ix
text messaging 163, 165
“third retirement” 173, 179–80
Todd, S. 66
Tomeny, T. S. 109
transcendence 34
transition years 174
transportation, to meetings at school 163
traumatic brain injury (TBI) 22
treatment compliance 154
trustees 178–9, 180–1, 212
22q3 Deletion Syndrome (genetic disorder) 37–8

United States of America, expenditure on healthcare 134; health insurance in 141–2

vaccination 144–5; records 138
vocational rehabilitation 194

wages 190, 191, 192
Walsh, F. 34, 35
Wehmeyer, M. L. 64
Weibel-Orlando, J. 123
Werner, E. E. 33
wills, legal 211–12, 219
workshops, sheltered 189, 190, 191–2, 192–3
World Health Organization 4
World War II 64, 190

For Product Safety Concerns and Information please contact our EU representative GPSR@taylorandfrancis.com
Taylor & Francis Verlag GmbH, Kaufingerstraße 24, 80331 München, Germany

www.ingramcontent.com/pod-product-compliance
Ingram Content Group UK Ltd.
Pitfield, Milton Keynes, MK11 3LW, UK
UKHW022203190926
475702UK00003B/182
* 9 7 8 1 1 3 8 6 7 2 4 5 1 *